ABHANDLUNGEN DER DEUTSCHEN AKADEMIE DER WISSENSCHAFTEN ZU BERLIN

Klasse für Medizin

Jahrgang 1964 Nr. 4

STRUKTUR UND FUNKTION DES GENETISCHEN MATERIALS (STRUCTURE AND FUNCTION OF THE GENETIC MATERIAL)

ERWIN-BAUR-GEDÄCHTNISVORLESUNGEN III 1963

Veranstaltet vom Institut für Kulturpflanzenforschung Gatersleben
der
Deutschen Akademie der Wissenschaften zu Berlin
25. bis 29. August 1963

Herausgegeben von
H. STUBBE
Redaktion
H. BÖHME

Mit 117 Abbildungen, davon 31 Abbildungen auf 19 Kunstdrucktafeln, und 42 Tabellen

AKADEMIE-VERLAG · BERLIN
1964

Vorgelegt von Hrn. KRAATZ in der Klassensitzung vom 19. 12. 1963

Zum Druck genehmigt am gleichen Tage, ausgegeben am 26. 8. 64

Erschienen im Akademie-Verlag GmbH, Berlin W 8, Leipziger Straße 3–4

Lizenznummer: 202 · 100/420/64
Gesamtherstellung: IV/2/14 · VEB Werkdruck Gräfenhainichen · 2229
Bestellnummer: 2001/64/IV/4 · ES 18 G 1 · Preis: DM 53,–

INHALTSVERZEICHNIS

Die biologische Organisation des genetischen Materials

Die Primäre Funktion des genetischen Materials

Die Funktion des genetischen Materials in der Proteinsynthese

Die Realisierung der genetischen Information durch spezifische Enzyme

Die Funktion des genetischen Materials auf chromosomaler Ebene

EINLEITENDE WORTE

Die beiden Erwin-Baur-Gedächtnisvorlesungen, die wir in den vergangenen Jahren durchgeführt haben, waren den Problemen der Mutagenese gewidmet. Die Veranstaltung im Jahre 1959 behandelte die „Chemische Mutagenese", die darauffolgende im Jahre 1961 die „Strahleninduzierte Mutagenese". Hauptgegenstand dieser beiden Gedächtnisvorlesungen waren die Vorgänge und Beziehungen zwischen der Einwirkung des mutagenen Agens und der erfolgten Mutation. Beim Studium dieser Beziehungen trat die Frage nach der Struktur des genetischen Materials immer mehr hervor.

An diesem Punkt knüpft nun unsere diesjährige Veranstaltung an. Wir wollen nicht nur wissen, wie ein bestimmtes Agens auf das genetische Material einwirkt und welche Veränderungen hierdurch eintreten. Uns beschäftigt in gleichem Maße die Frage, welche Struktur und Organisation das genetische Material hat, wie es seinen Informationsgehalt in den aufeinanderfolgenden Generationen erhält und, vor allem auch, wie es Stoffwechsel und Entwicklung kontrolliert und bestimmt.

Die Fortschritte unseres Wissens über die Struktur und die Organisation des genetischen Materials verdanken wir vor allem zwei Forschungsrichtungen.

Das eine Gebiet ist die Nukleinsäureforschung. Untersuchungen an Bakterien, Bakteriophagen und Viren haben uns im Verlaufe der letzten 20 Jahre den Beweis geliefert, daß die Nukleinsäuren das genetische Material darstellen; in den meisten Fällen spielt die DNS diese Rolle, in anderen Fällen die RNS (so bei zahlreichen Viren, z. B. dem Tabakmosaikvirus, und den RNS-Phagen). Die Aufstellung des WATSON-CRICK-Modells der DNS im Jahre 1953 markiert einen ersten Höhepunkt in der Entwicklung dieses Forschungszweiges. Seitdem hat sich dieses Gebiet in erstaunlicher Geschwindigkeit weiterentwickelt und uns viele neue Erkenntnisse gebracht. Darüber hinaus hat sich aber eine Fülle von Problemen aufgetan, die noch der Lösung harren. Bei der Klärung der offenen Fragen zeigt sich in besonderem Maße, wie unbedingt erforderlich die enge Zusammenarbeit zwischen Physikern, Chemikern, Biochemikern und Genetikern ist.

Der andere Forschungszweig, der uns wesentliche, neue Einsichten brachte, analysiert die Feinstruktur des Gens. Untersuchungen, die vor allem an Bakteriophagen, Bakterien und Pilzen durchgeführt wurden, haben uns gezeigt, daß Funktions-, Rekombinations- und Mutations-Einheit des Genotyps verschiedene Größen sind. Das hat uns veranlaßt, den Genbegriff neu zu durchdenken. Heute steht daher vor uns die Aufgabe, den Begriff des Gens unter Berücksichtigung auch solcher Erscheinungen wie der interallelen Komplementierung exakt zu fassen und genau zu definieren. Die Auswertung der Ergebnisse beider Forschungszweige hat es schließlich erlaubt, die genetischen Werte (etwa kleinste Rekombinationswerte) mit bestimmten biophysikalischen Größen (etwa den Nukleotidabständen) in Parallele zu setzen. Nicht zuletzt haben uns die Arbeiten an Mikroorganismen mit ganz neuen Wegen der Übertragung und der Rekombination von Erbanlagen bekannt gemacht, deren Entdeckung die Bedeutung der Genetik für die allgemeine Biologie erneut unterstreicht.

Die Frage, wie die Gene in die Stoffwechsel- und Entwicklungsprozesse eingreifen, hat die Genetiker schon immer beschäftigt. Bereits in den zwanziger Jahren wurde, nicht zuletzt unter dem Einfluß der Arbeiten RICHARD GOLDSCHMIDTS, die Vorstellung entwickelt, daß die Gene als Enzyme oder über Enzyme auf die Stoffwechselprozesse einwirken. Aber es verging eine lange Zeit, bis diese allgemeine Formulierung genetisch-biochemisch präzisiert werden konnte. Die Bearbeitung geeigneter Augenfarbmutanten von *Ephestia* und *Drosophila* stimulierte die Weiterentwicklung dieses Forschungszweiges. Die entscheidenden Fortschritte brachte dann die Analyse der biochemischen Mangelmutanten von *Neurospora* und verschiedener Bakterien. Sie erlaubten BEADLE und TATUM die Formulierung der „Ein Gen – Ein Enzym"-Hypothese. Die letzten Jahre schließlich haben in ganz erstaunlicher Geschwindigkeit und in ganz überraschendem Ausmaß Einblicke in die Einzelheiten dieser Beziehungen gebracht, die wohl nur noch derjenige erfassen und verfolgen kann, der selbst aktiv im Bereich der Molekular-Genetik tätig ist.

Es wurde klar, daß die DNS durch Vermittlung von RNS die Struktur der Enzyme und anderer Proteine festlegt. Die verschiedenen RNS-Formen (Messenger-, Transfer- und Ribosomen-RNS) konnten erfaßt werden. Damit und mit der Verwendung synthetischer Polynukleotide war ein wesentlicher Ansatzpunkt für die Arbeiten zur Aufklärung des genetischen Codes gegeben. Andererseits ergab sich nach der Konstitutionsaufklärung verschiedener Proteine die Möglichkeit, die als Folge von Mutationen auftretenden Aminosäure-Austausche exakt zu erfassen, und auf diesem Wege Aussagen über den genetischen Code zu machen.

Die weitere Aufklärung des genetischen Codes und der Mechanismen seiner Realisierung sowie die genaue Analyse von Struktur und Funktion der verschiedenen RNS-Formen sind wesentliche Aufgaben der gegenwärtigen Forschung.

Bei Bakterien enthüllte die Analyse von Induktions- und Repressions-Erscheinungen innerzellige Regulationsmechanismen, deren Aufdeckung notwendige Vergleiche mit den Regulationssystemen mehrzelliger Organismen anregte. Bei Mehrzellern spielen ja Regulationssysteme eine außerordentlich wichtige Rolle. Die cytologische, genetische und biochemische Bearbeitung solcher geeigneten Systeme wie z. B. der Riesenchromosomen der Dipteren mit ihren Strukturmodifikationen hat schon wesentliche Ergebnisse zu diesem Problem beigesteuert und verspricht für die Zukunft zweifellos weitere wichtige Einsichten.

Diese hier nur angedeuteten Probleme, die alle zum Thema „Struktur und Funktion des genetischen Materials" gehören, werden im Verlaufe unserer Tagung ausführlich und dem neuesten Stand der Forschung entsprechend behandelt werden.

Wir Gaterslebener sind glücklich darüber, eine so große Zahl von Gästen bei uns begrüßen zu können. Wir freuen uns, daß viele ausländische Wissenschaftler unserer Einladung gefolgt sind und daß wir auch zahlreiche Kollegen aus der Bundesrepublik begrüßen können. Sie alle sind uns herzlich willkommen!

Manche von Ihnen haben das Opfer einer langen und beschwerlichen Reise nicht gescheut, um zu uns zu kommen. Die meisten von Ihnen sind zum erstenmal in diesem kleinen und entlegenen Ort, in dem wir 1945 mit dem Aufbau dieses Instituts begonnen haben. Ihnen allen wünschen wir, daß Sie sich in diesen Tagen bei uns wohl fühlen, daß feste menschliche und wissenschaftliche Brücken geschlagen werden und daß Sie bereichert am Ende der Tagung von uns scheiden.

Leider ist es uns nicht vergönnt, zwei Kollegen hier bei uns zu haben, deren Besuch wir erwartet hatten: Francis Ryan und Bernard Nebel. Der Tod hat sie uns überraschend, vorzeitig und unerbittlich entrissen. Hier ist nicht der Ort, Leben und Werk beider Persönlichkeiten umfassend zu würdigen. Ich will nur sagen, daß uns allen der plötzliche Tod von Francis Ryan ganz unfaßbar ist. Ich hatte leider nur einmal Gelegenheit, ihn persönlich zu treffen. Seine kraftvolle und naturnahe Persönlichkeit strömte unerschütterliche Gesundheit, Güte und Menschlichkeit aus. Francis Ryan hat sich durch seine Arbeiten, die er mit seinem Team vom Zoologischen Institut der Columbia University durchführte, große Verdienste um die Aufklärung der molekularen Grundlagen des Mutationsprozesses erworben. Er hat gemeinsam mit Ruth Sager das Buch „Cell Heredity" verfaßt, das zu den besten Lehrbüchern der Genetik gehört. Die Herausgeber der „Zeitschrift für Vererbungslehre" trauern um einen sehr aktiven Mitarbeiter bei der Gestaltung dieser alten genetischen Zeitschrift.

Bernard Nebel war von uns eingeladen worden, um seine Vorstellungen über Struktur und Feinbau der Chromosomen näher kennenzulernen. Er schrieb mir aus dem Krankenhaus, daß er wohl nicht kommen werde, weil er sich nur langsam von einer Nierenentzündung erholen könne. Ich kannte ihn und Mabel Ruttle Nebel seit 1928, als wir zusammen an das neugegründete Kaiser-Wilhelm-Institut für Züchtungsforschung in Müncheberg kamen. Ein Jahr lang war er uns Anfängern ein Vorbild in der Strenge seiner Arbeitsdisziplin und der Weite und Unabhängigkeit seines Denkens. Er hat nach seiner endgültigen Übersiedlung in die USA viele Arbeiten über Chromosomenstruktur, über Bestrahlungswirkungen, über die polyploidisierende Wirkung von Colchicin und manche anderen Fragen veröffentlicht. Er war ein vielseitig interessierter und gebildeter Mann, der auf dem Umweg über die Medizin wieder zu seinem Hauptgebiet, der Cytologie, zurückkehrte. Kurz vor seinem Tode formulierte er neue Vorstellungen über die Struktur der Chromosomen, wie sie ihm das elektronenoptische Bild zeigte.

Es liegt nicht im Sinne dieser beiden ausgezeichneten Menschen und Forscher über den großen Verlust zu klagen, den ihr früher Tod uns allen brachte. Wir wollen uns glücklich schätzen, daß sie als gute Menschen unter uns waren und ihnen danken für ihr wissenschaftliches Werk, das sie uns hinterlassen haben und das lange bestehen bleiben wird.

Wir werden jetzt mit den Vorträgen unserer Tagung beginnen. Möge die Veranstaltung, die uns hier zu wissenschaftlichem Gedankenaustausch zusammenführt, recht fruchtbar sein. Möge sie den wissenschaftlichen und persönlichen Kontakt zwischen den Teilnehmern dieser Tagung über alle Grenzen der Länder und Kontinente hinweg fördern.

Im Namen des Herrn Präsidenten der Deutschen Akademie der Wissenschaften zu Berlin und im Namen des Herrn Vorsitzenden der Forschungsgemeinschaft der Akademie heiße ich Sie alle herzlich willkommen und eröffne hiermit die dritten Erwin-Baur-Gedächtnisvorlesungen.

H. Stubbe

Structural Modifications of DNA: Crosslinking, Circularization and Single-strand Interruptions

WACLAW SZYBALSKI

McArdle Memorial Laboratory, University of Wisconsin, Madison, Wisconsin, U.S.A.

The main features of the secondary DNA structure are now well established. As first proposed by WATSON and CRICK (1953), the native DNA molecule consists of two complementary strands held together by hydrogen bonds between adenine and thymine or guanine and cytosine. In addition to hydrogen bonding, other forces must be involved in stabilization of this double helical structure, including $\pi - \pi$ electron interaction between the stacked heterocyclic rings, hydrophobic bonds, and other long range forces. No covalent bonds between the complementary strands have been postulated, since these seem to be incompatible with the semiconservative mode of DNA replication. Some other speculations on the basic secondary structure of DNA (CAVALIERI and ROSENBERG, 1962; DONOHUE and TRUEBLOOD, 1960) were not corroborated by others and thus did not gain any general acceptance.

Although the double-helical complementary structure of native DNA is very prevalent among living organisms, a more primitive form of single-stranded DNA was first discovered in a small spherical bacteriophage, Φ X 174 (SINSHEIMER, 1959). The similar spherical phages S 13 and Φ R (TESSMAN, 1959; KAY, 1962)[1]) and the filamentous phages fl, fd and M 13 (ZINDER *et al.*, 1963; MARVIN and HOFFMANN-BERLING, 1963; HOFSCHNEIDER, 1963) also contain single-stranded DNA. It is not known, however, whether this type of DNA is only a relatively rare freak of nature, or whether it plays some role in all living cells. After all, single-stranded DNA seems to differ from double-stranded DNA in its mode of replication, being copied off the double-stranded „replicative" form (SINSHEIMER *et al.*, 1962), most probably by some new, as yet unidentified polymerase similar in action to the DNA-RNA polymerase (GEIDUSCHEK *et al.*, 1961), rather than to the conventional DNA polymerase (KORNBERG, 1961).

This review, however, will be restricted mainly to modifications of the secondary structure of double-stranded DNA, as occurring in nature or provoked by exposure of the cells to various lethal agents, some of natural origin. These additional structural features of DNA do not in any way invalidate the generality of its double-helical complementary structure, and refer only either to the structure of the ends of this enormously long molecule (*e.g.* circularity) or to rela-

---

[1]) The Φ X 174, S 1 3, and Φ R phages contain single-stranded DNA's indistinguishable as far as their buoyant densities in CsCl and Cs_2SO_4 are concerned (1.725 g/cm^3 and 1.447 g/cm^3, respectively). The densities of fl, fd and M 13 phage DNA's are again practically identical (1.723 g/cm^3 in CsCl and 1.446 g/cm^3 in Cs_2SO_4), indicating most probably that these three viruses are one and the same or very closely related. Heating to 100 °C followed by rapid cooling does not effect the buoyant density of any of these DNA's, confirming their single-stranded, non-complementary nature.

tively rare departures from the perfect double helix, including single-strand breaks and covalent links between the complementary strands (= crosslinks). Other modifications, *e.g.* glucosylation or deglucosylation of T-even phage DNA (Erikson and Szybalski, 1964), the halogen-for-methyl substitution in the thymine residue (Szybalski, 1962), and enzymatic methylation of preformed DNA (Gold and Hurwitz, 1963), which do not seem to change the topological properties of the classical double helix, will not be discussed at length here.

Crosslinking of the complementary DNA strands

(a) Effects of radiation

It was observed some time ago that massive doses of UV light (Setlow and Doyle, 1954; Baranowska and Shugar, 1960), X-rays, or electrons (Alexander and Stacey, 1959; Alexander *et al.*, 1959), when delivered to DNA, especially to highly concentrated solutions or dry material, cause the formation of insoluble gels. Covalent intermolecular linking was invoked to explain this observation, which was even recently applied to the preparation of DNA gels for analytical studies on specific thermal hybridization between nucleic acids (Britten, 1963).

In dilute DNA solutions, however, intermolecular linking was not recorded. Instead Marmur and Grossman (1961) observed crosslinking between the complementary DNA strands, in addition to dimerization between neighboring thymines on the same strand. The interstrand crosslinking of DNA by UV light requires large doses of UV and might or might not be of biological importance. On the other hand intrastrand thymine dimerization is not an efficient lethal process, since close to five thymine dimer molecules are found in the DNA complement of T 4 phage per one lethal hit (Wulff, 1963). The conditions of UV crosslinking were evaluated in some detail by Glisin and Doty (1962).

Thymine dimerization across the strands was postulated in the original study by Marmur and Grossman (1961) and in a later report by Wilson (1963), although the studies of Glisin and Setlow and Drake and Setlow (personal communications) indicated that this cannot be a cis-dimer of thymine similar to the interstrand thymine dimer, which is characterized by its instability to short-wave UV light. Incorporation of BUdR into native DNA was shown to enhance crosslinking by UV light (Opara-Kubinska *et al.*, 1963).

(b) Effects of reactive chemicals

About the same time that the crosslinking of the complementary DNA strands by UV light was discovered, a similar phenomenon was reported for DNA exposed to formaldehyde, nitrogen mustard, and nitrous acid (Geiduschek, 1961, 1962; Luzzati, 1962; Freifelder and Davison, 1963). Reversibility of thermal denaturation, as measured by the regain of hypochromicity and sedimentation properties was the principal criterion employed in these studies. The chemistry of crosslinking was not studied in detail, although it was postulated that diazo bonds might be involved in the case of nitrous acid, and a methylene bridge between the 6-amino groups of adenine in the case of formaldehyde (Alderson, 1960).

The bifunctional nitrogen mustards çonstitute another group of reactive chemicals which cause intermolecular (ALEXANDER *et al.*, 1959) and interstrand linking of DNA. Actually covalent linking of DNA either to itself or to other cell components was already postulated in the late forties by ELMORE *et al.* (1948) and GOLDACRE *et al.* (1949), but it was not expressed in more concrete chemical terms until the double-stranded nature of DNA became recognized (WATSON and CRICK, 1953). Chemical studies (LAWLEY and BROOKES, 1963) indicate that interstrand crosslinks are formed between the N-7 positions on the guanines, most probably across the deep groove of the double-stranded DNA molecule, which the N-7 positions face. Somewhat complementary physicochemical and biological studies employing spontaneous renaturation of DNA as a measure of crosslinking by nitrogen mustards were reported at about the same time (KOHN *et al.*, 1963; JONES *et al.*, 1963).

(c) Crosslinking by mitomycin C

All the agents discussed up to this point, which include radiation and highly reactive laboratory chemicals and which react *in vitro* with purified DNA, could hardly be considered natural metabolic products with which DNA could come in contact during the normal cell life. It came as a surprise, therefore, to find that a natural metabolic microbial product, mitomycin C, is a very effective DNA crosslinking agent (IYER and SZYBALSKI, 1963). Besides being a natural metabolite, mitomycin differs in at least one other important aspect from the agents described in the preceding sections: mitomycin has no effect on purified DNA *in vitro*, but very actively crosslinks bacterial DNA *in vivo*, when added to the growth medium. Although inactive *in vitro* in its original form, mitomycin could be „activated" by exposure to cell extracts, and under these conditions it also crosslinks purified DNA *in vitro*. This activation most probably involves conversion of the quinone moiety to the corresponding hydroquinone, since mitomycin reduced either enzymatically in the presence of hydrogen donors or by a purely chemical step (sodium dithionate, sodium borohydride, or hydrogen gas in the presence of a palladium-charcoal catalyst) crosslinks purified DNA *in vitro* (IYER and SZYBALSKI, 1964).

The three experimental approaches utilized in the study of DNA crosslinking by mitomycin were outlined in the original communication (IYER and SZYBALSKI, 1963). These will be briefly summarized here: (1) Upon thermal denaturation followed by rapid cooling the buoyant density of denatured DNA changes to values higher by 0.013–0.017 or by 0.022–0.025 g/cm^3, when determined in CsCl or Cs_2SO_4 density gradients, respectively. The higher values correspond to DNA's with high A + T content. Since crosslinked DNA molecules denature reversibly, their density does not change appreciably. *E.g.*, when a mixture of non-crosslinked and crosslinked DNA molecules extracted from *E. coli* is thermally denatured and rapidly cooled, two bands are formed in the CsCl gradient, one of denatured density (1.725 g/cm^3), and one of density very close to that of native DNA (1.710 g/cm^3). The proportion of the latter crosslinked DNA could be measured by integrating the UV absorption of the bands and correcting for the change in absorbance of irreversibly denatured DNA. (2) Upon exposure to increasing temperatures, native DNA undergoes a sharp transition to a denatured form with a 40–50% increase in absorbance at 260 μm within a narrow temperature range (melting temperature = t_m). Upon rapid cooling denatured normal DNA regains only a part of its hypochromicity, while the original low absorbance of crosslinked DNA is almost completely restored. A second exposure to heating distinguishes clearly between crosslinked and normal DNA: the former shows again a sharp increase in absorbance over a narrow temperature range, while the absorbance of the latter increases only gradually. By comparing the absorbance increases within the sharp transition region during the first and the second heatings, it is possible to calculate the proportion of crosslinked molecules, assuming again that one crosslink is sufficient to render the molecule spontaneously renaturable, even upon rapid cooling. (3) For biologically active, genetically transforming DNA the sharp thermal transition (denaturation) could be measured as the accompanying approximately 100-fold drop in transforming activity. Mitomycin crosslinked transforming DNA from *B. subtilis* cells, however, does not show this precipitous loss of activity upon brief heating over a narrow temperature range, followed by rapid cooling and assay with indole-requiring receptor cells. All three of these methods were described by IYER and SZYBALSKI (1963).

Employing all these different types of assays, it was determined that the extent of crosslinking by mitomycin increases with the G + C content of the DNA (IYER and SZYBALSKI, 1964). Crosslinking seems to be less pronounced in the case of unusual types of DNA, including the glucosylated and 5-hydroxymethylcytosine containing DNA of T-even phages and the glucosylated and uracil-containing DNA of *B. subtilis* phage PBS-2. Also ,,normal" DNA's in vegetative pools of T 1 and T 5 phage seem to escape partially the crosslinking, which affects more the DNA of the *E. coli* host. As in the case of pure DNA, mitomycin has no effect on extracellular phage particles, unless the cell extract is added. When mitomycin is added to growing mammalian cells, a roughly one hundred times higher concentration is required for comparable crosslinking of the chromosomal DNA in the human cell line D 98 S than of bacterial DNA. A similar comparison of the sensitivities of chromosomal versus viral DNA, both located in the same cell nucleus, was made for rabbit kidney cells infected with pseudorabies virus, in a cooperative study with Dr. A. S. KAPLAN. Under these conditions mitomycin crosslinking of the ,,naked" viral DNA was 10–20 tmes more efficient than that of the chromosomal DNA, even after correction for the intrinsically higher reactivity of the pseudorabies DNA inherent in its higher G + C content.

Although it was not determined by direct chemical analysis, mitomycin molecules most probably form the crosslinking bridge, since they have at least two reactive groups necessary for this bifunctionality (Fig. 1). The most probable ,,alkylating" centers are indicated by the arrows. These two centers would be activated in the following chain of events (IYER and SZYBALSKI, 1964): Enzymatic or chemical reduction of rhe quinone to hydroquinone configuration should increase the basicity of the ring nitrogen, since its free electrons cannot by any more withdrawn into the resonating quinone system. Therefore, the reductive step results in loss of the methoxy group and in the formation of the fully aromatic indole system. This new configuration would favor (a) the opening of the aziridine ring and (b) the fission of the carbon-oxygen bond in the carbamate side chain with simultaneous stabilization of the positive charges by the indole ring in the transition states of the reactions, thus providing highly reactive carbonium ions at the positions indicated by the arrows (Fig. 1). It should be pointed out, that the aziridine ring is not reactive in the normal oxidized form of mitomycin, since it does not seem to give a characteristic reaction with γ-(4-nitrobenzyl) pyridine (SCHWARTZ *et al.*, 1963; LOVELESS, personal communication), reacts poorly with thiosulfate at acid pH (SCHWARTZ

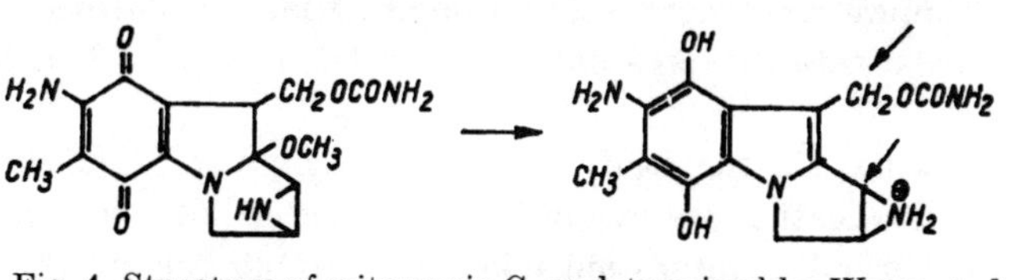

Fig. 1. Structure of mitomycin C, as determined by WEBB *et al.* (1963) (left side), and postulated structure of ,,activated" mitomycin obtained through an enzymatic reductive step, followed by the spontaneous elimination of the methoxy group.

et al., 1963), and lacks a titrable pK_a in the range 8–9 (GARRETT, 1963), all properties characteristic of other ethyleneimine derivatives.

Since mitomycin is a natural microbial metabolite, one wonders how the *Streptomyces* cell which produces it could escape its lethal DNA crosslinking effect. Since destruction of this antibiotic or impermeability to it could not be invoked to explain this resistance, lack of the activating enzyme or extremely aerobic conditions during biosynthesis of mitomycin might serve as a tentative explanation. One might wonder also whether this natural product might have some regulatory significance in the process of DNA replication, since crosslinking would obviously prevent strand separation, while secondary enzymatic „unlinking" should restore the replication. This problem will be taken up again in the following sections. Another phenomenon observed during mitomycin action on certain cells, extensive breakdown of DNA, will also be discussed later. This breakdown of DNA is considered only a secondary effect of mitomycin, since it does not occur with all mitomycin-sensitive species and since it is not correlated with the lethal action of this antibiotic.

(d) Natural occurrence of crosslinking

CsCl or Cs_2SO_4 density gradient centrifugation in conjunction with genetic transformation assay provides an extremely sensitive tool for detecting rare crosslinks in naturally occurring DNA. With highly polymerized DNA (average M.W. of 25×10^6 for *B. subtilis* transforming DNA), one crosslink per 40,000 nucleotide pairs would result in a molecule with a totally reversible denaturation behavior and banding therefore at a native-like buoyant density in the equilibrium density gradient. Since as little as one per 20 of such molecules could easily be detected by comparing the absorbances of the native-like versus the denatured band after centrifugation in the analytical centrifuge, one crosslink per up to 800,000 nucleotide pairs (per 500×10^6 M.W.) could be determined. This assay for crosslinks could be made even more sensitive by another factor of 50 to 100 by biological genetic transformation assay of the denatured and native-like fractions, taking advantage of the fact that the native-like DNA has a 50 to 100 times higher specific transforming activity than the denatured DNA molecules. Thus the sensitivity of this method is so enormously high that one crosslink per average bacterial DNA complement (M.W. of $1000–2000 \times 10^6$) could easily be determined.

Applying these methods we have come upon several cases where the presence of „renaturable" DNA is indicated:

(1) *B. subtilis* DNA was the first example of partially renaturable DNA (OPARA-KUBINSKA and SZYBALSKI, as quoted by SZYBALSKI *et al.*, 1963a). When thermally denatured and rapidly cooled transforming DNA is fractionated by preparative CsCl gradient centrifugation, the residual transforming activity bands almost exclusively at the density of native DNA[1]). With very gently extracted and deproteinized DNA, analytical CsCl or Cs_2SO_4 gradient centrifugation of similarly denatured DNA reveals a low percentage of material banding at the native-like density (OPARA-KUBINSKA *et al.*, 1963: Fig. 2c). These results indicate that some of the DNA fragments obtained during the extraction procedure might have a crosslink between the complementary strands. This crosslink might correspond to the „swivel

[1]) Similar results for *B. subtilis* DNA were reported by ROWND *et al.* (1963). On the other hand, the residual transforming activity of denatured DNA extracted from *Hemophilus influenzae* or pneumococci banded exclusively at the density of the denatured DNA (GUILD, 1961; ROWND *et al.*, 1961; MARMUR *et al.*, 1963b). Apparently the transforming activity in the latter case was associated with DNA fragments of much lower molecular weight or quite free of any crosslinks.

point" postulated by CAIRNS (1963) on the basis of his autoradiographic data, although our quantitative data indicate that there might be more than one crosslink per *B. subtilis* genome [1]). Since some markers, upon heating and rapid cooling, renature spontaneously with higher efficiency than others (MAHLER *et al.*, 1963), this might indicate that their position on the genome is much closer to the postulated crosslinks.

It is also possible that the small fraction of renaturable DNA is not of bacterial origin but belongs to some defective temperate phages contaminating the *B. subtilis* culture. The transforming activity associated with the renaturable material renders this explanation unlikely, although it was found that some defective *B. subtilis* phages, which could be obtained only upon UV induction and for which no indicator strain was found, carry DNA endowed with transforming activity for bacterial markers (ROMIG, personal communication). The renaturability of DNA from small viruses associated with circularity of the DNA molecule will be discussed later.

(2) Somewhat similar results were obtained with highly polymerized non-RNase-treated DNA extracted from the D 98 human cell line (SZYBALSKA and SZYBALSKI, 1962). Upon thermal denaturation and rapid cooling, followed by analytical CsCl gradient centrifugation, 3 to 5% of the DNA formed a rather broad peak at a density somewhat higher (1.700 g/cm^3) than the density of native human DNA (1.697 g/cm^3), but quite distinct from the bulk of the denatured DNA (1.714 g/cm^3). It is difficult to tell whether this special fraction represents DNA fragments close to the centromere portion of each chromosome or to another portion of the DNA complement characterized by covalent links, or whether it represents some lysogenic viral contaminant similar to those discussed in the following sections of this paper. The pronounced heterogeneity of mammalian DNA leaves wide room for a variety of speculations.

(3) Fowlpox virus DNA was shown to contain approximately 15% renaturable DNA (SZYBALSKI, *et al.*, 1963a). This property would most probably indicate a natural crosslink, since the conditions of extraction would not have permitted the isolation of a circular molecule intact (if fowlpox virus DNA is circular at all), a configuration which has an inherent thermal reversibility as discussed for polyoma and other small viruses in the next section. The DNA complement of fowlpox virus seems to be at least 20 to 30 times larger than that of polyoma virus and thus very sensitive to shear degradation .

(4) The double-stranded native DNA's of several small oncogenic viruses, including polyoma, SV 40, and myxoma, and of the „replicative" form of Coliphage Φ X 174 were shown to have at least three properties in common: very low molecular weight of the whole DNA complement (in the neighborhood of 3×10^6), circular configuration, and spontaneous thermal renaturability (WATSON and LITTLEFIELD, 1960; DULBECCO, 1963; WEIL and VINOGRAD, 1963; KLEINSCHMIDT *et al.*, 1963; BURTON and SINSHEIMER, 1963). It is not clear whether in addition there are some covalent interstrand links, but the difficulty in separation of two plectonemic and circular DNA strands is sufficient explanation for the spontaneous renaturability of the DNA.

(5) Another example of spontaneously renaturable DNA is the synthetic DNA produced by the *in vitro* enzymatic reaction mediated by *E. coli* DNA polymerase (RICHARDSON, *et al.*, 1963) or by calf thymus polymerase (BOLLUM, 1963b). In the first case covalent crosslinks are observed only between newly synthesized strands, while in the second case the primer strands seem to be linked to the newly synthesized strands.

---

[1]) One exponentially growing *B. subtilis* cell contains on the average three nuclei, amounting together to 6.6 ($\pm$ 0.3) $\times 10^{-9}$ μg DNA. Thus, one nucleus contains approximately 2.2×10^{-9} μg DNA *i.e.*, 2,150,000 nucleotide pairs (M.W. $= 1.3 \times 10^9$), which should correspond to a partially replicated genome (CAIRNS, 1963) of about 10^9 molecular weight.

(f) Biological properties of crosslinked DNA and biological function of crosslinking

Since some naturally occurring DNA's extracted from viable organisms appear to carry covalent crosslinks, linking of the complementary DNA strands does not seem to be associated only with an irreversible lethal event. The existence of many crosslinks along the DNA molecule would obviously be incompatible with the semiconservative mode of DNA replication, unless there was some accessory mechanism to open these links when the replication approached those special points. Thus the crosslink might even have some regulatory significance, especially when present at the initiation point of the postulated DNA „replicon" (JACOB *et al.*, 1963). The terminal crosslinks could well be the 3'-5' phosphate bonds, the pyrophosphate bonds, or some protein or hydroxyamino acid linkers. Their relative rarity might make precise chemical identification difficult.

In bacteria natural DNA crosslinks might be associated with the DNA „swivel" point (CAIRNS, 1963), or „closing" of the circle, as discussed below. For chromosomal DNA the centrosomal regions might be visualized as containing transiently crosslinked DNA.

Artificially imposed crosslinks, *e.g.* by mitomycin, result in death of the cell and inhibition of DNA synthesis, since apparently this type of crosslink cannot readily be opened by the innate cell enzymes. The transforming activity of such crosslinked, high-molecular weight DNA, however, is relatively little impaired. This fact could be readily explained as follows: one crosslink is sufficient to result in the spontaneous renaturability of the entire DNA molecule of the usual M.W. (20–30 $\times$ 10^6), whereas only a small fragment (M.W., 0.2–0.3 $\times$ 10^6) is actually incorporated into the recipient genome during the transformation process (SZYBALSKI, 1961; HUTCHINSON and ARENA, 1960), and this fragment only very rarely (1/100) carries the lethal crosslink. It is obvious that the majority of the small transforming DNA fragments excised from the donor DNA and incorporated into the recipient cells would not have any reason „to remember" that they originated from large molecules with one or very few crosslinks.

On the other hand this „excision" process, its kinetics, and the size of the excised fragments could be studied by following the loss of the spontaneous renaturability of the markers located on the crosslinked molecules, since upon separation from the crosslink they would lose the renaturability property. Some attempts to study this problem have been made in our laboratory and in the laboratory of Dr. Geiduschek (BECKER, personal communication).

Circularity of DNA

There are several lines of evidence pointing to the circularity of some DNA molecules. These will be briefly discussed, since circularity and crosslinking might be closely related.

(a) Genetic analysis has provided overwhelming evidence for the circularity of the DNA genome in *E. coli* K 12 (*c.f.*, JACOB and WOLLMAN, 1961). This genetic evidence is convincingly corroborated by autoradiographic visualization of the total *E. coli* genome by CAIRNS (1963). His data bear also on two additional important points: (1) unidirectional synthesis of DNA, and (2) the presence of a „swivel" point which permits free rotation of the duplicating strands, the joined ends of which most probably have to turn in opposite directions. The unidirectional DNA synthesis is in agreement with some genetic and physico-chemical experiments (NAGATA, 1963; YOSHIKAWA and SUEOKA, 1963a and b), but is difficult to comprehend from the point of view of the unitary chemical and enzymatic mechanism of DNA replication, as discussed by Atwood (1960) and Bollum (1963a), unless one assumes that each of the two new strands is synthesized by a different mechanism. *E.g.*, the first strand could be copied off the „intact" double helix in a manner postulated for the synthesis of single-stranded Φ X 174 DNA (Sinsheimer *et al.* 1962), while the complementary strand would be synthesized by a mode similar to that observed for polymerase-mediated DNA synthesis (Kornberg, 1961; Bollum, 1963a). Thus at least two polymerizing enzymes coupled into a special unit might be involved in the *in vivo* DNA replication process, which might explain why this reaction is many times more efficient than the *in vitro* synthesis of DNA (Kornberg, 1961). The „swivel" point, the chemical nature of which is not known but which has to consist of only a *single, freely rotating* chemical bond, might also be the point of terminal crosslinking of the DNA molecule. A single-strand break in the DNA double helix, with one or a few bases removed (most likely by depurination), would act also as a „swivel".

(b) There is good genetic evidence for the circularity of the T-even phage genome, but this fact was not corroborated by any physico-chemical evidence for circularity of the DNA molecules extracted from T-even heads (*c.f.* Thomas, 1963a). Explanation of the genetic circularity seems to rest in the circular permutations of the T-even genome (Thomas, 1963b). We did not observe any crosslinks in T-even phage DNA.

(c) A somewhat similar situation prevails in the case of the phage λ. Whereas genetic evidence suggests a circular permutation during the change from the vegetative to the prophage condition (Campbell, 1963; Calef and Licciardello, 1960), the DNA molecules extracted from the phage are linear molecules. They have, however, „sticky" ends, which cause the circularization of λ DNA molecules during storage in salt solutions of high ionic strength. At higher DNA concentrations the end-to-end aggregation plays a more prominent role (Hershey *et al.*, 1963). Although the exact nature of the „sticky" ends is not known, it seems probable that these represent single-stranded regions on one terminus of the molecule complementary to a single-strand terminal region on the other end. Closing of the circle is inhibited by low salt concentration, low temperature (Hershey *et al.*, 1963), and formaldehyde (Szybalski, unpublished), all these conditions indicating the complementary hydrogen bonding nature of these end-to-end links. The formation of circular λ DNA can be convincingly observed by electron microscopy . The „joining point" of each circle is recognized as a small discontinuity (Ris and Chandler, 1963).

(d) The clearest cases of DNA circularity are the single-stranded phage Φ X 174 DNA (Fiers and Sinsheimer, 1962), the double-stranded „replicative" form of this phage (Kleinschmidt *et al.*, 1963; Burton and Sinsheimer, 1963), and the double-stranded DNA of polyoma virus (Dulbecco, 1963; Weil and Vinograd, 1963). In the case of Φ X 174 DNA the circle-closing link might not be the usual DNA phosphate bond, since it is resistant to exonucleases (Fiers and Sinsheimer, 1962). As discussed earlier, it is not clear whether the end-to-end link acts also as a terminal crosslink of the complementary DNA strands (Weil and Vinograd, 1963).

Operationally, the DNA circles are easily recognized by their very high increase ($2.5 \times$) in sedimentation constant upon denaturation, and by electron microscopic visualization (Appendix by Stoekenius in Weil and Vinograd, 1963; Kleinschmidt *et al.*, 1963).

(e) There have been attempts to postulate that all chromosomal DNA is composed of interlocked circles (Stahl, 1961), but this bold idea has no real experimental foundation at the present time.

Function of DNA circularity

It is not easy to speculate on the function of DNA circularity, but at least two possibilites might be considered: (1) Closing of the circle eliminates the free ends of the DNA molecule and thus renders it resistant to all sorts of exonucleolytic activity. Exonucleases seem to be present in all cells and thus are potentially dangerous to any DNA which contains free and susceptible end groups. It is notable that under a variety of conditions, including the action of some phages, irradiation, and several inhibitors, rapid exonucleolytic DNA breakdown is provoked. One could postulate that this reaction might be initiated by the opening of the DNA circle. One should not, however, overlook several other potential methods of protecting the ends of the linear DNA molecule, including specific glucosylation, methylation, reaction with polypeptides, etc. This protection of DNA against nucleolytic attack might be closely related to the phenomenon of host-induced specificity observed with several phage-bacteria systems, including T-even Coliphages (Luria and Human, 1952; Erikson and Szybalski, 1964; Hatman and Fukasawa, 1963) and Coliphage λ (Dussoix and Arber, 1962). In all these cases complete or partial exonucleolytic breakdown of DNA is associated with penetration of host-modified DNA into the restrictive host (Dussoix and Arber, 1962; Erikson and Szybalski, 1964), although no breakdown of glucoseless DNA was observed in the preliminary experiments of Shedlovsky and Brenner (1963).
(2) Closing of the circle might result in polarized transcription of the DNA code into the messenger RNA, since it was found that *in vivo* only one of the two DNA strands is copied by the DNA-RNA polymerase (Spiegelman and Hayashi, 1963; Marmur *et al.*, 1963a), while no such limitation is imposed upon *in vitro* RNA synthesis primed by broken DNA fragments (Geiduschek *et al.*, 1961).

Single-strand interruptions

Breakage of a single (or of a few widely separated) phosphate ester bonds along the double-stranded DNA molecule would have little effect on its properties in the native state. Most probably there exists an enzymatic mechanism in the cell for repair of such damage (Kozinski and Kozinski, 1963). The action of very many agents, including radiation, cytotoxic drugs, low pH, and endonucleases, results in single-strand breaks. Single-strand breaks were found also in DNA extracted by very gentle techniques from perfectly viable phages (Freifelder and Davison, 1963a). Thus a rare single-strand break need not necessarily be equated to a lethal event. Breaks in the DNA molecule have to be postulated in order to explain genetic recombination (Meselson and Weigle, 1961) and fragmentary DNA replication (Kozinski and Kozinski, 1963) in several phages.

Single-strand breaks, which seem to have little effect on native DNA, could be easily detected after thermal denaturation of the DNA molecules. Since thermal strand separation eliminates the „splicing" effect of the hydrogen bonds, the denatured molecule would break up into *many* single-stranded fragments rather than into only *two* single strands. This change could be followed either by measuring the widening of the DNA bands in the CsCl gradient (Opara-Kubinska *et al.*, 1963), or by boundary-velocity or band-centrifugation analysis (Freifelder and Davison, 1963a; Vinograd *et al.*, 1963; Studier, personal communication).

Only a few examples of externally provoked single-strand breaks in DNA will be discussed here:

(a) Mitomycin has been reported to cause extensive breakdown of DNA (KERSTEN, 1962; SHATKIN *et al.*, 1962). This phenomenon seems to occur only with some species; it was not found with *B. subtilis* (IYER and SZYBALSKI, 1963). Since the latter cells are killed by mitomycin, it is obvious that breakdown of DNA is not correlated with the lethal action of mitomycin. The relationship of MC-induced breaks or crosslinks to the mutagenic effects of mitomycin (SZYBALSKI, 1958) is not known. Most probably the extensive breakdown of DNA is restricted to cells which contain an RNA-inhibited DNA endonuclease, similar to that described by LEHMAN (1964). It is quite possible that mitomycin, by attacking RNA bases, might cause destruction of some RNA organelles and thus release this endonuclease, which in turn would degrade the DNA. Some aspects of this hypothesis were discussed by KERSTEN (1962).

With long exposures to mitomycin, we have observed a widening of *B. subtilis* DNA bands in CsCl or Cs_2SO_4 gradients, especially after denaturation, indicating single-strand DNA breaks even in this bacterium. The crosslinking effect of mitomycin could mask some of the simultaneous single-strand breaks, as usually detected by spreading of the DNA band in the CsCl gradient after thermal denaturation.

(b) Streptonigrin (RAO *et al.*, 1963) and phleomycin (TANAKA *et al.*, 1963) were found to be much more effective in causing single-strand breaks in *B. subtilis* DNA than mitomycin (IYER and SZYBALSKI, *unpublished*). Streptonigrin is related to mitomycin in having an aminoquinone group, but is otherwise devoid of any obviously reactive configuration, like *e.g.* the aziridine ring, which is characteristic of the mitomycins.

Streptonigrin, as could also be inferred from its structure (RAO *et al.*, 1963), shown in Fig. 2, and phleomycin were not found to crosslink the DNA strands. When, however, *B. subtilis* cells are exposed for as short a period as 5 minutes to these antibiotics, the isolated DNA is found to be partially degraded and to carry many single-strand breaks. After longer exposure no high-molecular weight fibrous DNA can be extracted from the cells (IYER and SZYBALSKI, *unpublished*). None of these agents seem to induce any new DNases (*c.f.*, LEHMAN, 1964), although some increase in the DNase activity was reported by NAKATA *et al.* (1961). The mechanism of the DNA breakdown, as initiated by these drugs, is not known, but might be related to the indirect effect discussed for mitomycin.

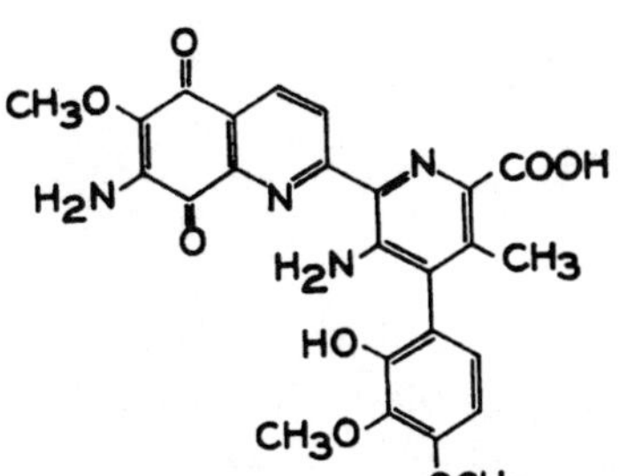

Fig. 2. Structure of streptonigrin, as determined by RAO *et al.* (1963).

(c) Radiation effects seem often to be associated with single-strand DNA breaks. Many types of radiation were studied in this context, including DNA-incorporated P^{32} decay (STENT and FUERST, 1960; LEVINTHAL and DAVISON, 1961), X-rays (ALEXANDER *et al.*, 1959; FREIFELDER and DAVISON, 1963b), UV, and visible light, in conjunction with halogenated deoxyuridine analogs or photodynamic sensitizers (OPARA-KUBINSKA *et al.*, 1963; WACKER *et al.*, 1963; FREIFELDER *et al.*, 1961; SMITH, 1964). It is possible that many so-called „dark repair" mechanisms for irradiated cells might be equated to the enzymatic repair of shattered phosphate ester bonds.

(d) Most of the agents discussed in sections (a) to (c) could be considered as DNA synthesis inhibitors. It might be interesting, therefore, to determine whether any type of selective inhibition of DNA synthesis would result in enzymatic degradation of the DNA. This might be true in some cases, since MENNIGMANN and SZYBALSKI (1962) observed an accumulation of single-strand DNA breaks concurrent with „thymineless death" of *B. subtilis* cells induced by 5-fluorodeoxyuridine (FUdR) inhibition of thymidylate synthetase. Under similar conditions TAYLOR (1963) observed a „shattering" effect of FUdR on the chromosomes of *Vicia faba*. On the other hand, FREIFELDER (*c.f.*, MAALØE, 1963) did not observe DNA breakdown during thymineless death of the 15 T^- strain of *E. coli*. Similarly, we have not seen any damage to DNA during DNA synthesis inhibition by phenethyl alcohol in *B. subtilis* cells (IYER and SZYBALSKI, *unpublished*). Activation of nucleases, therefore, seems to vary from species to species and from agent to agent, and it does not seem to be an obligatory consequence of DNA synthesis inhibition.

One might speculate as to what is the general role of nucleases within the living cell, how are the intracellular nucleic acids protected from these potentially lethal agents, and what is the mechanism of their activation. Several examples will be discussed here:

(a) Invading viruses or phages may activate the nucleolytic breakdown of host DNA, which later is utilized for the synthesis of viral DNA. T-even and T 5 phages serve as good examples. The breakdown of host DNA seems to be much earlier and not correlated with the appearance of phage-induced nucleases (*c.f.*, LEHMAN, 1964).

(b) Nucleases could form a defense mechanism against viral DNA. In the case of „restrictive" *E. coli* hosts the host-modified DNA is broken down upon penetration into the host, a phenomenon which seems to depend on the degree or mode of methylation of the DNA (ARBER, personal communication; GOLD and HURWITZ, 1963). A somewhat similar case is observed with the host-modified, deglucosylated DNA of T-even phages, which is partially degraded upon entry into the restrictive host B (*c.f.*, ERIKSON and SZYBALSKI, 1964). A small percentage, however, of intact deglucosylated DNA molecules can infect even the restrictive host, and once established can produce normal glucosylated DNA and viable phage. It appears therefore that partial degradation of deglucosylated DNA occurs only during the act of entry into restrictive cells and might be caused by surface-proximate nucleases. The reason for some host-modified nonglucosylated DNA molecules escaping this nucleolytic attack might be purely statistical, *e.g.*, if the number of nuclease molecules is limited, especially in a fraction of B cells which are in some special physiological state („old" cells are less restrictive than „young" cells: LURIA and HUMAN, 1952), or some nonglucosylated DNA-molecules might also be protected by the ancestral glucosylated DNA fragments strategically incorporated into the exonuclease-sensitive ends. The parental glucosylated DNA should be well dispersed among the glucoseless progeny produced in the $UDPG^-$ host (ERIKSON and SZYBALSKI, 1964; KOZINSKI and KOZINSKI, 1963).

There are many other examples of nucleolytic destruction of cell-invading DNA, and this defensive property might constitute one of the main biological roles of intracellular nucleases. On the other hand, nucleases, especially extracellular nucleases secreted into the surrounding medium, might be used for degrading nucleic acids in the medium prior to their utilization as nutrient by scavenger cells.

(c) Most of the agents which induce single-strand breaks in DNA also cause the induction of lysogenic phages. UV light, mitomycin, streptonigrin, and thymineless death are among the most common examples of inducing agents (LWOFF, 1953; OTSUJI *et al.*, 1959; LEVINE and BORTHWICK, 1963; MELECHEN and SKAAR, 1962). The molecular mechanism of lysogenic induction and its relation to single-strand DNA breaks is not known, but one could postulate that (1) breaks in DNA might free the lysogenic phage replicon from control by the host DNA, (2) host DNA represents a much larger target for attack by inducing agents, while the replication of the freed phage genome would not be affected, or (3) many of

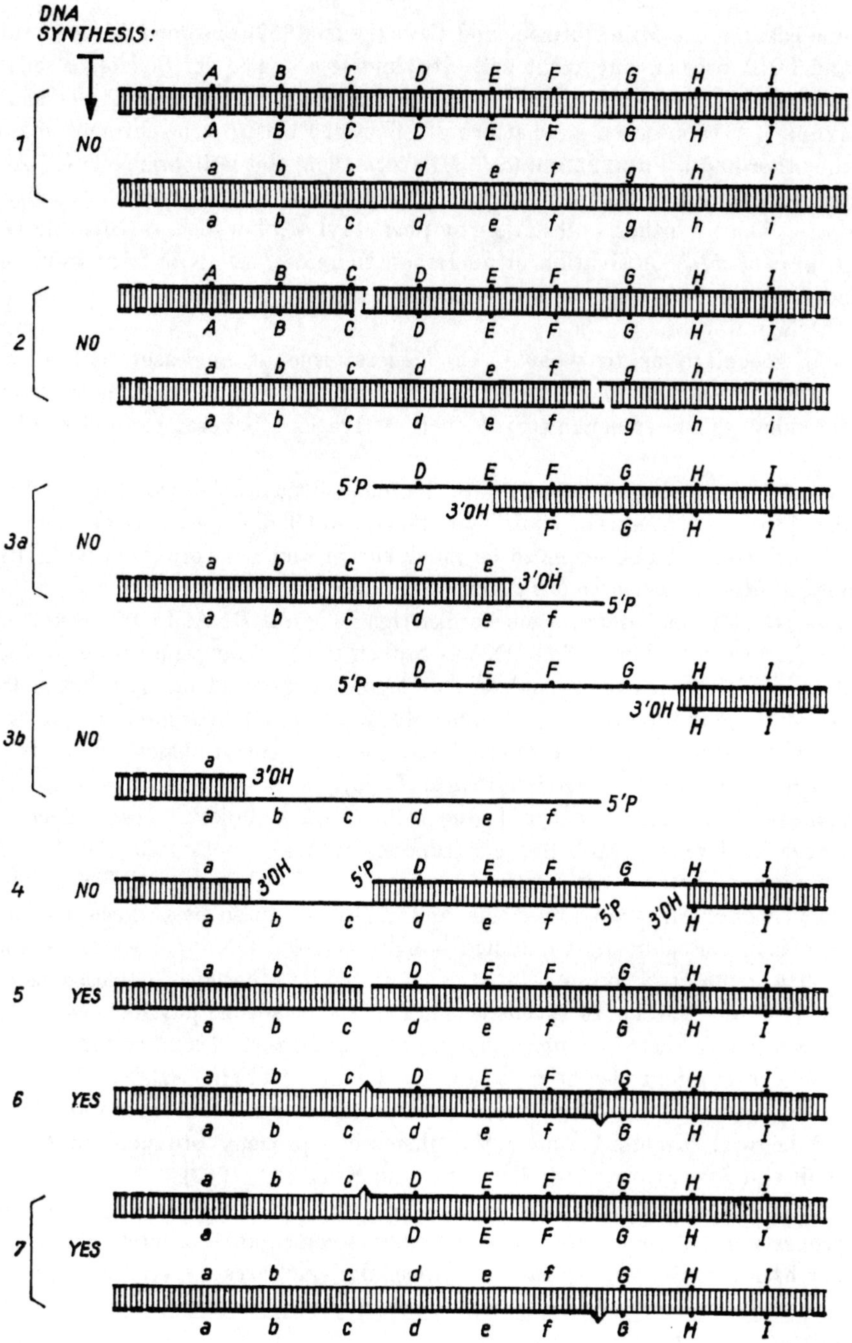

Fig. 3. Schematic representation of the genetic recombination act on the molecular level.

1. Two parental double-stranded DNA molecules, represented by heavy double lines, one with genetic markers indicated by capital letters (knobbed lines), and the other with markers in lower case letters.
2. Endonucleolytic double-strand breaks.

3a and 3b. Exonucleolytic hydrolysis of single strands which terminate with 3'OH (or 3'P) groups.

4. Pairing between complementary single-stranded regions. Events 1 to 4 are favored by the absence of DNA synthesis.
5. Polymerase-mediated DNA synthesis commencing at the 3'OH ends and filling the wide „gaps"; newly synthesized strands indicated by thin lines.
6. Closing of the final 3'OH-5'P link (kinked line); enzymatic mechanism unknown.
7. Replication of this partially „heterozygous" DNA molecule with production of two homozygous recombinant molecules.

the inducing agents inactivate the hypothetical repressor, presumably an RNA-containing substance, which normally interferes with the autonomous replication of lysogenic phage.
(d) Nucleases might also be involved in the ,,mysterious" process of genetic recombination between DNA molecules. One could imagine that recombination is a complex process mediated by several enzymes and consisting of many steps (Fig. 3), as hypothesized below for a nonreciprocal recombination between two phage DNA molecules.

The first step would consist of two breaks, somewhere in the homologous regions of two parental DNA molecules, as represented in Fig. 3, scheme 2. These double-strand breaks could be initiated by some intracellular endonuclease (LEHMAN, 1964) and should be considered as a chance event. The breaks could occur anywhere and only the overlapping longer segments will be considered here (D-E-F-G-H-I) and (a-b-c-d-e-f). Once the breaks occurred, the 3'OH (or 3'P) ends of the molecules would become sensitive to an exonuclease, similar in action to exonuclease III (DNA phosphatase-exonuclease) described by LEHMAN (1964). This exonuclease, which would act only on one strand of the double-stranded DNA molecule, would progressively expose the single-stranded complementary regions of the 5'P- (or 5'OH-) terminated strands (Fig. 3, schemes 3a and 3b), and thus permit homologous base pairing between the two parental strands (Fig. 3, scheme 4). The preparatory exonucleolytic action should be favored by the absence of DNA synthesis, since the action of the DNA polymerase would be counteracting the exonucleolytic ,,splicing", a necessary prerequisite to hydrogen bonding of the two molecules. That the act of recombination is inhibited during the active DNA synthesis period and involves the breakage and rejoining of parental molecules is indicated by the studies of WEIGLE (personal communication), KOZINSKI and KOZINSKI (1963) and MESELSON and WEIGLE (1961). The pursuant steps would require DNA synthesis, and would involve polymerase-mediated filling of the ,,gaps", left by the preceding step of exonucleolytic ,,splicing", which most probably would be carried beyond the homologous region D-F, in the manner indicated in scheme 3b (Fig. 3), until the time when polymerase-mediated DNA synthesis (scheme 5) intervened. The latter reaction is analogous to that described by RICHARDSON *et al.* (1963b). Closing of the last link between adjoining nucleotides (scheme 6) must be postulated in order to explain the results obtained by KOZINSKI and KOZINSKI (1963), although no enzyme capable of performing this function is known or was isolated. This re-formation of the last ester bond might be related to the so-called post-irradiation ,,dark" repair of single-strand breaks and other similar ,,repairs". There are no compelling theoretical reasons for the ,,closing of the last link", and in some other organisms this step might not take place.

The resulting double-stranded molecule, shown in scheme 6 (Fig. 3), is partially ,,heterozygous" for the D-G-F/d-g-f region, but upon subsequent replication (scheme 7) fully homozygous ,,recombinant" molecules would be produced.

The scheme outlined here is one of many possible, more-or-less complicated variations-on-a-theme, but its main virtue lies in presenting the whole recombination process in terms of already known chemical and enzymatic events. Deficiency in any one enzyme mediating this multistep process could be considered as a loss of a ,,recombinase", in analogy with the observations of KOZINSKI *et al.* (1963), who noted a decrease in DNA fragmentation caused by early inhibition of protein synthesis during T 4 phage DNA replication, and also isolated ,,non-fragmenting" T 4 phage mutants (KOZINSKI, personal communication). The problem of reciprocal recombination between DNA molecules is not considered here, although it would not be too difficult to design an appropriate molecular scheme for such an event, possibly following the general outlines proposed by WHITEHOUSE (1963).

Other secondary features of DNA

Throughout this discussion only the phosphate ester bonds between the bases have been considered as joining the fragments or „subunits" of the DNA molecule. Although other „linkers" have been postulated, including phosphoserine (Bendich and Rosenkrantz, 1963) or peptide bonds (Taylor, 1963), no critical evidence for such heterologous insertions was ever found, with the exception perhaps of the nuclease-resistant link of unknown structure which closes the circular Φ X 174 DNA molecule (Fiers and Sinsheimer, 1962) and the „swivel" of Cairns (1963), both of which were discussed earlier.

Although several small viruses are known to contain single-stranded DNA, there is very scant evidence for any accumulation of single-stranded DNA during the process of DNA replication in dividing cells. Some data based on the appearance of heavy, denatured-like DNA bands during CsCl gradient centrifugation of bacterial DNA (Rolfe, 1963; Lark, 1963) must be weighed with caution, since it was demonstrated by Erikson and Szybalski (1964) that deproteinization with improperly treated phenol can lead to the conversion of a small fraction of the DNA to a material which bands at higher density in the CsCl gradient. On the other hand, a denatured-like, somewhat denser DNA band transiently appears only during the early phases of the comparatively short period of DNA synthesis in naturally synchronized (Guttes *et al.*, 1961) nuclei of the slime mold *Physarum polycephalum*, when chloroform-butanol deproteinized or non-deproteinized DNA is banded in the CsCl gradient, in experiments performed in cooperation with Dr. W. Sachsenmaier.

Other natural and artificial features or modifications of DNA, including glucosylation and deglucosylation of T-even phage DNA (Erikson and Szybalski, 1964), the 5-halodeoxyuridine-for-thymidine substitution (Szybalski, 1962; Szybalski and Lorkiewicz, 1962; Erikson and Szybalski, 1963; Szybalski *et al.*, 1963b), intercalation of acridines (Lerman, 1963), interaction with actinomycin (Rauen *et al.*, 1960; Reich *et al.*, 1962), photochemical oxidation of DNA guanine (Simon and Van Vunakis, 1962), and DNA complexing with c-RNA (Opara-Kubinska and Szybalski, 1964) will not be discussed here.

Summary

Both under natural conditions and as an aftereffect of interaction with chemical or physical agents a double-stranded DNA molecule may exhibit several additional topological features, including crosslinks between the complementary DNA strands, end-to-end linking (circularization), and single-strand breaks. Nitrogen mustards, nitrous acid, and formaldehyde react with DNA directly *in vitro*, linking the complementary strands, while the naturally occurring antibiotic mitomycin has to undergo enzymatic or chemical activation (reduction a hydroquinone derivative) before performing a similar function. Naturally crosslinked DNA fractions have been found in some bacteria, human cells, and viruses. Circularity of DNA molecules seems not to be a rare feature in small viruses and bacteria and has been found in several systems amenable to genetic, radioautographic or physicochemical analysis. These structural features of DNA and also pre-existing single-strand breaks are discussed in relation to their possible biological significance, including the control of DNA synthesis, the mechanism of genetic recombination, and lethal or mutagenic effects.

Acknowledgements

This contribution is based partially on published and unpublished work carried out in this laboratory in cooperation with Dr. V. N. Iyer of the Canada Department of Agriculture, Ottawa, Canada, Dr. R. L. Erikson, presently at the Department of Pathology, the University of Colorado Medical Center, Denver, Colorado, and Mrs. Z. Opara-Kubinska, and partially on data from literature. The author is greatly indebted to all his colleagues, and also to Dr. Elizabeth H. Szybalka for helpful suggestions and editorial help, and to Mr. Larry Fenton for his able assistance with some phases of this work.

These studies were supported in part by grants No. CY-5215 and CA-07175 from the National Cancer Institute, U.S.P.H.S., Bethesda 14, Md.

References

ALDERSON, T., 1960: Mechanism of formaldehyde-induced mutagenesis. The uniqueness of adenylic acid in the mediation of the mutagenic activity of formaldehyde. Nature 187, 485—489.

ALEXANDER, P., J. T. LETT, H. MOROSON, and K. A. STACEY, 1959: Changes produced by ionizing radiations and some related agents in DNA *in vitro* and *in vivo*. in „Immediate and Low Levels Effects of Ionizing Radiations", Suppl. to the Int. J. Rad. Biol. pp. 47—69.

ALEXANDER, P., and K. A. STACEY, 1959: Cross-linking of deoxyribonucleic acid in sperm heads by ionizing radiation. Nature (London) 184, 958—960.

ATWOOD, K. C., 1960: Sequential deoxyribonucleic acid replication. Science 132, 617—618.

BARANOWSKA, J., and D. SHUGAR, 1960: Photochemistry of model oligo- and polynucleotides. III. Cross-linking and staining properties of ultraviolet irradiated films of nucleic acids and oligonucleotides. Acta Biochem. Polonica 7, 505—520.

BENDICH, A., and H. S. ROSENKRANZ, 1963: Some thoughts on the double-stranded model of deoxyribonucleic acid. Progress in Nucleic Acid Research 1, 219—230.

BOLLUM, F. J., 1963a: „Primer" in DNA polymerase reactions. Progress in Nucleic Acid Research 1, 1—26.

BOLLUM, F. J., 1963b: Intermediate states in enzymatic DNA synthesis. J. Cell. Comp. Physiol. 62 Suppl., 61—71.

BRITTEN, R. J., 1963: Complementary strand association between nucleic acids and nucleic acid gels. Nature 142, 963—965.

BURTON, A., and R. L. SINSHEIMER, 1963: Process of infection with Φ X 174: Effect of exonucleases on the replicative form. Science 142, 962—963.

CAIRNS, J., 1963: The bacterial chromosome and its manner of replication as seen by autoradiography. J. Mol. Biol. 6, 208—213.

CALABRESI, P., and A. D. WELCH, 1962: Chemotherapy of neoplastic diseases. Ann. Rev. Med. 13, 147—202.

CALEF, E., and G. LICCIARDELLO, 1960: Recombination experiments on prophage host relationship. Virology 12, 81—103.

CAVALIERI, L. F., and B. H. ROSENBERG, 1962: Observations on the replication of DNA, in „The Molecular Basis of Neoplasia", Univ. of Texas Press, Austin, 44—58.

CAMPBELL, A., 1963: Segregants from lysogenic heterogenotes carrying recombinant lambda prophages. Virology 20, 344—356.

DONOHUE, J., and K. N. TRUEBLOOD, 1960: Base pairing in DNA. J. Mol. Biol. 2, 363—371.

DULBECCO, R., 1963: Evidence for a ring structure of polyoma virus DNA. Proc. Natl. Acad. Sci. U.S. 50, 236—243.

Dussoix, D., and W. Arber, 1962: Host specificity of DNA produced by *Escherichia coli*. II. Control over acceptance of DNA from infecting phage λ. J. Mol. Biol. **5**, 37–49.

Elmore, D. T., J. M. Gulland, D. O. Jordan, and H. R. W. Taylor, 1948: The reaction of nucleic acids with mustard gas. Biochem. J. **42**, 308–316.

Erikson, R. L., and W. Szybalski, 1963: Molecular radiobiology of human cell lines. V. Comparative radiosensitizing properties of 5-halodeoxycytidines and 5-halodeoxyuridines. Radiation Research **20**, 252–262.

Erikson, R. L., and W. Szybalski, 1964: The Cs_2SO_4 equilibrium density gradient and its application for the study of T-even phage DNA: glucosylation and replication. Virology **22**, 111–124.

Fiers, W., and R. L. Sinsheimer, 1962: The structure of the DNA of bacteriophage Φ X 174. III. Ultracentrifugal evidence for a ring structure. J. Mol. Biol. **5**, 424–434.

Freifelder, D., and P. F. Davison, 1963a: Physicochemical studies on the reaction between formaldehyde and DNA. Biophys. J. **3**, 49–63.

Freifelder, D., and P. F. Davison, 1963b: „Letters to Editor", Biophys. J. **3**, 97–98.

Freifelder, D., P. F. Davison, and E. P. Geiduschek, 1961: Damage by visible light to the acridine orange-DNA complex. Biophys. J. **1**, 389–400.

Garrett, E. R., 1963: The physical chemical characterization of the products, equilibria, and kinetics of the complex tranformations of the antibiotic porfiromycin. J. Med. Chem. **6**, 488–501.

Geiduschek, E. P., 1961: „Reversible" DNA. Proc. Natl. Acad. Sci. U.S. **47**, 950–955.

Geiduschek, E. P., 1962: On the factors controlling the reversibility of DNA denaturation. J. Mol. Biol. **4**, 467–487.

Geiduschek, E. P., Nakamoto, T., and S. B. Weiss, 1961: The enzymatic synthesis of RNA: complementary interaction with DNA. Proc. Natl. Acad. Sci. U.S. **47**, 1405–1415.

Glišin, V. R., and P. Doty, 1962: The effect of temperature on the cross-linking of deoxyribonucleic acid strands by ultraviolet radiation. Biochim. Biophys. Acta **61**, 458–460.

Gold, M., and J. Hurwitz, 1963: The enzymatic methylation of the nucleic acids. Cold Spring Harbor Symp. Quant. Biol. **28**, 149–156.

Goldacre, R. J., A. Loveless, and W. C. Ross, 1949: Mode of production of chromosome abnormalities by the nitrogen mustard. The possible role of crosslinking. Nature **163**, 667–669.

Guild, W. R., 1961: Transformation by denatured deoxyribonucleic acid. Proc. Natl. Acad. Sci. U.S. **47**, 1560–1564.

Guttes, E., S. Guttes, and H. P. Rusch, 1961: Morphological observations on growth and differentiation of *Physarum polycephalum* grown in pure culture. Develop. Biol. **3**, 588–614.

Hershey, A. D., E. Burgi, and L. Ingraham, 1963: Cohesion of DNA molecules isolated from phage lambda. Proc. Natl. Acad. Sci. U.S. **49**, 748–755.

Hofschneider, P. H., 1963: Untersuchungen über „kleine" *E. coli* K 12 Bakteriophagen. Z. f. Naturforsch. **18b**, 203–210.

Hutchinson, F., and J. Arena, 1960: Destruction of the activity of deoxyribonucleic acid in irradiated cells. Rad. Res. **13**, 137–147.

Iyer, V. N., and W. Szybalski, 1963: A molecular mechanism of mitomycin action: linking of complementary DNA strands. Proc. Natl. Acad. Sci. U.S. **50**, 355–362.

Iyer, V. N., and W. Szybalski, 1964: Mitomycins and Porfiromycin: Chemical mechanism of activation and crosslinking of DNA. Science **145**, 55–58.

Jacob, F., S. Brenner, and F. Cuzin, 1963: On the regulation of DNA replication in bacteria. Cold Spring Harbor Symp. Quant. Biol. **28**, 329–348.

Jacob, F., and E. L. Wollman, 1961: „Sexuality and the Genetics of Bacteria", Academic Press, Inc., New York.

Jones, J., R. H. Golden, and R. J. Rutman, 1963: The reversible denaturation of mammalian DNA after bifunctional alkylation. Feder. Proc. **22**, 582.

Kay, D., 1962: The nucleic acid composition of bacteriophage Φ R. J. Gen. Microbiol. **27**, 201–207.

Kersten, H., 1962: Zur Wirkungsweise von Mitomycin C. I. Einfluss von Mitomycin C auf den Deoxyribonucleinsäure-Abbau in ruhenden Bakterien. Hoppe-Seyler's Z. physiol. Chem. **329**, 31–39.

Kleinschmidt, A. K., A. Burton, and R. L. Sinsheimer, 1963: Electron microscopy of the replicative form of the DNA of the bacteriophage Φ X 174. Science **142**, 961.

KOHN, K., D. GREEN, and P. DOTY, 1963: Interstrand crosslinking of DNA by nitrogen mustard (HN 2) and its effect on transforming activity. Feder. Proc. **22**, 582.

KORNBERG, A., 1961: „Enzymatic Synthesis of DNA", J. Wiley & Sons Publ., New York.

KOZINSKI, A. W., and P. B. KOZINSKI, 1963: Fragmentary transfer of P^{32}-labeled parental DNA to progeny phage. II. The average size of transferred parental fragment. Two-cycle transfer. Repair of the polynucleotide chain after fragmentation. Virology **20**, 213—229.

KOZINSKI, A. W., P. B. KOZINSKI, and P. SHANNON, 1963: Replicative fragmentation in T4 phage: Inhibition by chloramphenicol. Proc. Natl. Acad. Sci. U.S. **50**, 746—753.

LARK, K., 1963: Cellular control of DNA biosynthesis, in „Molecular Genetics". J. H. Taylor, Ed., Academic Press, Part 1, pp. 153—206.

LAWLEY, P. D., and P. BROOKES, 1963: The action of alkylating agents on deoxyribonucleic acid in relation to biological effects of the alkylating agents. Exper. Cell Research, Suppl. **9**, 512—520.

LEHMAN, I. R., 1964: The nucleases of *Escherichia coli*, Progress in Nucleic Acid Research **2**, 83—123.

LERMAN, L. S., 1963: The structure of the DNA-acridine complex. Proc. Natl. Acad. Sci. U.S. **49**, 94—102.

LEVINE, M., and M. BORTHWICK, 1963: Induction of phage production in lysogenic bacteria with streptonigrin. Bacteriol. Proc. **1963**, 153.

LEVINTHAL, C., and P. F. DAVISON, 1961: Degradation of deoxyribonucleic acid under hydrodynamic shearing forces. J. Mol. Biol. **3**, 674—683.

LURIA, S. E., and M. L. HUMAN, 1952: A nonhereditary, host-induced variation of bacterial viruses. J. Bacteriol. **64**, 557—569.

LUZZATI, D., 1962: The action of nitrous acid on transforming deoxyribonucleic acid. Biochem. Biophys. Res. Comm. **9**, 508—516.

LWOFF, A., 1953: Lysogeny. Bacteriol. Rev. **17**, 269—337.

MAALØE, O., 1963: Role of protein synthesis in the DNA replication cycle in bacteria. J. Cell. Comp. Physiol. **62** Suppl. 1. 31—44.

MAHLER, I., J. NEWMANN, and J. MARMUR, 1963: Studies of genetic units controlling arginine biosynthesis in *Bacillus subtilis*. Biochim. Biophys. Acta **72**, 69—79.

MARMUR, J., C. M. GREENSPAN, E. PALECEK, F. H. KAHAN, J. LEVINE, and M. MANDEL, 1963a: Specificity of the complementary RNA formed by *B. subtilis* infected with bacteriophage SP8. Cold Spring Harbor Symp. Quant. Biol. **28**, 191—199.

MARMUR, J., R. ROWND, and C. L. SCHILDKRAUT, 1963b: Denaturation and renaturation of deoxyribonucleic acid. Progress in Nucleic Acid Research **1**, 231—300.

MARVIN, D. A., and H. HOFFMANN-BERLING, 1963: Physical and chemical properties of two new small bacteriophages. Nature **197**, 517—518.

MELECHEN, N. E., and P. D. SKAAR, 1962: The provocation of an early step in induction by thymine deprivation. Virology **16**, 21—29.

MENNIGMANN, H. D., and W. SZYBALSKI, 1962: Molecular mechanism of thymine-less death. Biochem. Biophys. Res. Comm. **9**, 398—404.

MESELSON, M., and J. J. WEIGLE, 1961: Chromosome breakage accompanying genetic recombination in bacteriophage. Proc. Natl. Acad. U.S. **47**, 857—868.

NAGATA, T., 1963: The molecular synchrony and sequential replication of DNA in *Escherichia coli*. Proc. Natl. Acad. Sci. U.S. **49**, 551—559.

NAKATA, Y., K. NAKATA, and Y. SAKAMOTO, 1961: On the action mechanism of mitomycin C. Biochem. Biophys. Res. Comm. **6**, 339—343.

OPARA-KUBIŃSKA, Z., Z. BOROWSKA, and W. SZYBALSKI, 1963: Genetic transformation studies. III. Effect of UV light on the molecular properties of normal and halogenated DNA. Biochem. Biophys. Acta **72**, 298—309.

OPARA-KUBIŃSKA, Z., and W. SZYBALSKI, 1964: „Complexing RNA" (c-RNA) isolated from Bacilli. Abstracts, Biophysical Soc. Eight Ann. Meeting, Chicago, p. WA 9.

OTSUJI, N., M. SEKIGUCHI, T. IIJIMA, and T. TAKAGI, 1959: Induction of phage formation in the lysogenic *Escherichia coli* K-12 by mitomycin C. Nature **184**, 1079—1080.

RAO, K. V., K. BIEMANN, and R. B. WOODWARD, 1963: The structure of streptonigrin. J. Am. Chem. Soc. **85**, 2532—2533.

RAUEN, H. M., H. KERSTEN, and W. KERSTEN, 1960: Zur Wirkungsweise von Actinomycinen. Hoppe-Seyler's Z. physiol. Chem. **321**, 139—147.

REICH, E., I. H. GOLDBERG, and M. RABINOWITZ, 1962: Structure-activity correlations of actinomycins and their derivatives. Nature 196, 743—748.

RICHARDSON, C. C., C. SCHILDKRAUT, and A. KORNBERG, 1963: Studies on the replication of DNA by DNA polymerases. Cold Spring Harbor Symp. Quant. Biol. 28, 9—19.

RIS, H., and B. L. CHANDLER, 1963: The ultrastructure of genetic systems in prokaryotes and eukaryotes. Cold Spring Harbor Symp. Quant. Biol. 28, 1—8.

ROLFE, R., 1963: Changes in the physical state of DNA during the replication cycle. Proc. Natl. Acad. Sci. U.S. 49, 386—392.

ROWND, R., D. M. GREEN, and P. DOTY, 1963: The origin of the residual biological activity of thermally denatured *B. subtilis* DNA. Abstract, Biophys. Soc. 7th Ann. Meeting, TB7.

ROWND, R., J. LANYI, and P. DOTY, 1961: The biological and physical heterogeneity of thermally denatured and renatured deoxyribonucleic acid. Biochim. Biophys. Acta 53, 225—227.

SCHWARTZ, H. S., J. E. SODERGREN, and F. S. PHILIPS, 1963: Mitomycin C: Chemical and biological studies on alkylation. Science 142, 1181—1183.

SETLOW, R., and B. DOYLE, 1954: The action of radiation on dry deoxyribonucleic acid. Biochim. Biophys. Acta 15, 117—125.

SHATKIN, A. J., E. REICH, R. M. FRANKLIN, and E. L. TATUM, 1962: Effect of mitomycin C on mammalian cells in culture. Biochim. Biophys. Acta 55, 277—289.

SHEDLOVSKY, A., and S. BRENNER, 1963: A chemical basis for the host-induced modification of T-even bacteriophages. Proc. Natl. Acad. Sci. U.S. 50, 300—305.

SIMON, M. I., and H. VAN VUNAKIS, 1962: The photodynamic reaction of methylene blue with deoxyribonucleic acid. J. Mol. Biol. 4, 488—499.

SINSHEIMER, R. L., 1959: A single-stranded deoxyribonucleic acid from bacteriophage Φ X 174. J. Mol. Biol. 1, 43—53.

SINSHEIMER, R. L., B. STARMAN, C. NAGLER, and S. GUTHRIE, 1962: The process of infection with bacteriophage Φ X 174. I. Evidence for a „replicative form". J. Mol. Biol. 4, 142—160.

SMITH, K. C., 1964: Photochemistry of nucleic acids. Photophysiology (A. C. Giese, Ed.), Academic Press, New York 2, 329—388.

SPIEGELMAN, S., and M. HAYASHI, 1963: The present status of the transfer of genetic information and its control. Cold Spring Harbor Symp. Quant. Biol. 28, 161—181.

STAHL, F., 1961: A chain model for chromosomes. J. Chimie Physique Physico-Chim. biol., 58, 1072—1077.

STENT, G. S., and C. R. FUERST, 1960: Genetic and physiological effects of the decay of incorporated radioactive phosphorus in bacterial viruses and bacteria. Advances in Biol. Med. Physics, 7, 1—75.

SZYBALSKI, W., 1958: Observations on chemical mutagenesis in microorganisms. Annals N. Y. Acad. Sci., 76, 475—489.

SZYBALSKI, W., 1961: Molecular fate of transforming DNA. J. Chimie Physique Physico-Chim. biol., 58, 1098—1099.

SZYBALSKI, W., 1962: Properties and applications of halogenated deoxyribonucleic acids, in „The Molecular Basis of Neoplasia", (A Collection of Papers Presented at the 15th Ann. Symp. on Fundamental Cancer Research). pp. 147—171, University of Texas Press, Austin.

SZYBALSKI, W., and Z. LORKIEWICZ, 1962: On the nature of the principal target of lethal and mutagenic radiation effects. Abh. Dtsch. Akad. Wiss. Berlin, Kl. Med., Jahrg. 1962, Nr. 1, 63—71.

SZYBALSKI, W., R. L. ERIKSON, G. A. GENTRY, L. G. GAFFORD, and C. RANDALL, 1963a: Unusual properties of the fowlpox virus DNA. Virology, 19, 586—589.

SZYBALSKI, W., N. K. COHN, and C. HEIDELBERGER, 1963b: Effects of 5-trifluoromethyl-2′-deoxyuridine (F_3TdR) on the biochemical and radiobiological properties of human cells. Feder. Proc. 22, 532.

TANAKA, N., H. YAMAGUCHI, and H. UMEZAWA, 1963: Mechanism of action of phleomycin a tumor-inhibitory antibiotic. Biochem. Biophys. Res. Comm., 10, 171—174.

TAYLOR, J. H., 1963: DNA synthesis in relation to chromosome reproduction and the reunion of breaks. J. Cell. Comp. Physiol. 62 Suppl., 73—86.

TESSMAN, I., 1959: Some unusual properties of the nucleic acid in bacteriophages S 13 and Φ X 174. Virology 7, 263—275.

THOMAS, JR., C. A., 1963a: The organization of DNA in bacteriophage and bacteria, in „Molecular Genetics", J. H. Taylor, Ed., Part 1, pp. 113—151.

THOMAS, JR., C. A., 1963b: The arrangement of nucleotide sequences in T2 and T5 DNA molecules. Cold Spring Harbor Symp. Quant. Biol. 28, 395—396.

VINOGRAD, J., R. BRUNER, R. KENT, and J. WEIGLE, 1963: Band-centrifugation of macromolecules and viruses in self-generating density gradients. Proc. Natl. Acad. Sci. U.S. **49**, 902–910.

WACKER, A., H. D. MENNIGMANN, and W. SZYBALSKI, 1962: Effects of „visible" light on 5-bromouracil-labelled DNA. Nature **196**, 685–686.

WATSON, J. D., and F. H. C. CRICK, 1953: A structure for deoxyribose nucleic acid. Nature **171**, 737–738.

WATSON, J. D., and J. W. LITTLEFIELD, 1960: Some properties of DNA from Shope papilloma virus. J. Mol. Biol. **2**, 161–165.

WEBB, J. S., D. B. COSULICH, J. H. MOWAT, J. B. PATRICK, R. W. BROSCHARD, W. E. MEYER, R. P. WILLIAMS, C. F. WOLF, W. FULMOR, C. PIDACKS, J. E. LANCASTER, 1963: The structures of mitomycins A, B and C and porfiromycin. Parts I and II. J. Am. Chem. Soc. **84**, 3185–3187.

WEIL, R., and J. VINOGRAD, 1963: The cyclic helix and cyclic coil forms of polyoma viral DNA. Proc. Natl. Acad. Sci. U.S. **50**, 730–738.

WHITEHOUSE, H. L. K., 1963: A theory of crossing-over by means of hybrid deoxyribonucleic acid. Nature **199**, 1034–1040.

WILSON, R., 1963: Ultraviolet light induced cross linking in native and heat denatured DNA. Feder. Proc. **22**, 582.

WULFF, D. L., 1963: The role of thymine dimer in the photo-inactivation of the bacteriophage $T4v_1$. J. Mol. Biol. **7**, 431–441.

YOSHIKAWA, H., and N. SUEOKA, 1963a: Sequential replication of *Bacillus subtilis* chromosome, I. Comparison of marker frequencies in exponential and stationary growth phases. Proc. Natl. Acad. Sci. U.S. **49**, 559–566.

YOSHIKAWA, H., and N. SUEOKA, 1963b: Sequential replication of the *Bacillus subtilis* chromosome, II. Isotopic transfer experiments. Proc. Natl. Acad. Sci. U.S. **49**, 806–813.

ZINDER, N. D., R. C. VALENTINE, M. ROGER, and W. STOECKENIUS, 1963: f 1, a rodshaped male-specific bacteriophage that contains DNA. Virology **20**, 638–640.

The Production of Breaks in the Deoxyribonucleic Acid of *Bacillus subtilis*[1])

BERNARD S. STRAUSS[2])

Department of Microbiology, The University of Chicago, Chicago 37, Illinois, U.S.A.

For the past several years we have been interested in the mechanism of the mutagenic action of the alkyl methanesulfonates and in processes which cleave the DNA molecule[3]). It is our hope that the study of such processes will eventually lead to a chemical description of the process of genetic recombination. Recombination involves breakage of polynucleotide chains and the restoration of an unbroken chain without inactivation of the DNA. A great deal of genetic experimentation has gone into the description of the recombination process but we are still ignorant of its mechanism. An indirect approach involving separate study of breakage processes may be the best available tactic. In this report I would like to discuss two new deoxyribonucleases as well as some studies with a transducing bacteriophage of *Bacillus subtilis* in which fragments of bacterial DNA are inserted into phage heads without necessary inactivation and without integration with the phage DNA. As a byproduct of our studies with one of the nucleases we have been able to reach some tentative conclusions about the mode of action of the methanesulfonates as mutagens.

When a solution of *B. subtilis* DNA is treated with either ethyl- or methyl methanesulfonate the residual transforming activity becomes sensitive to an enzyme found in extracts of *Micrococcus lysodeikticus* and *B. subtilis* (Table 1). These extracts will reduce the viscosity of alkylated salmon sperm DNA more readily than that of non-alkylated control DNA (Fig. 1) but this reduction in viscosity is not accompanied by the release of acid soluble material from the DNA. Since this failure to produce acid soluble materials is similar to the action of pancreatic deoxyribonuclease at low concentrations, we assume that the enzyme is an endonuclease.

Ultraviolet irradiation also sensitizes transforming DNA to the action of this nuclease (STRAUSS 1962) which will be called the „differential endonuclease“ because of the restric-

[1]) This work has been supported in part by grants from the National Science Foundation and from the National Institutes of Health. The support of the Abbott Fund of the University of Chicaco is gratefully acknowledged.

[2]) Public Health Service Research Career Development Award (GM-K3-823) from the National Institute of General Medical Sciences.

[3]) This work represents the joint efforts of a number of collaborators. I should like to acknowledge the help of Dr. S. OKUBO, Mr. M. STODOLSKY and Dr. K. BOTT with the work on phage Sp10, Miss R. WAHL and Mrs. J. COSTON for their help with the transformation studies on alkylated DNA and Mr. Y. TSUDA and Miss B. DICPINIGAITIS for their help with the ATP stimulated nuclease. The study on the reversion of lac⁻ mutants is primarily the work of Dr. N. SCHWARTZ. Mr. M. MAILLIS contributed to our studies on the differential endonuclease.

Table 1
Sensitization of DNA by Alkylation

Treatment	Heat Sensitivity N_h/N_o	Specific Transforming Activity No. × 10^{-5} Before Enzyme Treatment (N_o)	After Enzyme Treatment (N)	Ratio N/N_o
None	1.06	5.3	3.7	0.70
Ethyl methanesulfonate (0.2 M)				
15 min.	0.87	5.2	1.2	0.23
60 min.	0.35	4.7	0.31	0.066
Methyl methanesulfonate (0.025 M)				
15 min.	0.51	2.3	0.157	0.068
60 min.	0.033	1.2	0.0053	0.0044

Alkylation was at 37° in 0.05 M phosphate buffer for the time indicated. The reaction was stopped by pouring the reaction mixture onto a Sephadex G-75 column and separating the reactants. DNA was washed off the column with 0.15 M NaCl. Heat sensitivity: N_h represents the residual transforming activity after 6 hours at 50°. One part of DNA in saline was diluted with 2 parts of 0.1 M phosphate buffer before heating. N_o represents the activity of non-heated DNA. Inactivation was exponential for an $8^1/_2$ hour heating period at 50°. Specific transforming activity represents the transformants per µg of DNA in the linear portion of the transformation response curve.
Enzyme treatment: 0.25 ml of DNA (approx. 30 µg/ml) was incubated with 10 µmoles $MgCl_2$, 11 µmoles of potassium phosphate buffer, pH 7.5 and 0.1 ml of enzyme in one ml of reaction mixture. The enzyme was a protamine sulfate eluate of an extract of *Micrococcus lysodeikticus* (Strauss, 1962). Incubation was for 15 min at 37° and the reaction was stopped with sodium lauryl sulfate and chloroform as previously described (*loc. cit.*).

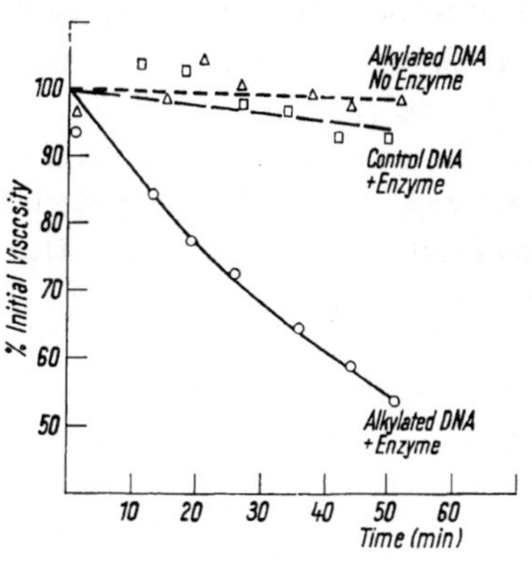

Fig. 1. Effect of an extract of *Micrococcus lysodeikticus* on the viscosity of alkylated salmon sperm DNA.
Commercial salmon sperm DNA in 0.15 M NaCl was alkylated for 90 minutes at 37° with 0.075 M methyl methanesulfonate. The reaction was terminated by precipitating the DNA with ethanol and winding the precipitated DNA on a glass rod. After passage through ethanol: water mixtures and through ethanol to remove adhering methyl methanesulfonate the DNA was dissolved in 0.15 M NaCl to give a solution of 850 µg/ml. The reaction mixture contained either 850 µg of alkylated or 983 µg of control DNA, 30 µmoles of $MgCl_2$, 20 µmoles of phosphate buffer pH 7.5 and 0.2 ml of enzyme in a total of 3 ml of reaction mixture in an Ostwald Viscometer maintained at 37°. The enzyme was a preparation from *Micrococcus lysodeikticus* eluted from protamine sulfate, precipitated with ammonium sulfate and passed through a column of Sephadex G-75. Viscosity was determined at the indicated intervals.

tion in its action to alkylated or irradiated DNA. Thermal denaturation of DNA, followed by annealing until most of the hyperchromicity is lost, sensitizes the transforming activity of the annealed DNA to enzyme action. The residual activity is reduced by a factor of four on incubation of annealed DNA with differential endonuclease. This reduction in activity is slight compared to the effect of alkylation or ultraviolet irradiation.

Alkylated DNA can replicate (STRAUSS, 1963) and DNA treated with methyl methanesulfonate is still capable of transformation (Table 1). We know that the transforming DNA is alkylated because of its sensitivity to heating at 50° in contrast to the control DNA. It has been adequately demonstrated (YOUNG and SPIZIZEN, 1961) that denatured DNA will not transform *B. subtilis* because it is not taken up by the organism. DNA alkylated with methyl methanesulfonate is taken up by *B. subtilis* (STRAUSS, 1963) and therefore can not be denatured. In addition, full hyperchromicity characteristic of native DNA is obtained on heating alkylated DNA (see Fig. 6). The specificity of the differential endonuclease can not be directed at alkyl groups *per se* because the enzyme will inactivate ultraviolet irradiated DNA. It seems likely that alkylation or ultraviolet irradiation produces some sort of local denaturation in the vicinity of a reacted site which introduces sufficient deformation of the secondary DNA structure to permit the enzyme to act.

ATP-requiring nuclease

The differential endonuclease activity may be contrasted with a second nuclease activity present in these extracts of *M. lysodeikticus*. This second nuclease requires ATP (or other nucleoside triphosphate) to act and the DNA is degraded to acid soluble products. Mg^{++} is absolutely required for the reaction. The ATP plays a stoichiometric role in the reaction and does not act, for example, merely to chelate some inhibitory metal ion. Liberation of inorganic phosphate is stimulated by DNA and it appears that one mole of ATP is split for each mole of DNA phosphorus liberated. When P-32 labeled DNA is used as a substrate it is found that about 60 per cent of the acid soluble P-32 released as a result of enzyme action is

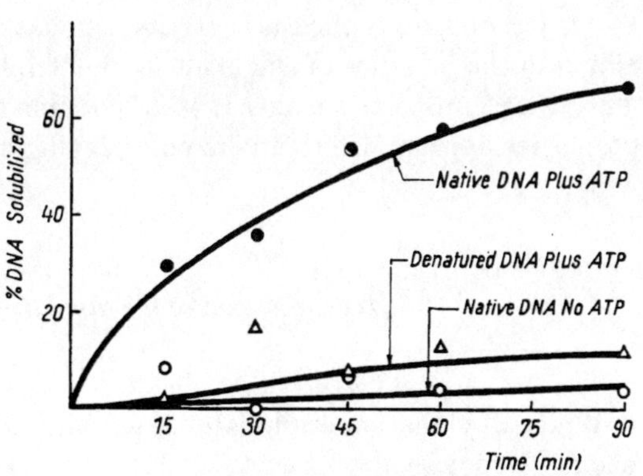

Fig. 2. Release of acid soluble material from native and heat denatured *B. subtilis* DNA by an extract from *M. lysodeikticus*. The incubation mixtures (1.0 ml) contained 20 µmoles of glycine buffer, pH 9.5, 10 µmoles of $MgCl_2$, 5 µmoles of mercaptoethanol, 0.2 µmoles of disodium ATP (where added), 0.05 ml of *M. lysodeikticus* extract (7.1 mg protein per ml) and 129 µg of *B. subtilis* DNA (0.340 µmoles). Denatured DNA was prepared by heating the DNA dissolved in 0.15 M NaCl + 0.015 M sodium citrate for 15 minutes in a boiling water bath. Incubation was at 37° in separate tubes. At the times indicated a sample was removed, chilled and the DNA precipitated and determined.

sensitive to alkaline phosphatase, a monoesterase. Therefore mononucleotides are produced by enzyme action but since there is a significant increase in the amount of acid soluble, monoesterase insensitive, P-32 liberated from the start of the reaction it is unlikely that this is a pure exonuclease. The ATP requiring nuclease requires native rather than denatured DNA (Fig. 2), does not distinguish between alkylated and non-alkylated DNA and produces considerable amounts of acid soluble nucleotides without great loss in transforming activity of the DNA substrate. About 50 per cent of the DNA must be degraded in order to produce one lethal hit in the transforming activity (Fig. 3); this is in contrast to the effect of pancreatic deoxyribonuclease on DNA. We therefore conclude that this reaction splits DNA at or near the end of the molecule in contrast to pancreatic deoxyribonuclease which can cause breaks throughout the DNA. Since the extract used is still quite crude we do not know whether one or several enzymes is responsible for the effect. It seems unlikely that the reaction can be due simply to reversal of the Kornberg polymerase (Kornberg 1961) since pyrophosphate will not substitute for ATP or for deoxy ATP and in fact the preparation contains an active pyrophosphatase.

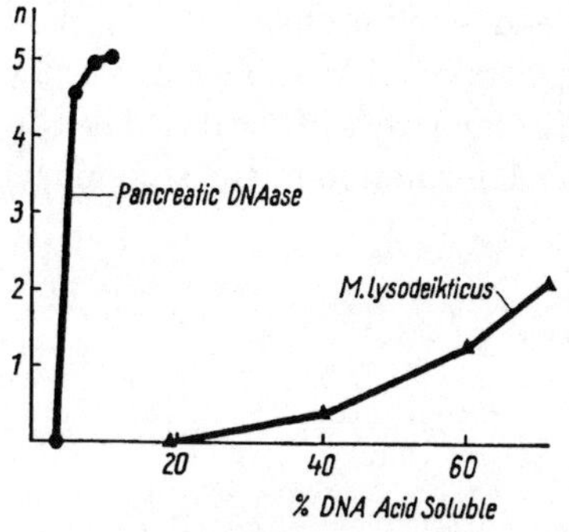

Fig. 3. Inactivation of transforming DNA by pancreatic deoxyribonuclease and by an extract of *M. lysodeikticus*. The incubation mixture (2.0 ml) for pancreatic deoxyribonuclease contained 40 μmoles potassium phosphate buffer pH 6.8, 20 μmoles of $MgCl_2$ and 0.05 μg of pancreatic deoxyribonuclease (Worthington Biochemical Company). The incubation mixture for the extract from *M. lysodeikticus* contained 40 μmoles of glycine buffer, pH 9.5, 20 μmoles of $MgCl_2$, 10 μmoles of mercaptoethanol, 0.4 μmoles of ATP and 0.1 ml of extract (7.1 mg protein per ml) in 2.0 ml total volume. Incubation was at 37°. All reaction mixtures contained 280 μg of *B. subtilis* DNA. The reaction was stopped by heating for 10 minutes at 60° after the addition of 0.2 ml of 1.5 M NaCl + 0.15 M sodium citrate. The transformation assay was for transformants to indole independence, DNA was determined by the diphenylamine reaction. The ordinate, *n*, indicates the number of hits calculated from the relationship $P(0) = N/N_0 e^{-n}$ where N/N_0 is the fraction of the original transforming activity surviving treatment.

Crude extracts of *M. lysodeikticus* contain but little deoxyribonuclease activity of the pancreatic type since transforming DNA can be incubated with such extracts without loss of activity (Table 1). We have incubated such extracts with ribonuclease in an effort to dissociate any ribonucleic acid inhibitor of „standard“ nuclease action (Lehman *et al.*, 1962) but without success. However as already shown it has been possible to demonstrate at least two types of special nuclease activity, one acting on partially denatured DNA and the other acting in the presence of single nucleoside triphosphates. The presence of such nucleases with unexpected properties makes it seem possible that further study will disclose a nuclease with properties appropriate to an enzyme playing a role in the reactions of recombination.

Mode of action of the alkylating agents in in vitro *reactions*

When alkyl methanesulfonates react with DNA *in vitro* the following sequence of reactions begins (Brookes and Lawley, 1961): a) alkylation of the purines, particularly the 7-position of guanine, b) depurination of the alkylated deoxyguanylate, c) single strand breakage of the apurinic strands and d) scission of the DNA when single strand breaks occur on opposite strands close to one another.

Single strand breaks can be detected by a method based on the difference in the reversible and irreversible thermal denaturation temperatures of DNA (Fig. 4) (Geiduschek, 1962). Reversible denaturation assays require the measurement of absorbance (260 mμ) at ambient temperature; irreversible denaturation is assayed by measuring the absorbance of heated DNA samples after quenching in an ice bath and equilibration at room temperature. Introduction of single strand breaks into the DNA reduces the difference in the thermal denaturation temperatures (T_m) of the two assays. If $T_{1/2,d}$ and $T_{1/2,i}$ stand for the points of half

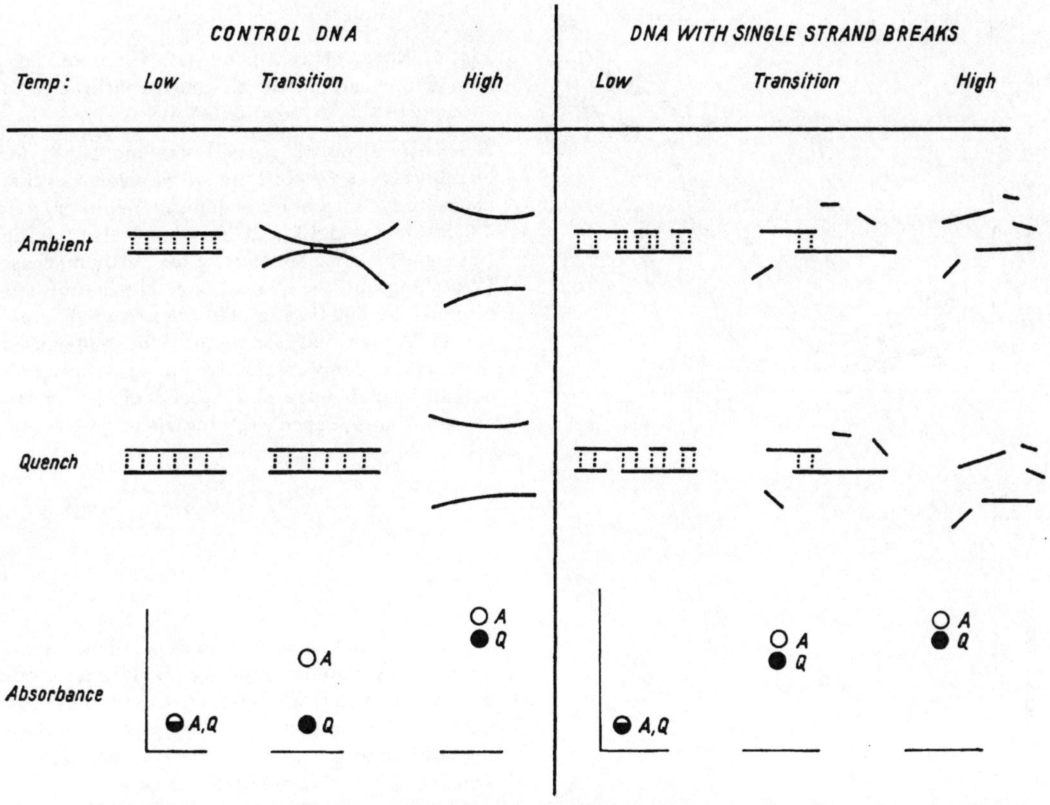

Fig. 4. Principle of the method for detecting single strand breaks for reversible (d) and irreversible (i) thermal denaturation curves.

maximal hyperchromicity in both assays, then we define $\Delta T = T_{1/2,i} - T_{1/2,d}$ (Geiduschek, 1962). The method may be calibrated by comparing the number of breaks measured from residual transforming activity with the ΔT measured in thermal denaturation assays after treatment of *B. subtilis* DNA with pancreatic deoxyribonuclease. Single strand breaks inactivate transforming DNA (Lerman and Tolmach, 1957). The average number of breaks can be calculated by setting the fraction of surviving transforming activity after DNase action equal to the $P(O)$ term of the Poisson distribution. $P(O) = e^{-n}$ where n is the average number of breaks per marker. ΔT values of 1.1° and 4.9° correspond to 8.9 and 0.08 hits respectively (Fig. 5); untreated *B. subtilis* DNA has a ΔT of about 6.5°.

DNA alkylated with either methyl- or ethyl methanesulfonate is inactivated by heating at 50° (Table 1) but the mechanism of this inactivation is not completely understood. It is not due to thermal denaturation since complete hyperchromicity is obtained with alkylated DNA heated for 6 hours at 50° (Fig. 6). It is unlikely that the inactivation is due to the insertion of breaks in the DNA since the ΔT of DNA alkylated and heated so that it behaves as though it had 2.9 hits per marker was not greatly decreased compared to control DNA (Table 2) although the shape of the i curve was somewhat altered. No change in the viscosity of salmon sperm DNA occurred during a 90 min alkylation period at 37° with 0.075 M methyl methanesulfonate nor did heating the alkylated DNA (after removal of unreacted methanesulfonate) for 5 hours at 50° result in a measurable viscosity change. The same sample of alkylated DNA responded to the differential endonuclease, which does produce breaks, with a large drop in viscosity (Fig. 1). If the inactivation for transformation is not due

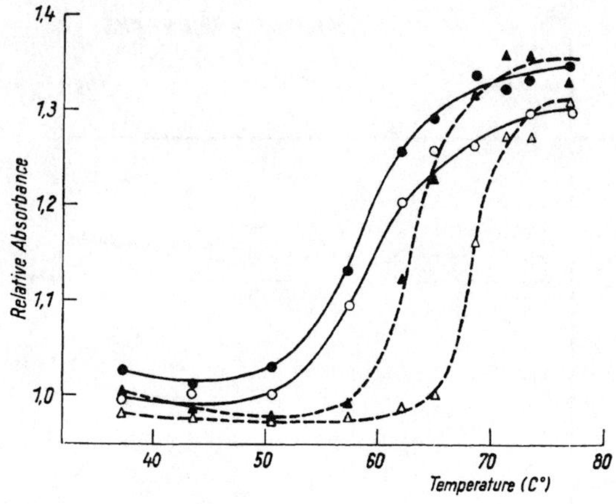

Fig. 5. Effect of treatment with pancreatic deoxyribonuclease on the thermal denaturation of *B. subtilis* DNA.

B. subtilis DNA (95 μg/ml) was incubated for 30 minutes at 37° in 2 ml of reaction mixture containing 115 μmoles of phosphate buffer, pH. 7.0, 20 μmoles $MgCl_2$ and 20 μg (circles) or 0.02 μg (triangles) of pancreatic deoxyribonuclease (Worthington Biochemical Co.). The reation was stopped by heating for 10 minutes at 60° and the DNA was dialyzed against the buffer used for thermal denaturation by passage through a column of Sephadex G-75. Solid circles or triangles—*d* assay: open circles or triangles—*i* assay.

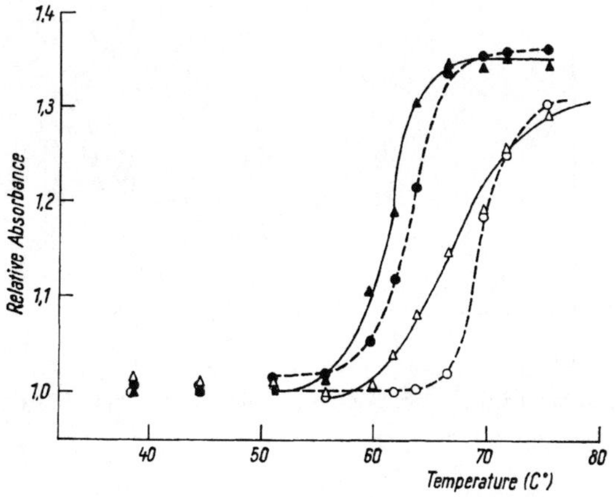

Fig. 6. Thermal denaturation of *B. subtilis* transforming DNA inactivated by alkylation for one hour with 0.025 M methyl methanesulfonate and heating 6 hours at 50°. Solid circles; control DNA heated 6 hours at 50° — *d* curve; Open circles — *i* curve. Solid triangles; DNA treated for 60 minutes with 0.025 M methyl methanesulfonate at 37° and then heated 6 hours at 50° after removal of the alkylating agent — *d* curve: open triangles — *i* curve.

Table 2

Summary of Thermal Denaturation Data

Treatment of DNA	Lethal Hits per Marker	Measured $\Delta T°$
control, non-alkylated	—	6.1–6.5
alkylated and heated 6 hr at 50°	2.9	5.6
pancreatic deoxyribonuclease	0.08	5.
,, ,,	8.9	1.

to breaks then it is most likely due to depurination reactions, assuming that the sequence of reactions is as outlined above. Storage of DNA with apurinic sites will eventually lead to breaks at the site of the depurination but these data make it unlikely that such breaks would be the primary cause of the inactivation.

Miss Wahl in this laboratory is now studying this particular problem in greater detail. She is determining whether alkylation and heating causes breaks by studying the sedimentation coefficients of alkylated DNA preparations. Since we are interested in single strand breaks and since the alkylated DNA is heat sensitive the DNA is denatured at 37° by formamide (Marmur and Grossman, 1961). The denaturation is preserved during sedimentation with 2 per cent formaldehyde (Freifelder, Davison and Geiduschek, 1961; Freifelder and Davison, 1962). It is already apparent that alkylated and heated DNA does contain breaks but we doubt (on the basis of preliminary data) that these are sufficient to account for the inactivation obtained.

If apurinic DNA will not transform then we assume that it will not replicate. Methylated DNA will transform and will replicate (STRAUSS, 1963), DNA with single strand breaks will not transform (LERMAN and TOLMACH, 1957) and will not replicate (STRAUSS, 1963) and it seems reasonable to suppose that DNA with apurinic sites will not replicate if it does not transform. Apurinic DNA will not serve as a substrate for the Kornberg polymerase (BOLLUM, 1963).

If depurination inactivates it is likely that only a single event is required. We have observed (STRAUSS, 1963) that heat inactivation of alkylated DNA at 50° follows exponential kinetics for more than one decade but of course some preliminary depurination may have occurred during the initial alkylation reaction. BROOKES and LAWLEY (1961) showed that when 2.5×10^{-3} M methyl methanesulfonate reacted with 10^{-2} M DNA (P) a total of 4 per cent of reagent combined with DNA with a half life for the reaction of 8 hours. In one hour 0.33 per cent of reagent would have combined. There would have been $3.3 \times 10^{-3} \times 2.5$ µmoles/ml = 8.25×10^{-3} µmoles of combined methyl groups per ml. In calf thymus DNA, guanylic acid makes up 21 per cent of the nucleotide phosphorus so that in 10^{-2} M DNA solution there will be 2.1 µmoles of guanine per ml. Combination of methyl methanesulfonate is primarily with guanine (BAUTZ and FREESE, 1960; BROOKES and LAWLEY, 1961) and therefore 8.25×10^{-3} µmoles of combined methyl groups per ml/2.1 µmoles of guanine per ml = 4×10^{-3} or about one in every 250 guanine rings will be alkylated. The base composition of *B. subtilis* DNA is identical with that of calf thymus (BELOZERSKY and SPIRIN, 1960) and our alkylation conditions with *B. subtilis* DNA were about 10^{-3} DNA and 2.5×10^{-2} M methyl methanesulfonate similarly at pH 7 and 37°. Since the product of the DNA and methyl methanesulfonate concentrations is the same in both experiments, a similar amount of reaction might be expected in the initial period; that is, one out of every 250 guanylic acids alkylated. Since guanine accounts for only 21 per cent of the nucleotides, 250 guanylic acids are found in a unit of about 1200 nucleotides or 600 nucleotide pairs, and this unit will have one alkylated, heat labile, purine. On the basis of current ideas (Crick, 1963) 600 nucleotide pairs would code for a protein of about 27,000 molecular weight which makes it possible that there is only one alkylated purine per locus.

If depurination inactivates DNA for replication, then mutations induced by the methanesulfonates probably occur by mispairing of the alkylated purine while still attached to the DNA as suggested by LAWLEY and BROOKES (1961) and by KRIEG (1963) rather than by mistake pairing with an apurinic site as suggested by BAUTZ and FREESE (1960) since the apurinic DNA would not be expected to replicate. Some mechanism for the addition of purines to apurinic sites would have to be postulated (STRAUSS, 1962b) to account for the mutagenicity of low pH and of heat for bacteriophage (FREESE, 1963), since both these treatments result in depurination.

The hypothesis of mispairing is supported by the results obtained in this laboratory by SCHWARTZ (1963) who studied the reversion patterns of mutants induced in the first instance by either ethyl methanesulfonate or by ultraviolet irradiation. A system was used which permitted visual distinction between partial reversion + suppressor mutations and reversions to wild-type enzyme levels. SCHWARTZ started with constitutive β galactosidase producing strains of *Escherichia coli*, i^-z^+, and he induced lac^- mutations, i^-z^-. When these double mutants were treated with mutagen and plated on a medium containing filter sterilized lactose as the sole carbon source, two types of revertants were distinguishable (Fig. 7). The first was like the wild-type surrounded by satellite colonies. This revertant type had normal β galactosidase activity and the reversion could be transduced to any *lac* mutant. The revertants with no satellites had low enzyme activity, and SCHWARTZ demonstrated that the enzymes produced by some strains had physical properties different from the normal. The partial reversion was allele specific – that is, it could only be transduced to the mutant from which it arose. The non-feeder revertants are, therefore, suppressors and Schwartz (1963) has evidence that these are suppressors very close to the *lac* locus.

When only the ability to induce revertants to the true wild type phenotype is determined it is found that there is a definite specificity in the revertibility of ethyl methanesulfonate induced mutations (Table 3). Aminopurine was able to induce true reversions of the 13

Table 3
Reversion Patterns of U.V. and EMS induced lac^- mutants

Strain	Number of mutants	Origin	Mutagen to Induce Reversion: None	UV	EMS	AP	
E. coli ML 308	23	EMS	1–29	1–28	150–830	+*	Range of Reversion frequency per 10^8
3.300	4	EMS	1–5	2.39 mostly non-feeder	2100–3200 mostly non-feeder	120–390 feeder and** non-feeder	Revertant Types
E. coli ML 308	5	UV	1–15	430–760	610–1190	–	Range of Reversion frequency per 10^8
3.300	4	UV	1–5	170–380 mostly feeder	170–500 mostly non-feeder	5–34 mostly non-feeder	Revertant Types

* Reversion frequencies not determined
** 13 mutants tested

independently obtained ethyl methanesulfonate induced strains tested indicating that the mutational change was a transition (Freese, 1963). Ethyl methanesulfonate itself induced only few true revertants in confirmation of the results of Krieg (1963). This behavior is exactly that predicted if ethyl methanesulfonate induced mutations were produced by mispairing while the alkylated purine was still attached to the parental DNA molecule. The depurination hypothesis suggests that a significant number of mutations should be non-transitions (transversions). The small number of ethyl methanesulfonate induced reversions of ethyl methanesulfonate induced primary mutants can be accounted for by the supposition of Krieg (1963) that this alkylating agent reacts with adenine at about one tenth the frequency of reaction with guanine.

In vivo action of the alkylating agents

In contrast to DNA alkylated *in vitro*, DNA extracted from *B. subtilis* organisms treated with methyl methanesulfonate behaves as though it contained numerous single strand breaks. This DNA has a much lower specific transforming activity than DNA alkylated *in vitro* under similar conditions (Table 4) but the transforming activity which does remain is relatively resistant to the action of the differential endonuclease. The product of enzyme sensitivity times specific transforming activity seems to be identical for DNA alkylated *in vitro* and *in vivo* (Table 4). The ΔT for DNA isolated from alkylated cells is lower than the 6.5° for non alkylated

Table 4
Properties of DNA alkylated *in vivo* and *in vitro*

Treatment	Relative Specific Transforming Activity	Heat Sensitivity $\frac{N_t}{N_o}$	Enzyme Sensitivity $\frac{N_i}{N_n}$
None	1.0	1.0	0.40
in vivo	0.03	0.164	0.14
in vitro	0.59	0.172	0.0082

Treatment *in vivo* was for 60 min at 37° with 0.025 M methyl methanesulfonate in salts solution (ANAGNOSTOPOULOS and SPIZIZEN, 1961). The suspension contained about 10^9 viable cells per ml. The *in vitro* treatment was for 60 min at 37° with 0.025 M methyl methanesulfonate in 0.05 phosphate buffer, pH 7, and containing 340 μg DNA per ml.
DNA was prepared by the MARMUR (1961) technique. The enzyme reaction mixture is as described in Table 1.
N_n not incubated, N_i incubated 15 minutes with a crude extract of *M. lysodeikticus*. N_0 not heated, N_t heated 6 hours at 50° in 0.15 M NaCl + 0.015 M sodium citrate.

DNA; ΔT values of 1.8°, 2.1° and 3.6° have been obtained from different preparations. Similar reduction in ΔT is produced by incubation of DNA *in vitro* with the differential endonuclease. Fifteen minutes of incubation with enzyme reduced the ΔT of alkylated DNA by 57 per cent compared to a non-incubated control; the ΔT of non-alkylated DNA was reduced by only 33 per cent on incubation with endonuclease.

We interpret these experiments as indicating that the alkylation of organisms has consequences for the DNA differing from the results of alkylation *in vitro*. Alkylation of the DNA does occur when organisms are treated with methyl methanesulfonate since the extracted DNA is heat sensitive at 50° (Table 4). This alkylation sensitizes the DNA to inactivation by endogenous differential endonuclease; DNA extracted from alkylated organisms is resistant because the enzyme has had a chance to act at all sensitive sites before and during the extraction process. DNA alkylated *in vivo* is therefore extracted at a lower specific activity than DNA alkylated *in vitro*.

Fragmentation of bacterial DNA as a result of virus infection

Not all processes leading to the fragmentation of *B. subtilis* DNA also lead to loss of transforming activity. Recently OKUBO, STODOLSKY and BOTT working in this laboratory have observed a process of DNA fragmentation which does not necessarily lead to its inactivation. They have been working with the *B. subtilis* transducing phage SP 10 (THORNE, 1962) which transduces strains derived from strain 168, indole-requiring. Sp 10 will not form plaques on the strain it transduces. Plaques formed on the Marburg strain are characteristically turbid although clear plaque mutants can be isolated and occur at a frequency of about 10^{-4} to 10^{-5}. Transforming DNA can be prepared from SP 10 carefully purified by treatment with pancreatic deoxyribonuclease, differential centrifugation and then isolation from a CsCl density gradient.

Transforming DNA isolated from the specialized transducing phage λdg contains bacterial DNA physically integrated into the viral DNA (KAISER and HOGNESS, 1960). λdg is a defective virus and the finding that generalized transducing phage of *E. coli* are also defective (ADAMS and LURIA, 1958) seems to suggest that there is a basic similarity between general and specialized transduction (JACOB & WOLLMAN, 1961). We have attempted to find out whether the transforming activity for *B. subtilis* strain 168 extractable from phage SP 10 is due to viral or bacterial DNA and whether the transforming activity is physically linked to the phage DNA.

It is possible to separate phage SP 10 DNA from *B. subtilis* DNA in a Cs_2SO_4 gradient (Fig. 8). SP 10 DNA is denser with a density equal to 1.437 compared to bacterial DNA with a reported density of 1.424 (ERIKSON and SZYBALSKI, 1963). The phage DNA has a lower thermal denaturation temperature than does *B. subtilis* DNA in both reversible and irreversible thermal denaturation assays

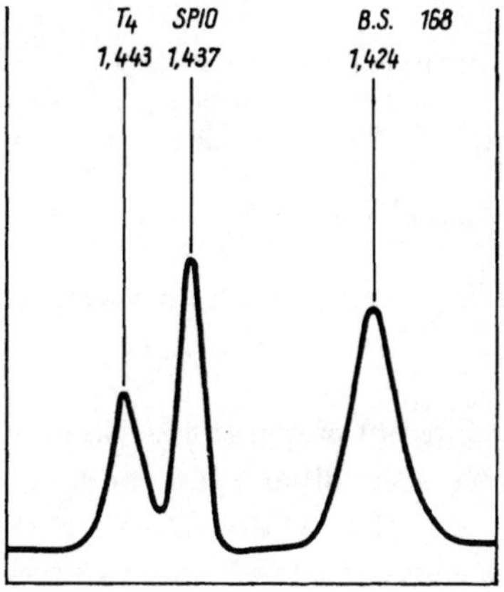

Fig. 8. Equilibrium banding of SP 10 and *B. subtilis* DNA in a Cs_2SO_4 gradient. A mixture of 0.75 μg of *B. subtilis* DNA, 0.3 μg of coliphage T4 DNA and 0.5 μg of SP 10 DNA in 0.4 ml of 0.01 M tris buffer, pH 8, with 2×10^{-3} M EDTA (final concentration) was added to 0.295 ml of saturated Cs_2SO_4 solution to give a density of 1.447. This mixture was added to a 12mm KelF cell and centrifuged 24 hours at 35,600 rpm in the analytical rotor of the Spinco Model E ultracentrifuge. The figure is a microdensitometer tracing of a photograph made with ultraviolet optics.

Fig. 9). However, the transforming activity for *B. subtilis* extracted from SP 10 is thermally denatured at temperatures characteristic of *B. subtilis* transforming DNA and characteristic of the irreversible thermal denaturation temperature for *B. subtilis* DNA rather than of SP 10 DNA (Fig. 9). We have invariably obtained an approximate doubling of transforming activity at the temperature at which SP 10 is irreversible denatured so long as the transformations were carried out at a DNA concentration of about 2 μg/ml, i.e. in the plateau region of DNA concentration.

The thermal denaturation experiments suggested that SP 10 transforming activity was carried by bacterial rather than by phage DNA. If this were so, then the denaturation of SP 10 DNA at temperatures below that at which *B. subtilis* DNA denatures would increase transforming activity since SP 10 DNA would be expected to act as an efficient competing material at high DNA concentrations and this competition would be removed by denaturation.

We next inquired whether the bacterial DNA occurred attached to phage DNA or as a separate piece. Insertion of a piece of bacterial DNA which denatured at a higher temperature than the phage DNA would be analogous to the insertion of a stable cross link. Such cross links cause an increase in the irreversible thermal denaturation temperature limited only by the stability of the cross link (GEIDUSCHEK, 1962). The presence of an inserted bacterial piece might make the irreversible denaturation temperature of phage DNA carrying an inserted piece of bacterial DNA identical with that of pure *B. subtilis* DNA even though the reversible thermal denaturation temperatures differ.

Since bacterial and phage DNA can be separated in a Cs_2SO_4 gradient , it was possible to test the separability of transforming activity from the bulk of the SP 10 DNA. For this experiment *ind*⁻ DNA prepared from *B. subtilis* 168 was used as a marker for bacterial DNA and was mixed with SP 10 DNA. The mixture was centrifuged in a Cs_2SO_4 gradient and successive drops were isolated and assayed for absorbance at 260 mμ and for transforming

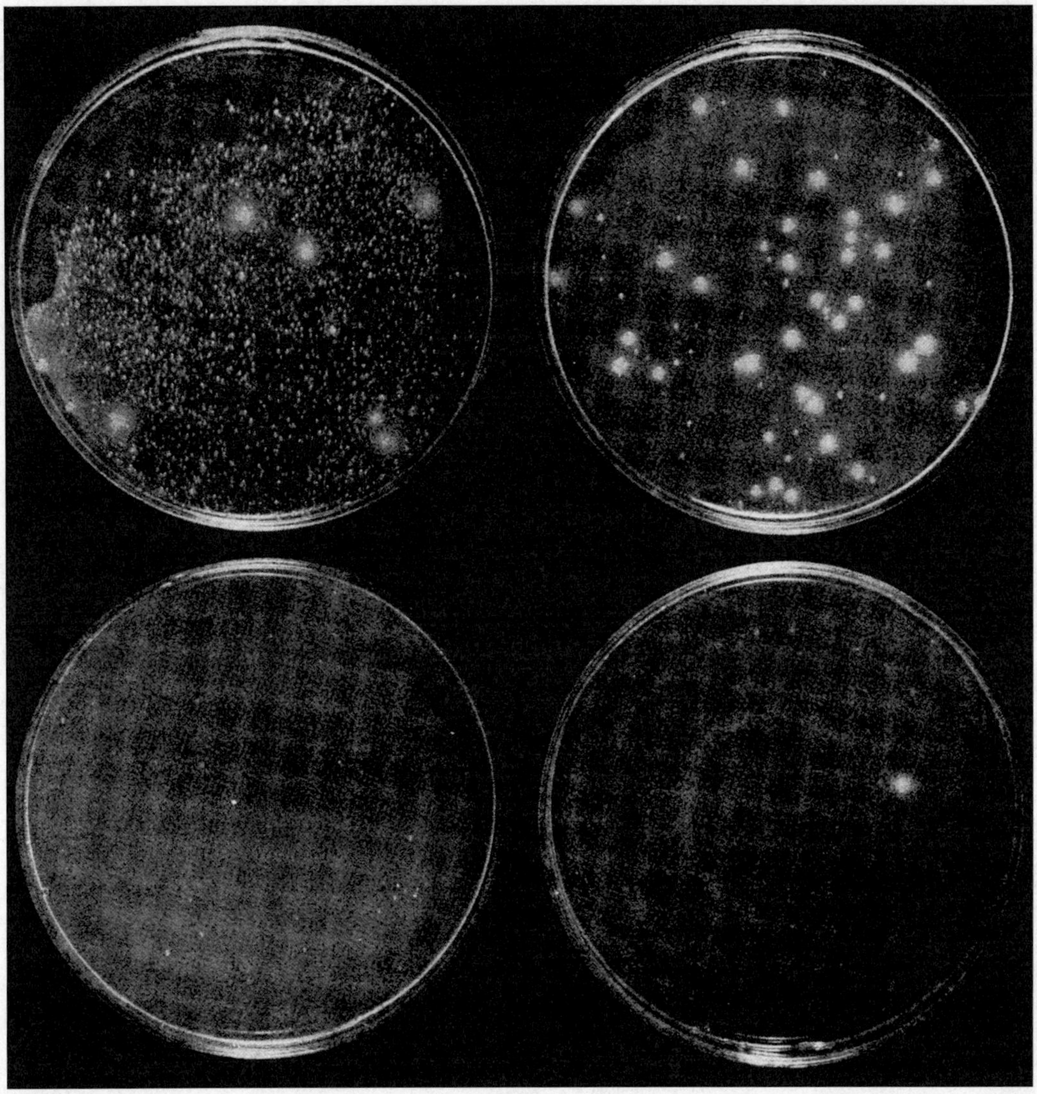

Fig. 7. Reversions of an ethyl methanesulfonate induced *lac*$^-$(i^-z^-) mutant of *E. coli*. Top left — induced by 2-aminopurine; top right–spontaneous mutants; bottom left–induced by ethyl methanesulfonate; bottom right — ultraviolet induced. The cultures were photographed after 5 days incubation on medium containing filter-sterilized lactose as a carbon source.

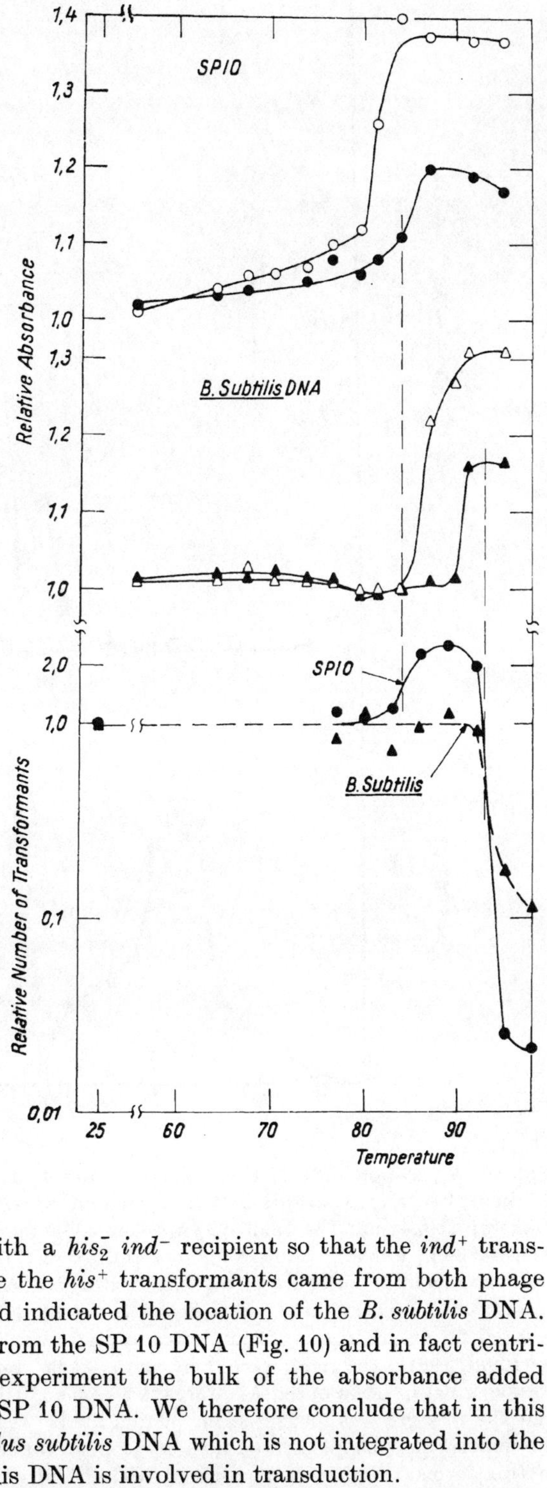

Fig. 9. Thermal denaturation and heat inactivation curves for DNA prepared from *B. subtilis* and from phage SP 10.
Thermal inactivation of transforming activity (bottom curve) was measured by heating 0.1 ml of DNA (dialyzed against 0.15 M NaCl + 0.015 M sodium citrate) in a small tube for 10 min at the indicated temperature. The sample was then quenched in an ice bath and equilibrated at 37°. One ml of competent cells of strain (*ind*$^-$) containing 2.3×10^8 viable organisms was added and the mixture was shaken for 30 min at 37°. The entire SP 10 sample was plated in 2.5 ml of soft agar. Dilutions of the *B. subtilis* DNA were made after treatment and 0.1 ml samples were plated. Transformations to *ind*$^+$ were scored after 2 days incubation at 37° on a mineral salts plus glucose medium.
Thermal denaturation (top curves) was measured by heating DNA dissolved in 0.15 M NaCl + 0.015 M sodium citrate for 20 min at the indicated temperature in a sealed cuvette. After the determination of absorbance at 260 mμ the sample was quenched in an ice bath for 5 minutes, equilibrated at room temperature and its absorbance was again determined. Absorbance taken at ambient temperature (open circles or triangles) gives the reversible denaturation profile, absorbances measured at room temperature (close circles or triangles) indicate irreversible denaturation (GEIDUSCHEK, 1962).

activity. Transformations were assayed with a *his*$_2^-$ *ind*$^-$ recipient so that the *ind*$^+$ transformants came only from SP 10 DNA while the *his*$^+$ transformants came from both phage and predominantly from bacterial DNA and indicated the location of the *B. subtilis* DNA. All of the transforming activity separated from the SP 10 DNA (Fig. 10) and in fact centrifuged along with *B. subtilis* DNA. In this experiment the bulk of the absorbance added to the centrifuge tube was contributed by SP 10 DNA. We therefore conclude that in this transducing phage there exists native *Bacillus subtilis* DNA which is not integrated into the viral DNA complement and we infer that this DNA is involved in transduction.

It would seem that small segments of the bacterial host DNA can be incorporated into virus in the course of maturation, as originally suggested by ZINDER (1953), without recombining with the phage DNA. We do not know what type of nuclease is responsible for the

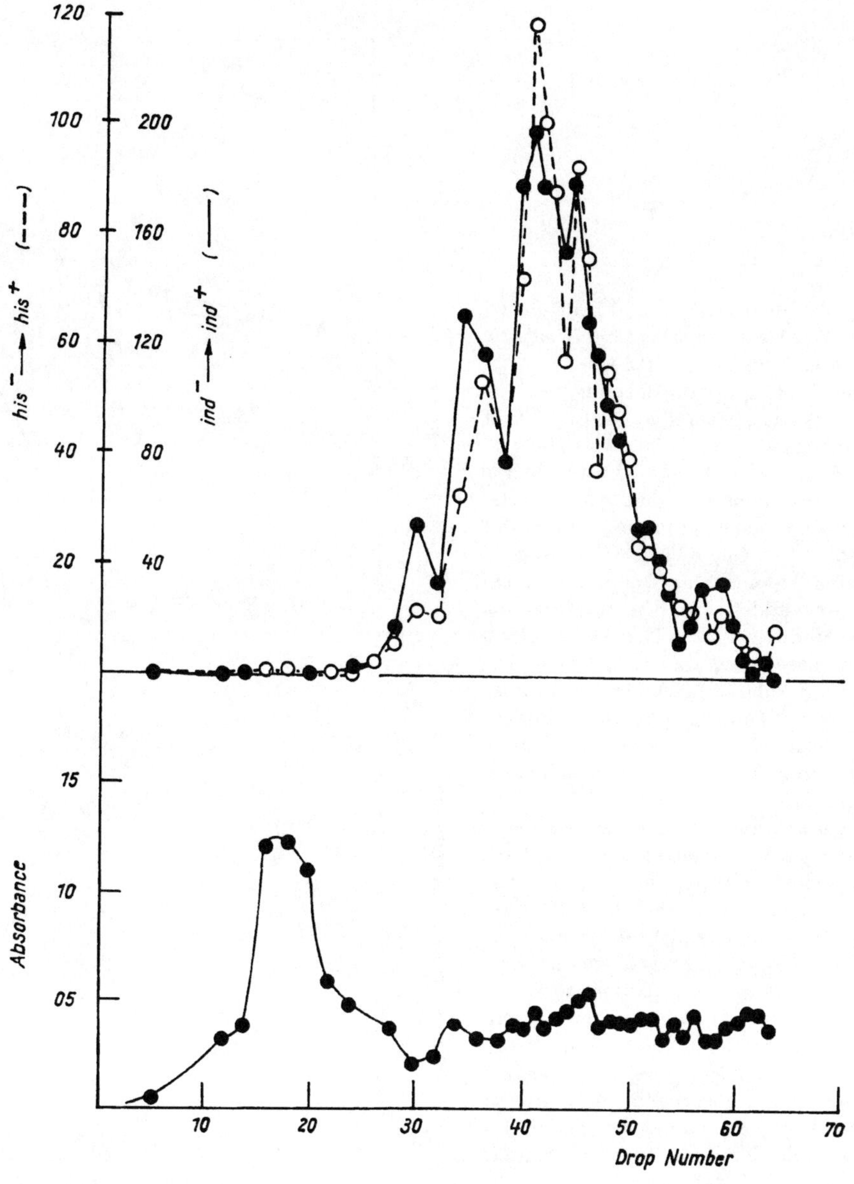

Fig. 10. Separation of SP 10 DNA and the transforming activity isolated from phage SP 10 in a Cs_2SO_4 gradient. 0.5 µg of *B. subtilis ind*⁻ DNA was mixed with 36 µg of DNA isolated from phage Sp 10 and made up to 0.44 ml. The final concentration of buffer was 0.01 M tris, pH 7.5. Saturated Cs_2SO_4 solution (0.33 ml) was then added to give a density of 1.447 as determined from the refractive index and the tube was filled with paraffin oil. The mixture was centrifuged in the Spinco SW 39 Swinging Bucket rotor (rotor temperature = 25°) for 36 hours at 30,000 rpm. Successive drops were collected and assayed for absorbance at 260 mµ after dilution with 0.5 ml of salts solution (Anagnostopoulos and Spizizen, 1961). The tubes were then heated at 60° for 10 min to sterilize their contents. One ml of a competent suspension of $ind^- his_2^-$ organisms (2.3 × 10^8/ml) was then added to the 0.5 ml DNA sample and the mixture was incubated for 30 min at 37° with shaking. Samples of 0.1 ml were plated on minimal medium supplemented with tryptophan for scoring his^+ transformants, the remaining 1.4 ml of transformation mixture was mixed with 2.5 ml of soft agar and plated on medium supplemented with histidine to score ind^+ transductants. Plates were scored after two days incubation at 37°. No ind^+ transformants were obtained when the 168 (ind^-) DNA was tested separately prior to centrifugation; 0.1 ml of a 10^{-2} dilution of the 168 DNA gave 376 his^+ transformants when 0.1 ml of transformation mixture was plated on medium supplemented with tryptophan.

breakup of the bacterial DNA in these infections but it is apparent that some of the fragments retain biological, i. e. transforming, activity.

The processes reported in the paper all involve the breakage of DNA strands. If carried far enough all of them undoubtedly lead to the inactivation of DNA. However the investigations with phage SP 10 imply that it is possible to stop the breakage process and still retain biological activity for portions of the genome. The process of genetic recombination is one which also appears to involve breakage of DNA and its subsequent rejoining (Meselson and Weigle, 1961; Kellenberger, Zichichi and Weigle, 1961). It is our hope that study of processes which lead to such breakage without irreversible inactivating the DNA may give information as to the nature of at least part of the recombination process.

References

Adams, J. N., and S. E. Luria, 1958: Transduction by bacteriophage P1: abnormal phage function of the transducing particles. Proc. Natl. Acad. Sci. U.S. **44**, 590—594.

Anagnostopoulos, C., and J. Spizizen, 1961: Requirements for transformation in *Bacillus subtilis.* J. Bacteriol. **81**, 741—746.

Bautz, E., and E. Freese, 1960: On the mutagenic effect of alkylating agents. Proc. Natl. Acad. Sci. U.S. **46**, 1585—1594.

Belozersky, A., and A. Spirin, 1960: Chemistry of the nucleic acids of microorganisms. In the Nucleic Acids, Vol. III. Chargaff and Davison, eds. New York, Academic Press.

Bollum, F. J., 1963: „Primer" in DNA Polymerase Reactions. Progress in Nucleic Acid Res. **1**, 1—26.

Brookes, P., and P. Lawley, 1961: The reaction of mono- and di-functional alkylating agents with nucleic acids. Biochem. J. **80**, 496—503.

Crick, F. H. C., 1963: The Recent Excitement in the Coding Problem. Progress in Nucleic Res. **1**, 163—217.

Erikson, R. L., and W. Szybalski, 1963: Natural and imposed variation in glucose content of phage DNA as determined by Cs_2SO_4 gradient centrifugation. Abstracts Biophysical Soc. p. WA 8.

Freese, E., 1963: Molecular Mechanism of Mutations in Molecular Genetics, Part I. J. H. Taylor, ed. New York, Acad. Press, pp 207—269.

Freifelder, D., P. Davison, and E. P. Geiduschek, 1961: Damage by visible light to the acridine orange DNA complex. Biophys. J. **1**, 389—400.

Freifelder, D., and P. Davison, 1962: Hyperchromicity and strand separation in bacterial DNA. Biophys. J. **2**, 249—256.

Geiduschek, E. P., 1962: On the factors controlling the reversibility of DNA denaturation. J. Mol. Biol. **4**, 467—487.

Jacob, F., and E. L. Wollman, 1961: Sexuality and the Genetics of Bacteria. Academic Press, New York.

Kaiser, A. D., and D. Hogness, 1960: The transformation of *Escherichia coli* with deoxyribonucleic acid isolated from bacteriophage λ dg. J. Mol. Biol. **2**, 392—415.

Kellenberger, G., M. L. Zichichi, and J. J. Weigle, 1961: Exchange of DNA in the recombination of bacteriophage λ. Proc Natl. Acad. Sci. U.S. **47**, 869—878.

Kornberg, A., 1961: Enzymatic synthesis of DNA. John Wiley & Sons, Inc., New York.

Krieg, D. R., 1963: Ethyl methanesulfonate-induced reversion of bacteriophage T4 rll mutants. Genetics **48**, 561—580.

Lawley, P. D., and P. Brookes, 1961: Acidic dissociation of 7 : 9 dialkylguanines and its possible relation to mutagenic properties of alkylating agents. Nature **192**, 1081—1082.

Lehman, I. R., G. G. Roussos, and E. A. Pratt, 1962: The deoxyribonucleases of *Escherichia coli.* III. Studies on the nature of the inhibition of endonuclease by ribonucleic acid. J. Biol. Chem. **237**, 829—833.

Lerman, L. S., and L. Tolmach, 1957: Genetic Transformation. I. Cellular incorporation of DNA accompanying transformation in pneumococcus. Biochim. et Biophys. Acta **26**, 68–82.

Marmur, J., and L. Grossman, 1961: Ultraviolet light induced linking of deoxyribonucleic acid strands and its reversal by photoreactivating enzyme. Proc. Natl. Acad. Sci. U.S. **47**, 778–787.

Meselson, M., F. Stahl, and J. Vinograd, 1957: Equilibrium sedimentation of macromolecules in density gradients. Proc. Natl. Acad. Sci. U.S. **43**, 581–588.

Meselson, M., and J. J. Weigle, 1961: Chromosome breakage accompanying genetic recombination in bacteriophage. Proc. Natl. Acad. Sci. U.S. **47**, 857–868.

Schwartz, N., 1963: Nature of ethyl methanesulfonate induced reversion of lac mutants of *Escherichia coli*. Genetis **48**, 1357–1375.

Strauss, B. S., 1962: Differential destruction of the transforming activity of damaged deoxyribonucleic acid by a bacterial enzyme. Proc. Natl. Acad. Sci. U.S. **48**, 1670–1675.

Strauss, B. S., 1963: Recovery of deoxyribonucleic acid from the effects of alkylation. J. Gen. Microbiol. **30**, 89–103.

Thorne, C. B., 1962: Transduction in *Bacillus subtilis*. J. Bacteriol. **83**, 106–111.

Young, F. E., and J. Spizizen, 1961: Physiological and genetic factors affecting transformation of *Bacillus subtilis*. J. Bacteriol. **81**, 823–829.

Zinder, N. D., 1953: Infective heredity in bacteria. Cold Spring Harbor Symposia Quant. Biol. **18**, 261–269.

The Chemical Changes of Phage DNA Involved in Host-induced Modification

K. A. STACEY, N. SYMONDS, S. W. GLOVER, and J. SCHELL*

Medical Research Council, Microbial Genetics Research Unit, Hammersmith Hospital, London W. 12

Certain viruses, notably bacteriophages, undergo a remarkable „sea-change" when grown in some hosts: they lose, or sometimes gain the capacity to infect other hosts. Moreover this change in infectivity is not due to a mutation nor is it inherited in the usual sense, for it can be lost or gained by a single cycle of growth in a suitable host. This change has therefore been called „host-induced modification" and several examples have been investigated (see LURIA, 1953). ARBER and DUSSOIX (1962) studied the growth of phage λ in strains of *Escherichia coli* K 12 (K) and the same strains lysogenic for phage P 1 (K(P 1)). Phage λ grown in K ($\lambda \cdot$ K) produce only one plaque when plated with K(P 1) for every 10^4 when plated with K, and is therefore said to be restricted by K(P 1). Phage from the few plaques formed on K(P 1) ($\lambda \cdot$ K(P 1)) now plate with equal efficiency on both strains and since they are no longer restricted, they are therefore said to be modified. As long as these phage are grown on K(P 1), the infectivity of $\lambda \cdot$ K(P 1) stays at this high level but is lost in one cycle of growth on K, the progeny from this host again plate only 1 in 10^4 on the lysogenic strain. P 1 also induces the modification of phages T 1 and P 2 (LEDERBERG, 1957). DUSSOIX and ARBER (1962) showed that K(P 1) cells survive infection with restricted λ, labelled with P^{32} and that some of the P^{32} appears after a time in the medium indicating that the restricted phage is ultimately broken down. Phage λ shows similar host-modification by B, C and K strains of *coli* (BERTANI and WEIGLE, 1953).

We have followed ARBER and DUSSOIX in studying the P 1 system, because it seemed possible that it might be easier to study only the biochemical changes imposed by the phage in otherwise identical bacteria. ARBER and DUSSOIX (1962) found that the P 1 modification was imposed upon phage λ, if the P 1 was introduced by superinfection, even after λ multiplication was already in progress. This result suggested to them that modification was a separate process from restriction. This we have confirmed by isolating mutants of P 1 which, while retaining the capacity to modify λ have lost the ability to restrict. K strains made lysogenic with such mutant P 1 phages plated $\lambda \cdot$ K with the same efficiency as non-lysogenic K, but released fully modified progeny. P 1 mutants which have lost both capacities, they neither restrict nor modify, have also been isolated. It seems likely that the two activities, restriction and modification, are under separate genetic control in phage P 1 (GLOVER *et al.*, 1963).

* Present address: Laboratory for Microbiology, Faculty of Sciences, State University, Ghent, Belgium.

ARBER (1962) has reported that both restriction and modification apply not only to phage, but to other ways in which DNA is transferred from cell to cell, transduction and conjugation. The efficiency of transfer of an early chromosomal marker from a non-lysogenic male to a lysogenic female was only one-tenth that obtained when neither were lysogenic. This result he generalized by suggesting that most, if not indeed all, DNA in a bacterial cell is modified. We have confirmed and extended his observations by showing that the transfer of the episomes F, Flac, Fgal and a colicin (Col I) are subject to the same rules of restriction and modification as λ, although it has become clear that the expression of restriction varies quantitatively with the system studied (GLOVER *et al.*, 1963).

Restriction is a complex process and depends for its expression not only on the genetic character of the strain and the system studied but also on the physiological state of the cells. In this paper only modification will be discussed.

ARBER and DUSSOIX (1962), in elegant experiments with isotope labelled phage, demonstrated that the modification is carried by the nucleic acid of the phage. This was confirmed by showing that pure $\lambda \cdot$ K DNA, isolated by phenol extraction did not cause the release of λ phage in the λ transformation system if the recipient was lysogenic for phage P 1: only when both helper phage and the λ DNA come from K · P 1 cells was any infectious λ produced (ARBER 1962).

It is clear since modification can lead either to a gain or loss in infective capacity that we must look, therefore, for chemical structures which can be added to the fundamental

Table I

C600 T^- were grown in a minimal medium (M-9) supplemented with 20 µg each of threonine and leucine, 1 µg of thiamine, and 40 µg of thymine per ml. Aliquots were filtered and suspended in one tenth the volume of 0.01 M $MgCl_2$ and incubated for 1 hour at 37° to increase the ability to absorb λ (ARBER 1958). A virulent mutant of $\lambda \cdot$ K, λ_v, was added to give a multiplicity of exposure of 10. After 10 mins fresh medium was added and the suspension aerated for 15 mins. The mixture was centrifuged, the pellet suspended in one tenth the volume 0.14 M NaCl containing 0.002 M $CaCl_2$ and P 1 added to give a multiplicity of 10. After 5 mins a 1 in 100 dilution was made into the media listed below and incubated at 37° for a further 60 mins. After the addition of $CHCl_3$ the lysates were assayed by plating with C 600 and C 600 (P 1). The ratio of the plaques formed on the two strains was a measure of the modification produced by phage P 1. Normally $\lambda_v \cdot$ K plates with a efficiency of only 2×10^{-4} on C 600(P 1).

Incubation medium post P 1 infection M 9-TLB containing:-		Burst	% plating on C 600
Expt. I	thymine	6	25
	no thymine	18	26
	no thymine + 20 γ/ml FUDR + 20 γ/ml uracil	2	21
	+ thymine + 10 γ/ml FO	2	20
	+ thymine + 100 γ/ml Azaguanine	5	30
	+ thymine + 100 γ/ml Azauracil	4	29

structure of DNA without impairing its capacity for replication or its role in genetic control. Three hypotheses are possible: one, the modification consists of the addition to the λ DNA of a special fraction of DNA; two, ribonucleotides might be added to the ends of the DNA chain; or three, that modification consists of the addition of some other chemical groupings. The first and second of these were made unlikely by experiments which stem from the demonstration that P 1 could still impose its modification after λ development had begun. A strain of K 12 was isolated unable to make its own thymine (C 600 T). Cultures were infected with λ and after 15 mins development, superinfected with P 1, and phage maturation completed in the absence of thymine. The fraction of the progeny able to form plaques when plated with K(P 1) was determined and used as a measure of the extent to which it is possible to alter modification. Some typical results are given in Table I. They show that although the burst size is greatly reduced from that obtained if the whole period of phage development is completed in the presence of thymine, its absence has not produced any alteration in the size of the fraction of modified phage. The addition of fluorouracil or fluorodeoxyuridine, both of which greatly interfere with the utilisation of thymine by this strain, do not alter or add to the effect of thymine deprivation. This suggests that little or no more λ DNA is made after the P 1 infection, and that the already synthesized λ DNA is modified without further DNA synthesis. Moreover the presence of the antimetabolites fluorouracil, azauracil and azaguanine had no effect, in the presence or absence of thymine, which can probably be taken to imply, since they all interfere with RNA synthesis, that the addition of ribonucleotides is not involved in modification.

The search must be made for some other chemical groupings. It should be possible, by the addition of various labelled precursors during the period of phage maturation in the absence of thymine, to obtain unambiguous chemical identification of any groups added during this time, and initial experiments indicate this to be a promising mode of approach.

A very likely candidate for the process of modification is that of methylation, which has recently begun to attract much attention; and HURWITZ and his collaborators have already evidence pointing in this direction (GOLD *et al.*, 1963). However, a series of attempts to alter the process of modification of phage λ by interference with methylation with aminopterin and with methionine analogues gave largely negative results. Aminopterin was used in conjunction with ethionine in experiments with coli C and with the methionine-requiring strain Hfr H(P 1), it was only necessary to substitute ethionine or nor-leucine for methionine. The plating efficiency of the burst in each case was measured on various indicator strains but no change in the modification was ever detected. In the absence of methionine no progeny phage were released but ethionine and nor-leucine seemed adequate substitutes. If, however, the met$^-$ Hfr H(P 1) was incubated without methionine for 1 hour before λ infection no phage were released if nor-leucine was substituted but almost the normal burst if ethionine was used. It would appear that if methylation is involved then ethionine can be used as an ethylating agent or it ,,spares" the small residual pool of methionine.

That a change in the groups attached to DNA is indeed a cause of host modification has been demonstrated in an entirely different system. LURIA and HUMAN (1952) discovered that certain strains of *coli* B resistant to phages T 3, T 4, and T 7 after infection with phage T 2 released few progeny phage capable of growing in coli B although the existence of a nearly normal burst of phage could be demonstrated by plating with *Shigella dysenteriae*. These host modified phage T 2, gave rise to normal T 2 in this host and under certain rather extreme physiological conditions in some *coli* B strains. T 6 was found to behave similarly.

The recent papers on *coli* strains unable to make uridine diphosphoglucose (UDPG) because of genetic defects in the production of the enzyme UDPG synthetase (UDPG pyrophosphorylase) (FUKASAWA *et al.*, 1962, SUNDARAJAN *et al.*, 1962) pointed to a single mutational event which would link T 4 resistance and the ability to produce T 2 phage. A block in UDPG synthetase could be expected to cause the production of an altered cell wall lipopolysaccharide, in which the T 4 receptors lie (Weidel 1957), because little or no glucose or galactose would be incorporated, and moreover the deficiency of UDPG would prevent the glucosylation characteristic of the DNA of T even phages. A deficiency in the supply of UDPG carries other consequences which are easily observed; such mutants are necessarily unable to ferment galactose and further, since this enzymic defect leaves the galactose kinase fully functional the cells should still be able to take up galactose and be „poisoned" by the accumulation within the cell of galactose 1-phosphate.

A number of T 4 resistant *coli* B strains were isolated and tested for their ability to plate the T phages and to ferment galactose. Many, the fraction varied with the method of isolation, were found to be resistant to T 3, T 4, T 7, and did not ferment galactose. All these $B/_{3,4,7}$ strains when grown in a minimal salts medium with glycerol as the energy source ceased dividing on the addition of 0.01 M galactose. After T 2 infection the phage plated 100 to 1000 times better with *Shigella* than with *coli* B. The phage grown in one of these strains was shown by direct analysis to be deficient in glucose compared with normal T 2 (Symonds *et al.*, 1963). Several strains show a great tendency to revert to regaining the capacity to ferment galactose: all of the revertants tested (4 separate strains) have also recovered the ability to produce normal T 2 + T 6.

While this work was in progress we learnt that the same conclusion, that the absence of glucose was the basis of the host induced modification of the T even phages, had already been reached in other laboratories. Fukasawa has studied the properties of T 4 released by a $UDPG^-$ mutant of K 12 (Fukasawa and Saito, 1963, Hattman and Fukasawa, 1963) and shown it to contain only 10% of the normal complement of glucose. Shedlovsky and Brenner (1963) have shown us, prior to publication, their manuscript in which they, too, report that T 4 grown in another $UDPG^-$ mutant of K 12 is deficient in glucose and is far less able to grow in *coli* B than in K 12.

We wish to thank Dr. S. Brenner for kindly sending us his manuscript.

References

Arber, W., 1958: Transduction des caractéres gal par le bacteriophage Lambba. Arch. Sci. (Genéve) **11**, 259–338.

Arber, W., 1962: Specificités de l'acide désoxyribonucléique. Path. Microbiol. **25**, 668–681.

Arber, W., and D. Dussoix, 1962: Host specificity of DNA produced by *Escherichia coli* I. Host controlled modification. J. Mol. Biol. 5, 18–36.

Bertani, G., and J. J. Weiglë, Host controlled variation in bacterial viruses. J. Bact. **65**, 113–121.

Dussoix, D., and W. Arber, 1962: Host specificity of DNA produced by *Escherichia coli* II. Control over acceptance of DNA from infecting phage **5**, 37–49.

Fukasawa, T., and Saito, 1963: Fed. Proc. **22**, 406.

Fukasawa, T., K. Jokura, and K. Kurahashi, 1962: A new enzymatic defect of galactose metabolism in *Escherichia coli* K 12 mutants. Biochem and Biophys. Res. Comm. **7**, 121–125.

Glover, S. W., J. Schell, N. Symonds, and K. A. Stacey, 1963: The control of host-induced modification by phage P 1. Genetical Res. (Camb.) **4**, 480–482.

Gold, M., J. Hurwitz, and M. Anders, 1963: The enzymatic methylation of RNA and DNA II. Proc. Nat. Acad. Sci. (Wash.) 164–169.

Hattman, S., and T. Fukasawa, 1963: Proc. Nat. Acad. Sci. (Wash.) **50**, 297–300.

Lederberg, S., 1957: Suppression of multiplication of heterologous phages in lysogenic bacteria. Virology **3**, 496–513.

LURIA, S. E., 1953: Host induced modifications of viruses. Cold Spr. Harb. Sym., 18, 237–244.

LURIA, S. A., and M. L. HUMAN, 1952: A nonhereditary host-induced variation of bacterial viruses. J. Bact. 64, 557–564.

SHEDLOVSKY, A., and S. BRENNER, 1963: Proc. Nat. Acad. Sci. (Wash.). 50, 300–306.

SUNDARAJAN, T. A., A. M. C. RAPIN, and H. M. KALCKAR, 1962: Biochemical observations on *E. coli* mutants defective in uridine diphosphoglucose. Proc. Nat. Acad. Sci. (Wash.) 48, 2187–2193.

SYMONDS, N., K. A. STACEY, S. W. GLOVER, J. SCHELL, and S. SILVER, 1963: A chemical basis for a case of host induced modification in phage T 2. Biochem. Biophys. Res. Comm. 12, 220–222.

WEIDEL, W., 1958: Ann. Rev. Microbiol. 12, 27–48.

Zur Sekundärstruktur ribosomaler Ribonukleinsäure aus Normal- und Tumorgewebe

H. Bielka

Institut für experimentelle Krebsforschung (Direktor Prof. Dr. A. Graffi) der Deutschen Akademie der Wissenschaften zu Berlin, Berlin-Buch

Im Rahmen der Frage über die Bedeutung von Nukleinsäuren für den Mechanismus der Carcinogenese und die maligne Verhaltensweise von Krebszellen beschäftigen wir uns z. Z. mit einigen Versuchen über optische Eigenschaften von Nukleinsäuren aus normaler Leber sowie Hepatomen, die durch Dimethylaminoazobenzol und Diäthylnitrosamin erzeugt worden waren.

Zwei Methoden wurden verwendet: 1. Der hyperchromatische Effekt einer RNS-Lösung beim Erwärmen und die Interpretation der Ergebnisse im Hinblick auf Wasserstoffbrückenbindungen; 2. die Reaktion von RNS mit Formaldehyd bei verschiedenen Temperaturen und die Interpretation dieser Befunde im Hinblick auf das Verhältnis freier Aminogruppen zu gebundenen im RNS-Molekül.

Nachfolgend wird über die Ergebnisse der Untersuchungen an ribosomaler RNS aus Leber und den genannten Hepatomen berichtet; die Ergebnisse sind in Tabelle 1 dargestellt.

Die *RNS aus Ribosomen normaler Leber* zeigt beim Erhitzen von 20° auf 90 °C eine einheitliche Phasentransition, die den Übergang eines durch Wasserstoffbrückenbindungen kontrahierten helicalen Polynukleotids zu einem gestreckten Molekül ohne geordnete Sekundärstruktur anzeigt. Der hyperchromatische Effekt beträgt 21%, $T_m = 52{,}8$ °C, $\Delta T = 51{,}1°$. Komplette Hydrolyse der RNS durch Alkali ergibt einen hyperchromatischen Effekt von 39%. Der thermisch bedingte hyperchromatische Effekt beträgt somit 55% der maximal möglichen Zunahme der optischen Dichte bei 260 nm. Daraus ergibt sich, daß etwa 55% des Polynukleotids Wasserstoffbrückenbindungen aufweisen, der Rest des Moleküls ist demnach ohne geordnete Sekundärstruktur. Die Veränderungen in der Sekundärstruktur durch Erhitzen sind vollständig reversibel; die O. D. bei 20 °C ist vor und nach dem Erhitzen und Wiederabkühlen die gleiche.

Die Versuchsergebnisse mit Formaldehyd stehen in guter Übereinstimmung mit den oben angeführten Versuchen bezüglich der Bedeutung von Aminogruppen für die Bildung von H-Brücken. Es ergibt sich eine Parallelität zwischen hyperchromatischem Effekt durch Erhitzen als Ergebnis der Spaltung von H-Brücken im Molekül und den mit Formaldehyd erfaßbaren freien Aminogruppen. Bei 20 °C sind etwa 45% aller Aminogruppen frei, 55% demnach in H-Bindungen einbezogen. Bereits beim Erhitzen auf 30 °C steigt der Anteil freier Aminogruppen, nämlich auf etwa 52%, parallel der Zunahme O. D. beim Erhitzen von 20 ° auf 30 °C. Beim weiteren Erhitzen auf 85 °C wird der Anteil H-Brücken-gebundener Basen fortlaufend kleiner; bei 85% sind alle Aminogruppen frei, das Polynukleotid ist vollständig gestreckt. Die zunehmende Reaktion der RNS mit Formaldehyd mit steigenden Temperaturen ergibt sich auch aus den Veränderungen der Quotienten 280/260 und 250/260 für die spektrale Absorption.

Ribosomale RNS aus Hepatomen zeigt beim Erhitzen ebenfalls eine einheitliche Phasentransition. Die UV-Hyperchromasie beträgt 19%, $T_m = 57{,}6°$, $\Delta T = 46°$. Auch hier sind die Temperatur-induzierten Veränderungen in der Sekundärstruktur voll reversibel. Aus dem Vergleich der hyperchromatischen Effekte durch Erhitzen sowie durch Alkali-Einwirkung ergibt sich weiterhin gleichfalls, daß etwa 55% des Moleküls H-Brücken aufweisen. Die Versuche mit Formaldehyd zeigen, daß bei 20 °C etwa 75% der Aminogruppen nicht mit Formaldehyd reagieren, d. h. gebunden sind. Dieser Prozentsatz ist höher als der Anteil an H-Bindungen im Molekül. Erhitzen von ribosomaler RNS aus Hepatomen von 20 auf 30 °C führt nicht zu einer Freisetzung von Aminogruppen. Das steht in Übereinstimmung mit dem Befund, daß auch die O. D. beim Erwärmen der Tumor-rRNS in dem genannten Temperaturintervall keine Änderung erfährt. Weiteres Erwärmen bis auf 85 °C führt auch hier zu einer Abnahme an gebundenen Aminogruppen der Basen.

Tabelle 1
Optische Eigenschaften ribosomaler RNS aus Leber- und Hepatomgewebe

		Leber		Hepatom
Thermisches Profil	O. I.	20.5 % ± 0.8		18.5 % ± 1.4
			p 0.01	
	T_m	52.8° ± 2.5		57.6° ± 1.2
			p 0.001	
	ΔT_{rr}	51.1° ± 2.8		46.0° ± 4.6
			p 0.05	
UV Hyperchromizität durch Formaldehyd bei	20°	2.9 ± 1.0		1.4 ± 1.5
	30°	3.9 ± 1.7		1.4 ± 1.6
			p 0.05	
	50°	9.4 ± 0.9		5.5 ± 2.9
			p 0.01	
	70°	18.0 ± 1.3		14.8 ± 2.5
			p 0.05	
	90°	27.5 ± 0.3		24.7 ± 2.7
			p 0,05	
% freie / gebundenen Aminogruppen bei	20°	45 / 55		25 / 75
	30°	52 / 48		25 / 75
UV-Spektren 280/260 ohne Formaldehyd	20°	0.462		0.472
+ 1% Formaldehyd	20°	0.472		0.474
+ 1% Formaldehyd	50°	0.495		0.492
+ 1% Formaldehyd	90°	0.590		0.588
250/260 ohne Formaldehyd	20°	0.920		0.923
+ 1% Formaldehyd	20°	0.910		0.913
+ 1% Formaldehyd	50°	0.898		0.906
+ 1% Formaldehyd	90°	0.855		0.904
Basen Zusammensetzung	G	32.5 ± 1.71		34.3 ± 1.59
	C	31.9 ± 2.02		31.3 ± 2.02
	A	18.7 ± 0.89		18.9 ± 1.02
	U	16.8 ± 2.06		15.6 ± 0.62

Beim *Vergleich der Ergebnisse von RNS aus Normal- und Tumor-Geweben* ergeben sich einige signifikante Unterschiede, die insgesamt für eine erhöhte Stabilität der Sekundärstruktur der ribosomalen RNS aus Tumoren sprechen. In der rRNS aus Hepatomen ist der T_m-Wert signifikant höher, ΔT niedriger. Bei 20° ist der Prozentsatz an gebundenen Aminogruppen in der RNS aus Hepatomen höher als in Normalgeweben und ist auch höher als dem in H-Brücken geordnetem Molekülanteil entspricht. In der RNS aus Ribosomen normaler Leber besteht dahingegen eine gute Übereinstimmung zwischen gebundenen Aminogruppen und H-Brücken-gebundenen Molekülanteilen. Im Gegensatz zur RNS aus Normalleber führt Erwärmen der rRNS aus Hepatomen von 20° auf 30 °C nicht zu einer Erhöhung der O. D. und Freisetzung von Aminogruppen. Weiterhin ist auch bei 50°, 70° und 85 °C der Anteil freier Aminogruppen in der rRNS aus Tumoren jeweils geringer als in rRNS aus Leber. Daraus ergeben sich auch Unterschiede in den Veränderungen der spektralen Quotienten nach Reaktion mit Formaldehyd bei verschiedenen Temperaturen für rRNS aus Normal- und Tumor-Geweben.

Wie aus der letzten Spalte der Tabelle 1 hervorgeht, bestehen in den Basenzusammensetzungen der rRNS aus beiden Gewebstypen keine signifikanten Differenzen.

Für die aufgezeigten Unterschiede in der Stabilität der Sekundärstruktur ribosomaler RNS aus normalen und neoplastischen Geweben gibt es unseres Erachtens zunächst drei Erklärungsmöglichkeiten. 1. Die Wasserstoff-Brücken-Bindungen in der rRNS aus Tumorgewebe sind fester als in der rRNS aus Normalgewebe. 2. Die Sequenz der Nukleotide ist alteriert, wodurch es in bestimmten Regionen der rRNS aus Tumorgeweben zur Ausbildung längerer helicaler und somit festerer Abschnitte im RNS-Molekül kommt bei gleichem Gesamtanteil helicaler Anordnungen im Molekül. 3. Neben Wasserstoffbrücken-Bindungen treten im Molekül noch andersartige Bindungen auf, die die H-Bindungen und somit die gesamte molekulare Struktur des Moleküls stabilisieren. Möglicherweise spielen dabei Aminogruppen eine besondere Rolle. Versuche zur Klärung dieser Frage werden von uns zur Zeit durchgeführt.

Stabilität der N-glykosidischen Bindung von Nucleosiden

H. Venner

Institut für Mikrobiologie und experimentelle Therapie, Jena,
der Deutschen Akademie der Wissenschaften zu Berlin

Im Zusammenhang mit unseren Arbeiten über die Synthese der Desoxynucleoside des Adenins, Guanins, Hypoxanthins und Xanthins beobachteten wir bereits 1959 die unterschiedliche Stabilität der N-glykosidischen Bindung der verschiedenen in Nucleinsäure vorkommenden Nucleoside. Bei der Papierchromatographie der verschiedenen Nucleoside, bei denen ein stark saures Lösungsmittelgemisch verwendet wurde, versuchten wir, die identische Lage von den mit UV-Lampen nachgewiesenen Flecken für die heterozyklische Komponente und der anschließend mit Hilfe von Anilinphthalat für Ribose bzw. Borsäure/Methanol für Desoxyribose gekennzeichneten Flecke als Beweis für die Einheitlichkeit der Nucleoside zu verwenden.

Die Ribonucleoside des Adenins und Guanins laufen dabei einheitlich und bei der Entwicklung des Chromatogramms ist keine Einwirkung des Lösungsmittelgemisches zu beobachten. Hier ist durch die Reaktion mit Anilinphthalat die Ribose als konzentrischer Fleck innerhalb des Fleckes der heterozyklischen Komponente nachweisbar. Bei Uridin und Cytidin reichen dagegen die hydrolytischen Bedingungen des Anilinphthalat-Testes nicht aus, um die Ribose nachweisbar zu machen.

Bei der Chromatographie der Desoxyribonucleoside konnten wir feststellen, daß die Pyrimidindesoxyribonucleoside Thymidin und Uridin- bzw. Cytidindesoxyribosid während des papierchromatographischen Laufes nicht gespalten werden, jedoch ist nach Anfärbung mit Borsäure-Reagens die Desoxyribose als konzentrischer Ring in dem durch UV-Lampe ermittelten Nucleosidfleck jeweils nachweisbar. Wesentlich anders ist dagegen das Resultat bei den beiden Purindesoxyribonucleosiden: Adenosindesoxyribosid und Guanosindesoxyribosid. Dabei ist die Desoxyribose nach genügend langer Laufzeit des Gemisches eindeutig während der papierchromatographischen Entwicklung abgespalten worden und hat die Vergleichs-Desoxyribose während des Laufes praktisch eingeholt. Solche Reaktionen müßten erwartungsgemäß sogenannte Straßen liefern, auf denen sich die Desoxyribose – mehr oder minder verteilt – befunden hätte. Offensichtlich stellt sich jedoch bei diesem Lösungsmittelgemisch ein solcher Gradient ein, daß die Desoxyribose in den jeweiligen Stadien der Wanderung stets beisammen bleibt. Dies konnten wir in hier nicht gezeigten Chromatogrammen sehen. Es wäre nun möglich gewesen, die Geschwindigkeit der Spaltung unter den hier verwendeten Bedingungen der Papierchromatographie aus der entsprechenden Fleckenlage: Base/abgespaltene 2-Desoxyribose bzw. Vergleichs-2-Desoxyribose zu ermitteln. Dies er-

Verwendete Abkürzungen: GR = Guanosin; GDR = Guanindesoxyribosid; AR = Adenosin; ADR = Adenindesoxyribosid; CR = Cytidin; UR = Uridin.

schien jedoch für die exakte Ermittlung der Reaktionsgeschwindigkeit der Spaltung nicht ausreichend genug.

In der Zwischenzeit wurde von Wacker und von Pollmann und Schramm ebenfalls über die Spaltung von Nucleosiden berichtet. Während sich Wacker und Mitarbeiter vor allen Dingen mit der Spaltung verschiedener Pyrimidindesoxyribonucleoside befaßten, wurde von Pollmann und Schramm mit Hilfe der potentiometrischen Titration insbesondere die Spaltung der Glykosidbindung bei Hefe-RNA untersucht. Von den erwähnten Autoren wurden keine quantitativen Untersuchungen über die pH-Abhängigkeit angestellt. Wir haben deshalb diese Untersuchungen wieder aufgegriffen mit dem Ziel, auch zu Aussagen über die Spaltgeschwindigkeit bei dem der Messung direkt nicht zugänglichen physiologischen pH-Bereich

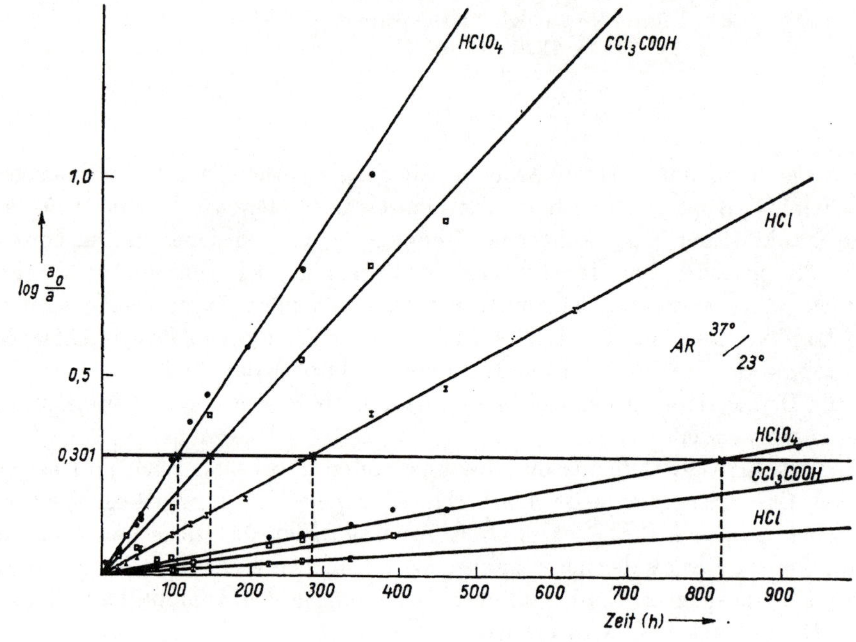

Abb. 1

von 5–7 zu gelangen. Als Technik für unsere weiteren Arbeiten benutzten wir zur Trennung wiederum die Papierchromatographie, jedoch wurde die vorangehende Spaltung in Meßkolben unter definierten Bedingungen bei 23° bzw. 37 °C bei verschiedenen pH-Werten vorgenommen. Alle Hydrolysen wurden im Dunklen durchgeführt. Es wurde jeweils die Konzentration an abgespaltener Base und umgesetztem Nucleosid ermittelt und in Abhängigkeit von der Zeit aufgetragen. Dabei ergaben sich die in den nachfolgenden Abbildungen gezeigten Resultate.

In Abb. 1 wurde der Logarithmus des Quotienten aus Ausgangskonzentration und der zum jeweiligen Zeitpunkt noch vorhandenen Konzentration an Nucleosid gegen die Zeit aufgetragen. Wie man sieht, werden für die jeweiligen pH-Werte – hier gleichbedeutend mit anderen Säuren – dabei Geraden erhalten. Die Streuung der Werte ist gering, die Geraden gehen alle vom Ursprung des Koordinatensystems aus. Aus der Darstellung ergeben sich die jeweiligen Halbwertszeiten als Schnittpunkte mit der waagerechten Linie, die dem Logarithmus 1/2: 0,3 entspricht. Die oberen 3 Geraden beziehen sich auf eine Temperatur von 37 °C, die unteren auf eine solche von 23 °C. Wie zu erwarten, liegen diese bei niederer Temperatur also niedriger. Die entsprechenden Daten für die Einwirkung von Ameisensäure und Essigsäure kann ich für Adeninribosid nicht zeigen, da wir wegen der sehr langen Spaltzeiten darüber noch keine Angaben machen können.

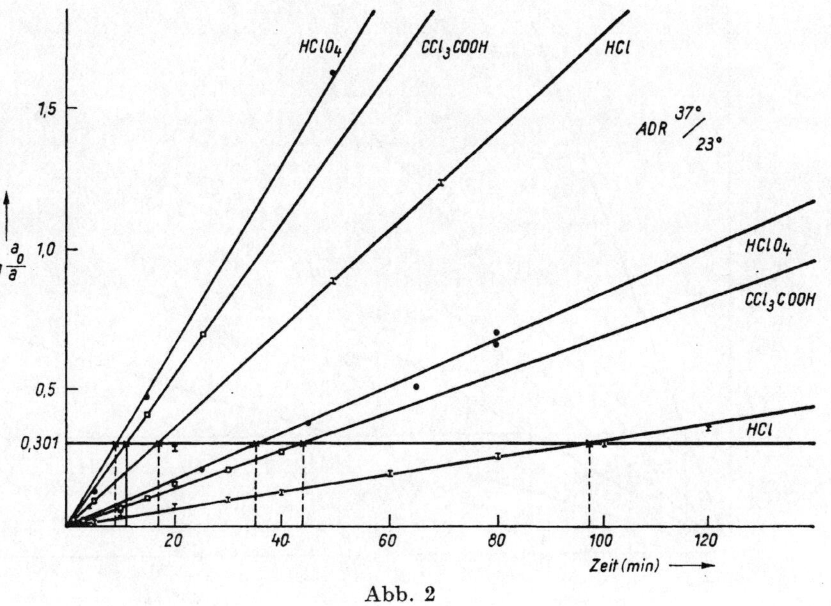

Abb. 2

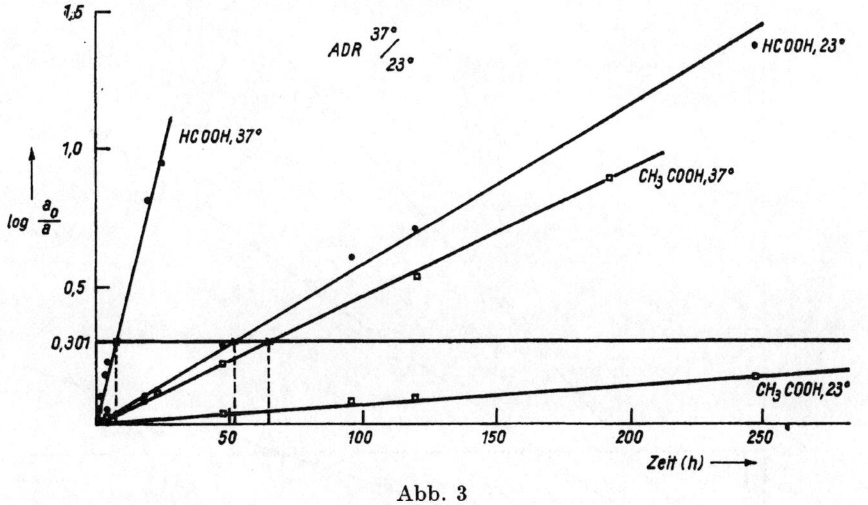

Abb. 3

Für ADR (Abb. 2) liegen die Verhältnisse für Perchlorsäure, Trichloressigsäure wieder ähnlich wie bei AR, jedoch sind die Zeiten wesentlich kürzer. Die Abszisse ist hier in Minuten angegeben. Bei Ameisensäure und Essigsäure (Abb. 3) beobachtet man im Prinzip den gleichen Tatbestand, d. h. Linearität, und die Geraden treffen sich im Ursprung des Koordinatensystems. Entsprechendes gilt auch für die in den Abbildungen 4 und 5 dargestellten Untersuchungen an GDR. Die Zeiten sind jedoch hier noch kürzer als beim Adenindesoxyribosid. Bei Guanosin ist die Spaltgeschwindigkeit aber erheblich langsamer im Vergleich zum Guanindesoxyribosid, wie Abb. 6 zeigt.

Aus den Geraden lassen sich die entsprechenden Konstanten berechnen, entweder nach folgender Formel (1):

$$K \cdot \tau = \ln 2 \quad \text{bzw.} \quad K = \frac{0{,}693}{\tau} \tag{1}$$

oder nach der Formel (2):

$$\log \frac{a_0}{a} = \frac{K}{2{,}303} \cdot t; \quad K = \log \frac{a_0}{a} \cdot \frac{2{,}303}{t}. \tag{2}$$

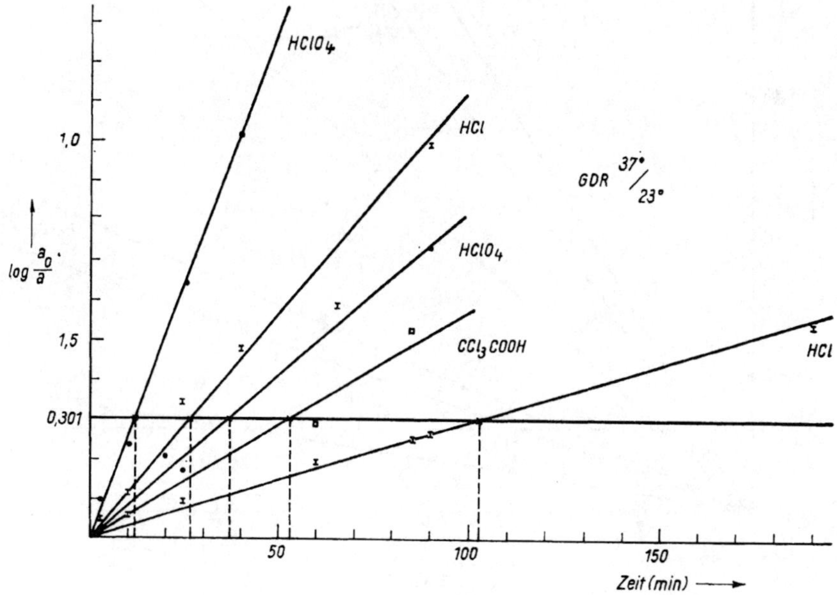

Abb. 4

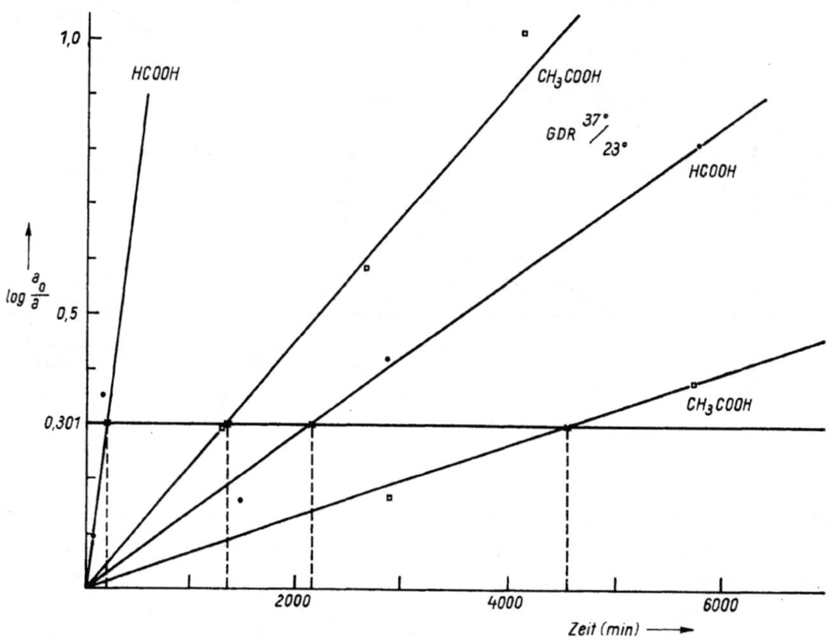

Abb. 5

Wie bei allen untersuchten Nucleosiden und Desoxynucleosiden handelt es sich demnach um eine pseudo-unimolekulare Reaktion, wie auch für eine Hydrolyse unter diesen Bedingungen zu erwarten ist, da das Wasser in sehr hohem Überschuß vorliegt. Aus der Temperaturabhängigkeit kann man die Aktivierungswärme errechnen nach der Formel (3):

$$\mu = \frac{R \cdot T_{II} \cdot T_{I}}{T_{II} - T_{I}} \cdot \ln \frac{K_{II}}{K_{I}} \; (T_{II} > T_{I}) . \tag{3}$$

Die μ-Werte liegen in den untersuchten Fällen im Bereich von 11–16 kcal. Dies deutet daraufhin, daß es sich um eine protonenenkatalysierte Reaktion handelt.

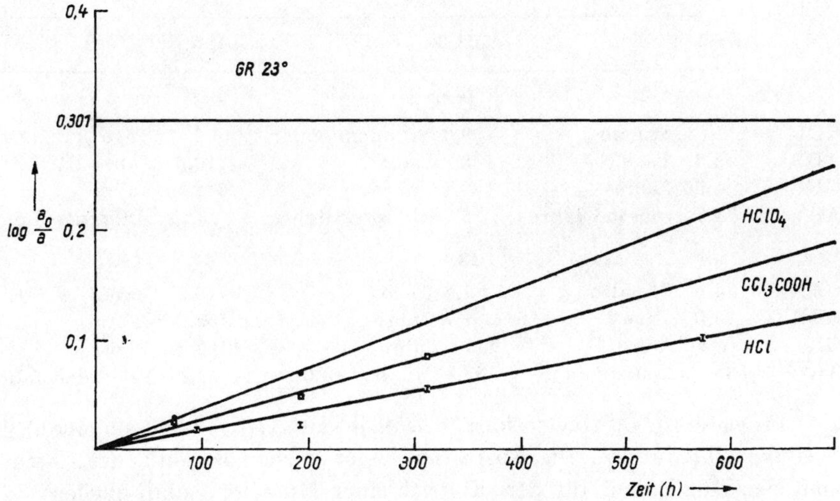

Abb. 6

In Abb. 7 ist nun die pH-Abhängigkeit der Nucleosidspaltung aufgetragen. Als Ordinate ist der Logarithmus der Konstanten angegeben, als Abszisse der entsprechende pH-Wert. Dabei erhält man für die jeweiligen Nucleoside für eine gleiche Temperatur Geraden unterschiedlicher Neigung. Es zeigt sich, daß die Stabilität der N-glykosidischen Bindung in den Desoxyribonucleosiden wesentlich geringer ist als bei den Ribosiden. Die entsprechenden Guanin- bzw. Adeninnucleosid-Kurven schneiden sich paarweise bei etwa pH 1, d. h. unterhalb von pH 1 wird Adenindesoxyribosid schneller gespalten als Guanindesoxyribosid und umgekehrt. Das Sinngemäße gilt für das Paar Guanin-/Adeninribosid. Aus den Kurven für die pH-Abhängigkeit kann man nun auch auf diejenigen pH-Werte extrapolieren, die der Messung aus zeitlichen Gründen nicht ohne weiteres zugänglich sind. Dabei interessiert vor allem der physiologische pH-Bereich von etwa 5–7. Sofern die Extrapolation zulässig ist, was durch weitere Untersuchungen noch erhärtet werden soll, ergeben sich für die pH-Werte von 5–7 für die einzelnen Nucleoside folgende Daten, wenn man eine Abspaltung von 1 Mol Base pro 2.500 Mole Nucleoside annimmt.

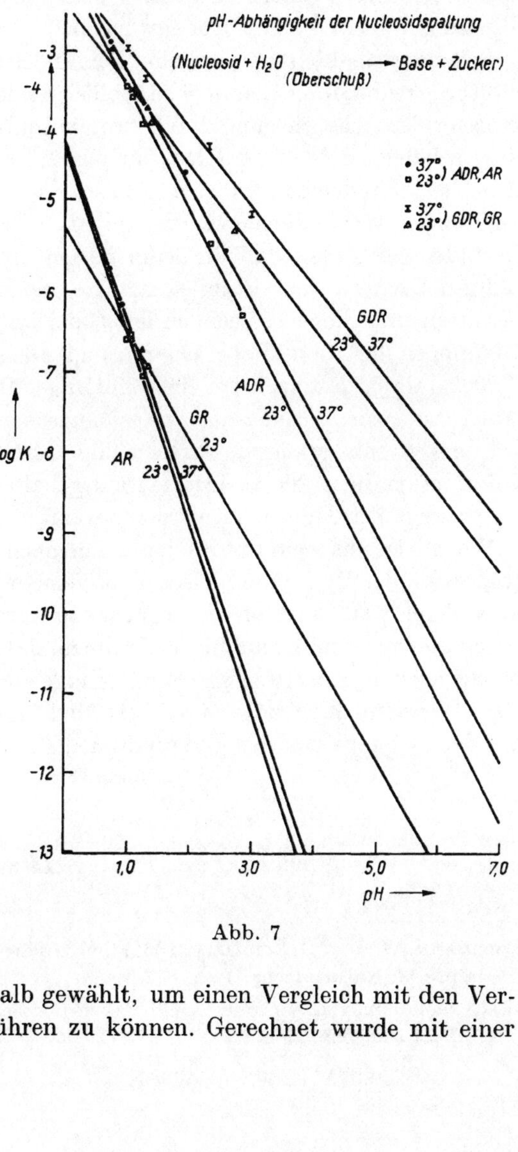

Abb. 7

Das Spaltverhältnis von 1/2.500 wurde deshalb gewählt, um einen Vergleich mit den Verhältnissen, wie sie in DNA vorliegen, durchführen zu können. Gerechnet wurde mit einer

	pH 5		pH 6		pH 7	
			37 °C			
GDR	1	Stunde	9,9	Stunden	4	Tage
ADR	5,2	Tage	138	Tage	10,3	Jahre
GR	1,56	Jahre	29,1	Jahre	542	Jahre
AR	71,5	tausend Jahre	15	Millionen Jahre	3,27	Milliarden Jahre
			23 °C			
GDR	24,1	Stunden	1,8	Tage	18,9	Tage
ADR	18,5	Tage	1,7	Jahre	55	Jahre
GR	9,4	Jahre	206	Jahre	4510	Jahre
AR	136	tausend Jahre	32,7	Millionen Jahre	7,8	Milliarden Jahre

Fadenlänge von etwa 10.000 Nucleotiden, davon jeweils $1/4 = 2.500$ als eine der 4 Basen, respektive Glykosidbindungen. Die Abspaltung einer solchen Base aus der Kette ist gleichzusetzen mit der Möglichkeit für den Eintritt einer Mutation, und insofern können die angegebenen Werte als maximale Häufigkeiten des Eintritts einer Mutation gewertet werden, wobei keinerlei weitere chemische oder physikalische Effekte auf diese N-glykosidische Bindung in irgendeiner Form einwirken.

Selbstverständlich können in der DNA noch stabilisierende Effekte auftreten durch Wasserstoffbrückenbindung, andere stabilisierende Wechselwirkung zwischen benachbarten Nucleotiden, Abschirmung durch Protein und dergleichen. Zumindest aber für den Zustand der einfädigen DNA und RNA dürften die Betrachtungen ohne weiteres übertragbar sein. Aus den Untersuchungen geht hervor, daß bei pH 5 die relativ labilen N-glykosidischen Bindungen des Guanins und Adenins mit 2-Desoxyribose in einem solchen Zeitbereich liegen (Stunden bis Tage), daß die Information insbesondere bei Mikroorganismen in einer einfädigen DNA zu wenig stabilisiert wäre und mit dem Auftreten von solchen spontanen Ereignissen unbedingt zu rechnen ist. Ganz im Gegensatz dazu liegen für die glykosidischen Bindungen der Riboside bei Guanin und Adenin die Werte bei solch langen Zeiten ($\sim$ 2 bis 70.000 Jahre), daß auch bei einer einfädigen RNA ohne zusätzliche stabilisierende Kräfte die Ablösung einer Purinbase in physiologischen Zeiträumen überhaupt nicht eintritt. Dies würde weiterhin erklären, daß es völlig ausreicht, wenn RNA, die als Zwischenträger einer Information dient, diesen Informationsgehalt auf Grund solcher Reaktionen für die fragliche notwendige Zeitdauer nicht verlieren kann.

Wir haben uns weiterhin Gedanken gemacht, wie die größere Stabilität der Purinriboside, respektive der Pyrimidinnucleoside allgemein, aus der Struktur zu erklären ist. Darauf soll an anderer Stelle ausführlich eingegangen werden.

Ich möchte zum Schluß noch erwähnen, daß durch entsprechende Untersuchungen an den Nucleinsäuren mit etwas anderer Technik ebenfalls genaue Werte ermittelt werden sollen. Es müßte dann auch möglich sein, ein Maß für die stabilisierenden Kräfte innerhalb der DNA aus der Differenz zur rein glykosidischen Bindung in den Nucleosiden errechnen zu können.

Literatur

Pollmann, W., und G. Schramm, 1961: Säurehydrolyse von Ribonucleinsäure und Desoxyribonucleinsäure. Z. Naturforschg. **16** b, 673.

Wacker, A., und L. Träger, 1963: Über die Säurehydrolyse der Desoxyriboside und Riboside. Z. Naturforschg. **18** b, 13.

Organization of Genetic Material in *Salmonella*[1])

M. DEMEREC

Biology Department, Brookhaven National Laboratory, Upton, N. Y.

Evidence is rapidly accumulating that the genetic material carried in a chromosome is arranged in a highly organized manner. The nucleotides of DNA constituting a gene are grouped in sequences, like the letters of a word, and presumably each word uniformly consists of three letters. Successive words make up a sentence containing the information needed to build a protein molecule. Each word of the sentence is transcribed to form an amino acid of the protein for which the particular gene is responsible.

The available results support the hypothesis that different mutant alleles of a gene originate through either changes or rearrangements of the nucleotides within the sentence of the DNA molecule that specifies the gene. In work with microorganisms, there are very sensitive techniques for detecting recombinants in crosses involving different alleles. By means of these methods it has been possible to discover that recombination takes place between a large proportion of allelic mutants and therefore that the changes responsible for them have occurred at different sites of a gene locus. In *Salmonella typhimurium*, intercrosses between alleles of about 90 gene loci all give rise to recombinants, indicating that all the genes are similarly constructed.

Our studies of complex gene structure are carried out exclusively by means of the transduction technique. Since the same technique has been used in current experiments analyzing larger portions of the genetic material, I shall briefly mention the features of the method that are pertinent to this discussion.

The temperate phage P 22 serves as a vector to carry a chromosomal fragment from a donor to a recipient bacterium. Studies by ZINDER and LEDERBERG (1952) have shown that transduction is nonspecific, that is, that the whole bacterial genome is represented among transducing fragments. Results of OZEKIS (1959) experiments indicate that the ends of fragments are predetermined, so that fragments representing any particular segment of chromosome are always the same. It seems probable that the chromosome splits up into fragments and that a phage particle is able to transport any one of them to the bacterium that it infects. Therefore when a donor strain of bacteria carries a certain genetic marker, some of the phage particles grown in that strain will contain transducing fragments that have the marker. If the recipient bacteria infected with such phage carry a different genetic marker in the section homologous with the transducing fragment, then their progeny will include a new

[1]) Research carried out at Brookhaven National Laboratory under the auspices of the U.S. Atomic Energy Commission.

type, representing recombination between the two markers. Thus transduction between *Salmonella* strains is a very effective technique for genetic analysis and mapping of individual transducing fragments, although it cannot be used to map the whole chromosome. The fragments carried by phage P 22 are short. P. E. HARTMAN (personal communication) estimates that the *S. typhimurium* genome is represented by between 100 and 200 fragments. Our collection of 5000 different mutants includes markers located in about 70 transducing fragments.

Genetic analysis of the *Salmonella* genome has revealed that the genes are not distributed at random; genes controlling similar functions are often clustered in one transducing fragment, and occasionally their arrangement within a cluster corresponds to the sequence of the biochemical reactions they control. Twelve clusters have been discovered so far: two purine clusters, one consisting of 3 genes (*purC*, *I*, and *guaA*) and one of 2 genes (*purD*, *H*); an arginine cluster with 4 genes (*argA*, *C*, *F*, *H*); a cysteine with 5 genes (*cysC*, *D*, *H*, *I*, *J*); a histidine with 8 genes (*hisE*, *F*, *A*, *H*, *B*, *C*, *D*, *G*); an isoleucine and isoleucine-valine with 4 genes (*ile*, *ivaA*, *B*, *C*); a leucine with 4 genes (*leuA*, *B*, *C*, *D*); a methionine with 2 genes (*metB*, *F*); a pantothenic acid with 3 (*panA*, *B*, *C*); a proline with 3 (*proA*, *B*, *C*); a threonine with 4 (*thrA*, *B*, *C*, *D*); and a tryptophan with 4 (*tryA*, *B*, *D*, *C*). Evidence is accumulating that, in addition to this clustering of genes within transducing fragments, there is a similar grouping of genes located in adjacent fragments. For example, on the genetic map of the *Salmonella* chromosome prepared by hybridization studies three aromatic acid genes (aromatic *D*, phenylalanine, and tyrosine) appear to be close together. The phenomenon is seen frequently in *Salmonella*. Among 13 groups of mutants analyzed so far, 11 have all or some of their known loci arranged in clusters, while in the other 2 groups clustering has not been observed.

The existence of clusters of genes controlling related reactions shows that such arrangements must be beneficial to the species by conferring a selective advantage on individuals and populations that contain them. Whether or not adjacent loci have a common origin is irrelevant to the question of their ultimate position, as long as there is a mechanism capable of separating them. With such a mechanism in operation, only selective advantage – during a long series of evolutionary adjustments – could preserve a specific gene arrangement if the genes involved had a common origin, or bring about such an arrangement if they originated in different parts of a genome (DEMEREC and HARTMAN, 1959).

In our laboratory we are making a special effort to compile an extensive genetic map of the whole chromosome of *S. typhimurium*. Two methods are being utilized. One is the usual conjugation technique, in which fertile recipient strains are crossed with *Hfr* donor strains. The other is a newly developed technique which makes use of *S. typhimurium* × *E. coli* hybrids in transduction experiments. A brief outline of this technique follows.

In earlier work with *S. typhimurium* × *E. coli* hybrids (MIYAKE and DEMEREC, 1959) it was noted that, in transduction experiments between a hybrid strain and a *Salmonella* strain (phage grown in the hybrid strain), markers carried in a *Salmonella* part of the hybrid chromosome were readily incorporated in the recipient chromosome but those carried in an *E. coli* part were not. The potentiality of this observation for genetic mapping of the *Salmonella* chromosome was realized at the time, but work on other problems prevented its application until recently. An initial experiment was designed in order to map a section of the chromosome as well as to test the efficiency of the technique. We had done a considerable amount of work with the *cysC* region (DEMEREC, GILLESPIE, and MIZOBUCHI, 1963), which is carried in one transducing fragment and contains a cluster of 5 genes (*cysC*, *D*, *H*, *I*, *J*). In this region we had identified about 300 single-site markers and more than 90 deletions, so that a good supply of material was available for various genetic tests. Moreover, several other gene loci had been identified in the near vicinity of that region. A cross was made between the *Salmonella* mutant *cysDJ-109 mut* and *E. coli* strain *Hfr-101 met*. *Salmonella cys-109* carries two cysteine mutations, one in locus *cysD*, not far from one end of the cluster, and the other in locus *cysJ*, not far from the opposite end. Between them, in addition to the *cysH* and *cysI* loci, there lies a long „silent section". The strain also carries a mutator gene (*mut*), which is essential for the efficient production of hybrids. The *Hfr* strain carries the wild-type alleles of the mutant cysteine genes. When *Salmonella cysDJ-109 mut* and *E. coli Hfr-101* are crossed and selection is made for cys^+, it is reasonably certain that all the isolates will be hybrids. (The only other way in which cys^+ colonies could originate would be through simultaneous reversions at the *cysD* and *cysJ* sites carrying the changes responsible for *cysDJ-109*. The probability of occurrence of such double mutations is extremely low, and no cys^+ colonies were observed on control plates.) Furthermore, it is expected that in a large proportion of the hybrids the section between the two *cys-109* mutant sites will be *E. coli* in origin. This section comprises the entire *cysH* and *cysI* loci, a portion of locus *cysD*, and all of the silent section.

From the *S. typhimurium cysDJ-109* × *E. coli Hfr-101 met* cross, plated on enriched minimal medium (selection for cys^+ hybrids), 78 colonies were isolated, and broth cultures were established by passing the material through an additional single-colony isolation. P 22 phage was prepared in every one of the 78 hybrids. The phage titer varied greatly among the different hybrids, although all the material was handled in the same way. For 51 of the hybrids it was less than 5×10^7/ml, whereas for the other 27 it varied between 3×10^8 and 2×10^{11}/ml. The reasons for these variations in titer have not yet been investigated. It seems probable that they may be correlated with the proportions of *E. coli* chromosome present in the hybrids. In this experiment, however, we were primarily interested in the *cysC* region and therefore it was not important for us to know how many other sections of *E. coli* chromosome might be represented in the hybrids.

Twenty-five high-titer phages grown in the wild-type hybrid bacteria were used in transduction experiments. Presumably, all the phage cultures contained some phage particles with fragments of *E. coli* chromosome. The recipients were *Salmonella* strains carrying the mutant markers *cysC, D, H, I*, and *J*, *argB-69*, *argE-116*, *aroD-35*, *cysA-20*, *gly-1*, *lysA-8*, *metC-32*,

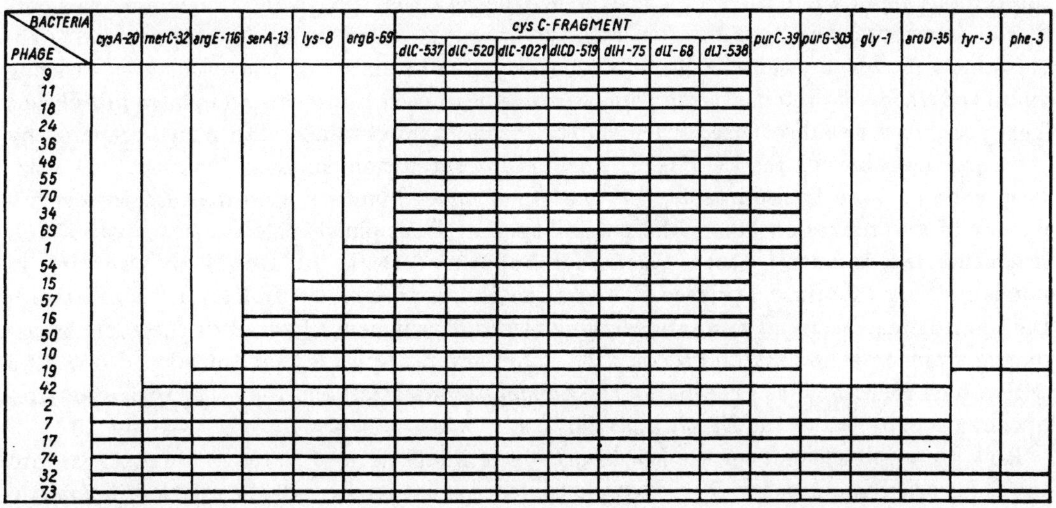

Fig. 1. Schematic diagram illustrating results of transduction crosses between *Salmonella* strains carrying closely linked genetic markers located in different transducing fragments and 25 *S. typhimurium* × *E. coli* hybrids. Horizontal lines indicate *E. coli* regions of the hybrid chromosomes.

purC-39, *purG-303*, *phe-3*, *serA-13*, and *tyr-3*. All the *cys* loci are located in one transducing fragment; each of the other loci is carried in a different fragment, but the results of conjugation experiments place them in the proximity of the *cysC* cluster. The findings of the transduction experiments are graphically presented in Figure 1. Absence of a horizontal line indicates that the number of transductants in experiments involving a *Salmonella* marker and phage from a hybrid was similar to the number obtained in control experiments with *Salmonella* phage. Presence of a line indicates that no transductants or only a few transductants were detected. No effort was made to enlarge the tests when no transductants were detected, and it seems likely that zero scorings were the result of small-scale testing.

Figure 1 shows clearly that every one of the 25 hybrid donors gave rise to a small number of transductants in the crosses with cysteine mutants representing the five loci of the *cysC* cluster. This result is in full agreement with the hypothesis that an *E. coli* chromosomal segment behaves differently in transduction than a *Salmonella* segment, recombining much less frequently with the *Salmonella* chromosome. The mutants represented by other transducing fragments can be arranged in order according to whether they produced large or small numbers of transductants with the hybrids. This is in agreement with the assumption that in different hybrids the *E. coli* segments differ in length, and that consequently the hybrids can serve in a fashion similar to overlapping deletions for genetic mapping of the *Salmonella* chromosome.

In the experiment reported here, the order of known genes was determined in 13 different transducing fragments. The position of *cysA-20* is still considered tentative because the conclusion is in partial disagreement with the conclusion reached in preliminary conjugation experiments. The material was not adequate to resolve the relative order of *purG* and *gly-1*, or of *tyr-3* and *phe-3*. Earlier transduction experiments had shown that the order of loci in the *cysC* cluster is *cysC*, *D*, *H*, *I*, *J* (DEMEREC *et al.*, 1963). The hybrid material was not adequate to determine the orientation of the cluster with respect to *argB* or *purG*.

The results of these experiments with hybrids indicate that a P 22 phage particle is able to transport a chromosome fragment consisting of *E. coli* material and deposit it in a *Salmonella* bacterium, and that recombination occurs with a low frequency between the *E. coli* fragment and the *Salmonella* chromosome. Before this conclusion was reached, several other interpretations of the data were considered. One was that phage P 22 does not transport *E. coli* fragments, and that the few wild-type variants observed in the experiments were transductants which originated from a relatively small number of phage particles carrying wild-type fragments retained from the parental phage used to prepare the phage in hybrids. This possibility was discounted when similar results were obtained with phage prepared by three passages through the hybrids. The second interpretation considered was that the wild-type variants were transductants, but that their small numbers were due not to low frequency of recombination but to the possibility that P 22 phage particles transport *E. coli* fragments less frequently than *Salmonella* fragments. Dr. R. B. MIDDLETON, working in uor laboratory, obtained evidence that eliminates this possibility. In transduction between the hybrids and bacterial mutants carrying two different genes located in the same transducing fragments (*ara-leu* and *thr-ser*), he found several hybrids that transduced one gene with a high frequency (as expected of the *Salmonella* material) and the other with a low frequency (as expected of the *E. coli* material).

How are we to account for the low frequency of integration of *E. coli* genic material into the *Salmonella* chromosome? The most plausible explanation seems to be a lack of homology at the subgenic (molecular) level. This divergence in homology could originate through changes within coding triplets, which, because of the degeneracy of the code, do not affect transcription of amino acid; or through changes that modify the transcription of amino acids of the nonfunctional regions of the protein; or through a combination of both. According to recently proposed hypotheses, the degeneracy of the amino acid code is so extensive that almost every amino acid can be coded by at least two different triplets (Woese, 1962; Wahba *et al.*, 1963). Thus two sentences could be composed which would transcribe exactly alike but differ in almost every consecutive word. If identity of words is essential for synapsis and consequent recombination, then two genes represented by two such sentences, although responsible for the same enzyme, would not recombine with each other.

Workers in several laboratories have devoted considerable effort to genetic mapping of the *S. typhimurium* and *E. coli* chromosomes. More than 90 gene loci have been placed on the *Salmonella* map and about 60 on the *E. coli* map. A very striking feature of the two maps is the almost complete homology, with respect to function and position, of comparable genes in these two genera of bacteria. There seems also to be a remarkable similarity in the enzymes controlled by homologous genes. Nevertheless, the evidence presented here indicates a high degree of divergence between the two genera in the molecular structure of homologous genes.

Summary

Transduction with bacteriophage P 22 has proved an extremely sensitive technique for detecting recombination between closely linked genetic markers in *Salmonella typhimurium*. Crosses made by this method between alleles of about 90 gene loci have produced frequencies of recombinants indicating that the genes are complex in structure and that complexity of structure is a general feature of all *Salmonella* genes. Thus we are able to identify mutational sites within gene loci and to determine their approximate order on a genetic map.

The limits of transducing fragments carried by phage P 22 are predetermined, so that for any one region of the chromosome all fragments are alike. Gene loci in *Salmonella* are non-randomly distributed on the chromosome: genes controlling similar functions are often clustered in one transducing fragment, and sometimes their arrangement within a cluster corresponds to the sequence of the biochemical reactions they control. Twelve clusters have been discovered so far.

Because the transducing fragments are predetermined, transduction between *Salmonella* strains is not a suitable method for chromosome mapping, since markers located in different fragments will be transduced independently even if they are close together. The conjugation technique is available, however, and more than 90 gene loci have thus been placed on the *S. typhimurium* genetic map. A comparison between this map and that of the *Escherichia coli* chromosome shows almost complete homology in arrangement of the known genes of the two genera.

S. typhimurium and *E. coli* can be crossed. Transduction studies with the hybrids produced by these crosses reveal that phage P 22 is able to transport fragments derived from either the *Salmonella* or the *E. coli* chromosome. Integration of *E. coli* genic material into the *Salmonella* chromosome, however, occurs with a very low frequency. The evidence obtained in our experiments indicates that a lack of homology at the subgenic level is responsible for the failure of integration. It suggests that the genes of *S. typhimurium* and *E. coli* are homologous with respect to function and position on the chromosome but not with respect to fine structure. This divergence in homology could originate from changes within coding triplets which, because of the degeneracy of the code, do not affect transcription; or from changes that modify the transcription of amino acids of the non-functional regions of the protein; or from a combination of both.

A sensitive new technique is described for mapping the *Salmonella* chromosome by transduction between *S. typhimurium* × *E. coli* hybrids as donors and genetically marked *S. typhimurium* mutants as recipients.

References

DEMEREC, M., D. H. GILLESPIE, and K. MIZOBUCHI, 1963: Genetic structure of the *cysC* region of the *Salmonella* genome. Genetics **48**, 997—1009.

DEMEREC, M., and P. E. HARTMAN, 1959: Complex loci in microorganisms. Ann. Rev. Microbiol. **13**, 377—406.

MIYAKE, T., and M. DEMEREC, 1959: *Salmonella-Escherichia* hybrids. Nature **183**, 1586.

OZEKI, H., 1959: Chromosome fragments participating in transduction in *Salmonella typhimurium* Genetics **44**, 457—470.

WAHBA, A. J., R. S. GARDNER, C. BASILIO, R. S. MILLER, J. F. SPEYER, and P. LENGYEL, 1963: Synthetic polynucleotides and the amino acid code. Proc. Nat. Acad. Sci. (Washington) **49**, 116—122.

WOESE, C. R., 1962: The nature of the biological code. Nature **194**, 1114—1115.

ZINDER, N. D., and J. LEDERBERG, 1952: Genetic exchange in *Salmonella*. J. Bacteriol. **64**, 679—699.

Restrictions and Host-induced Modifications of Phages λ and T_1 by certain Types of R Factors in *Escherichia coli* K-12

TSUTOMU WATANABE, HIROSHI NISHIDA, TOSHIHIKO ARAI, SACHIKO SATO and CHIZUKO OGATA

Department of Microbiology, Keio University School of Medicine, Tokyo, Japan

ARBER (personal communication) has recently found, in a series of studies on host-induced modifications (BERTANI and WEIGLE, 1953; LURIA, 1953) of phage λ, that an R factor (episomic drug resistance factor) (see WATANABE, 1963a) restricts phage λ in *Escherichia coli* K-12. The strain with this R factor had originally been supplied to him by the present authors and happened to be an fi^- type (or type 2 in our earlier terminology) (WATANABE, FUKASAWA, and TAKANO, 1962; WATANABE, 1963b). Another strain carrying an fi^+ (or type 1) R factor which we had supplied to ARBER did not show such an inhibitory effect against phage λ. The term *fi* (fertility inhibition) means the suppression of the functions of F of *E. coli* K-12. Male bacteria of K-12 carrying an fi^+ R factor have very much reduced abilities of mating, of synthesis of f phagespecific receptor (WATANABE, FUKASAWA, and TAKANO, 1962) and of synthesis of f^+ antigen (personal communication from F. ØRSKOV). fi^- R factors do not possess these inhibitory actions against F. We have undertaken to study the generality of the phenomenon, which was discovered by ARBER, employing more strains of R factors of independent origins. Preliminary results of our studies have already appeared in a Japanese journal (WATANABE and NISHIDA, 1963).

YOSHIKAWA and AKIBA (1962) have also found a similar fact with phages λ and P1 independently of ARBER's and our studies. In addition, YOSHIKAWA and AKIBA (1962) found that phage λ undergoes a host-induced modification in the host carrying fi^- R factors which restrict the growth of λ. We have confirmed their results of host-induced modification of λ using several fi^- R factors of independent origins. We have found, in addition, that an fi^- R factor restricts λ but does not modify it.

In parallel with the above studies with phage λ, we have also studied on the responses to the phages of T series of *E. coli* K-12 strains carrying various R factors. Phage T_1 among them was found to be restricted by fi^- R factors but not by fi^+ R factors and further some of the fi^- R factors were found to modify phage T_1.

The detail of these studies will be reported in the present paper.

Materials and methods

Bacterial strains

Strains CSH-2 (F^-) (*Meth*$^-$ λ^+) and W 3102 (F^-) (*Gal*$_2^-$ λ^-), both of which are the substrains of *E. coli* K-12, were used.

Phage strains

Phage λ wild type (λ^{wt}), a clear mutant of λ (λ^{cl}) and a virulent mutant of λ (λ^{vi}) were employed. The latter two phages and the phages of T series were kindly supplied by TOMIZAWA.

R factors

The R factors employed are listed in Table 1. These R factors had been carried by *Shigella* strains isolated from dysentery patients of independent epidemics.

Table 1
R factors employed in the present study

Strain number of R factor	Drug resistance markers*	*fi***
N-1	*Su, Sm, Tc*	−
N-3	*Su, Sm, Tc*	−
N-6	*Su, Sm, Tc*	+
N-9	*Su, Sm, Tc*	+
R-15	*Su, Sm*	−
222	*Su, Sm, Cm, Tc*	+

* Drug resistance markers: *Su*, *Sm*, *Cm*, and *Tc* are the abbreviations of sulfanilamide, streptomycin, chloramphenicol, and tetracycline respectively.
** *fi*$^+$ means the suppression of the functions of F of *Escherichia coli* K-12 and *fi*$^-$ means the absence of this suppression.

Culture media

Bacteria were grown in Penassay broth (Difco) or in LENNOX broth (LENNOX, 1955) at 37 C with aeration. For solid media, Penassay broth agar, nutrient agar and LENNOX agar were used. LENNOX agar was used either with or without enrichment with $CaCl_2$.

Results

Efficiencies of plating of phage λ and its mutants on W 3102

Phage λ^{wt} used was obtained by UV-induction of CSH-2 (F^-). Phages λ^{cl} and λ^{vi} were propagated on W 3102. The efficiencies of plating (e. o. p.) of λ^{wt} and its mutants are shown in Table 2. In the experiments shown in this table, nutrient agar was used without enrichment with $CaCl_2$. As seen here, no visible plaques were formed by these phages on the indicator strains carrying R factors N-1 and R-15. However, when Lennox agar containing M/400 $CaCl_2$ was employed, visible plaques of λ^{cl} and λ^{vi} were formed, although they were still smaller and more turbid than the plaques developed on the other strains (Table 3). On LENNOX agar containing M/400 $CaCl_2$, λ^{wt} still did not form visible plaques but when the concentration of $CaCl_2$ was increased to M/40, very turbid, small plaques of λ^{wt} were formed on W 3102 (N-1) although with reduced e. o. p.

Table 2
Efficiencies of plating of phage λ and its mutants on *Escherichia coli* W 3102* with and without R factors

Indicator	Efficiency of plating** of λ^{wt}	λ^{cl}	λ^{vi}
W 3102	10^0	10^0	10^0
W 3102 (N-1)	0 (< 3.0×10^{-8})	0 (< 3.0×10^{-8})	0 (< 3.0×10^{-8})
W 3102 (N-3)	5.0×10^{-3}	1.5×10^{-2}	3.9×10^{-2}
W 3102 (N-6)	10^0	10^0	10^0
W 3102 (N-9)	10^0	10^0	10^0
W 3102 (R-15)	0 (< 3.0×10^{-8})	0 (< 3.0×10^{-8})	0 (< 3.0×10^{-8})
W 3102 (222)	10^0	10^0	10^0

* W 3102 is a $Gal_2^-\lambda^-$ F^- substrain of *E. coli* K-12.
** Efficiencies of plating were determined on semisolid nutrient agar.

Table 3
Effect of $CaCl_2$ on plaque formation of phage λ^{vi} on *Escherichia coli* W3102* with and without R factors

Indicator	Efficiencies of plating on $CaCl_2$-free LENNOX agar	LENNOX agar with M/400 $CaCl_2$
W 3102	10^0	10^0
W 3102 (222)	10^0	10^0
W 3102 (N-1)	10^{-7}	ca. 10^{-1}**
W 3102 (R-15)	10^{-7}	ca. 10^{-1}**

* W 3102 is a Gal_2^- λ^- F^- substrain of *E. coli* K-12.
** The plaques developed on W 3102 (N-1) and W 3102 (R-15) are too obscure to count accurately.

Transduction of Gal^+ by an HFT lysate of λ into W3102 carrying various R factors

An HFT lysate of λ was prepared with the procedure of MORSE, LEDERBERG, and LEDERBERG (1956) and transduction of Gal^+ was carried out also with their procedure. The results are as shown in Table 4. It can be seen that the frequencies of Gal^+ transduction are reduced by the presence of fi^- R factors but not by the presence of fi^+ R factors in the recipient.

E. o. p. of phage T_1 on CSH-2 carrying various R factors

Phage T_1 used was propagated on W 3102 (F^-). The e. o. p. of phage T_1 on CSH-2 (F^-) carrying various R factors are shown in Table 5. It was noted that the plaques of T_1 developed on the indicators other than CSH-2 (N-1) were as large and as clear as those on the indicator without an R factor. The plaques developed on CSH-2 (N-1) were small and turbid as seen in Figure 1. Similar results were obtained when W 3102 was used instead of CSH-2.

Table 4

Frequencies of transduction of Gal^+ by an HFT lysate of phage λ into *Escherichia coli* W 3102* with and without R factors

Recipient	Frequency of Gal^+ transduction
W 3102	10^0
W 3102 (N-1)	3.0×10^{-3}
W 3102 (N-3)	5.4×10^{-2}
W 3102 (N-6)	10^0
W 3102 (N-9)	10^0
W 3102 (R-15)	3.1×10^{-2}
W 3102 (222)	10^0

* W 3102 is a Gal_2^- λ^- F^- substrain of *E. coli* K-12.

Adsorption of phages λ^{wt} and T_1 to W 3102 carrying various R factors

Nine ml of about 5×10^8 cells/ml of bacteria grown in Penassay broth were mixed with 1ml of each phage having a titer of 5×10^7/ml and aerated at 37 C for 10 min. One tenth ml aliquot was diluted with 10 ml ice-cold Penassay broth and then centrifuged at 5,000 r. p. m. for 5 minutes in the cold. The supernatant was treated with chloroform and the free phage was assayed. There was no significant difference in the adsorption rates of these phages to W 3102 carrying various R factors, although the data are not shown here.

Table 5

Efficiencies of plating of phage T_1 on *Escherichia coli* CSH-2* with and without R factors

Strain	Efficiency of plating**
CSH-2	10^0
CSH-2 (N-1)	8.7×10^{-3}***
CSH-2 (N-3)	1.3×10^{-4}
CSH-2 (N-6)	10^0
CSH-2 (N-9)	10^0
CSH-2 (R-15)	7.1×10^{-4}
CSH-2 (222)	10^0

* CSH-2 is a $Meth^-$ F^- substrain of *E. coli* K-12.

** Phage T_1 used was propagated on W 3102, a Gal_2^- λ^- F^- substrain of *E. coli* K-12.

*** The plaques developed on CSH-2 (N-1) were much smaller than those developed on the other strains as shown in Figure 1.

Host-induced modifications of phages λ^{vi} and T_1 in the strains carrying various R factors

The plaques of phages λ^{vi} and T_1 developed on W 3102 carrying various R factors in LENNOX agar containing M/400 $CaCl_2$ were scraped off and suspended in Penassay broth and homogenized. The homogenates were centrifuged at 5,000 r. p. m. for 10 minutes and the supernatants were plated for phage titrations on various indicator strains. The growth of phages λ^{vi} and T_1 on the strains carrying fi^- R factors resulted in the increase of their e. o. p. on the same indicator strains up to the e. o. p. on the indicators without R factors and with fi^+ R factors. A part of the results obtained with T_1 are shown in Table 6. The propagation of these modified phages in the host without an R factor again reduced their e. o. p. on the indicators with fi^- R factors, as a part of the results with T_1 are shown in Table 7. These results suggest that the observed phenomena are host-induced modifications of phages. Table 8 is a summary of the results of restrictions and host-induced modifications of phages λ and T_1 by fi^- R factors. As seen here, various types of host-induced modifications of phages λ and T_1 were observed with various fi^- R factors.

Table 6

Efficiencies of plating on *Escherichia coli* CSH-2* with and without R factors of phage T_1 grown on CSH-2 (N-3)

Indicator	Efficiency of plating
CSH-2	10^0
CSH-2 (N-1)	2.0×10^{-2}**
CSH-2 (N-3)	10^0
CSH-2 (N-6)	10^0
CSH-2 (N-9)	10^0
CSH-2 (R-15)	10^0
CSH-2 (222)	10^0

* CSH-2 is a *Meth*$^-$ F$^-$ substrain of *E. coli* K-12.

** The plaques developed on CHS-2 (N-1) were much smaller than those developed on the other strains as shown in Figure 1.

Effect upon the multiplications of phages λ and T_1 of fi^- transductant R factors obtained from an fi^+ R factor

Although a majority of drug-resistant transductants obtained by phage P-22 in *Salmonella typhimurium* LT-2 with a four-drug-resistant fi^+ R factor are unable to transfer their drug resistance by conjugation (Watanabe and Fukasawa, 1962 a), a few transductant R factors have recently been found to be transmissible by conjugation (Watanabe, 1963b). Some of them were found to be fi^- upon their conjugational transfer to male bacteria of *E. coli* K-12. The effects of these fi^- transductant R factors were investigated upon the e. o. p. of phages λ and T_1 on W 3102. It was found that these fi^- transductant R factors do not exert any inhibitory effect against the progeny formation of phages λ and T_1 unlike the naturally occurring fi^- R factors and like the original fi^+ R factor.

Table 7

Efficiencies of plating on *Escherichia coli* CSH-2* with and without R factors of phage T_1 grown on CSH-2 (N-3) and then on CSH-2

Indicator	Efficiency of plating
CSH-2	10^0
CSH-2 (N-1)	4.0×10^{-2}**
CSH-2 (N-3)	1.5×10^{-3}
CSH-2 (N-6)	10^0
CSH-2 (N-9)	10^0
CSH-2 (R-15)	1.5×10^{-3}
CSH-2 (222)	10^0

* CSH-2 is a *Meth*$^-$ F$^-$ substrain of *E. coli* K-12.

** The plaques developed on CSH-2 (N-1) are much smaller than those on the other strains as shown in Figure 1.

Discussion

It is reported in the present paper that fi^- R factors restrict the growth of phages λ and T_1, fi^+ R factors not possessing this inhibitory action. The results with λ are in accordance with those of Arber (personal communication) and Yoshikawa and Akiba (1962). Transduction of *Gal*$^+$ into a *Gal*$^-$ λ^- recipient was also reduced by the fi^- R factors possessed by the recipient. However, the adsorptions of phages λ and T_1 to the bacteria were not affected by any R factors in the recipient indicating that the restrictions of these phages are the events after the adsorption of these phages to the host bacteria. We are now studying on the nucleic acid injection of these phages into various strains to see if there is any suppression of the nucleic acid injection of these phages by fi^- R factors. Our preliminary results have

Table 8
Summary of restrictions and host-induced modifications of phages λ and T_1 by R factors

Strain of R factor	*fi*	Responses of	
		λ	T_1
N-6, N-9, 222	+	No restriction No modification	No restriction, No modification
N-1	-	Restriction, No modification	Restriction, No modification
N-3	−	Restriction, Modification to N-3	Restriction, Modification to N-3 and R-15
R-15	−	Restriction, No modification	Restriction, Modification to R-15 and N-3

indicated that there is no significant difference in the extent of nucleic acid injection of these phages.

In confirmation of the report of YOSHIKAWA and AKIBA (1962), we have found that phage λ undergoes a host-induced modification in the host bacteria carrying some fi^- R factor. In addition it was found that phage T_1 also undergoes a similar modification in the host bacteria carrying fi^- R factors as shown in Table 8. Furthermore, one of the fi^- R factors, N-1, which we used, did not cause such host-induced modifications of these phages. Some of the fi^- R factors, N-3, which caused the host-induced modifications of these phages modified phage T_1 to the host carrying the same R factor N-3 as well as to that carrying another fi^- R factor R-15. R factor N-3 modified phage λ only to the host with N-3 and not to the host with R-15. Finally, R factor R-15 did not modify phage λ but modified phage T_1 to the hosts with R-15 and with N-3.

R factor N-1 which does not modify phages λ and T_1 somehow caused the requirement of $CaCl_2$ for the formation of progeny phages of λ and T_1. The effect of $CaCl_2$ upon the growth of phages λ and T_1 could not be observed with any other R factors. The mechanism of the requirement of $CaCl_2$ for the progeny formation of phages λ and T_1 in the strains carrying R factor N-1 is now under investigation. Our preliminary results so far obtained indicate that the effect of $CaCl_2$ is exerted on the step following the adsorption of the phages to the host cells.

Several transmissible fi^- R factors were obtained by transduction of an fi^+ R factor with phage P-22 in *S. typhimurium* LT-2. They were found not to restrict phages λ and T_1 in *E. coli* K-12, suggesting that fi^- determinant(s) of R factors is not directly concerned with the restrictions of these phages.

The transfer of an fi^+ R factor to a recipient bacterial strain carrying an fi^+ R factor is markedly suppressed (WATANABE and FUKASAWA, 1962b). Our recent studies on the superinfection immunity of R factors have disclosed that the transfer of fi^- R factors to the strains carrying fi^- R factors are also suppressed, whereas the transfer of fi^- R factors to the strains with fi^+ R factors or the transfer of fi^+ R factors to the strains with fi^- R factors is not reduced (unpublished data). Furthermore, in the analysis of the strains carrying two types of R factors which were derived by superinfection, it was found that the strains with two types of fi^+ R factors are genetically very unstable, segregating one of the two types of R factors so frequently unless they are recombined (WATANABE and LYANG, 1962). To the contrary,

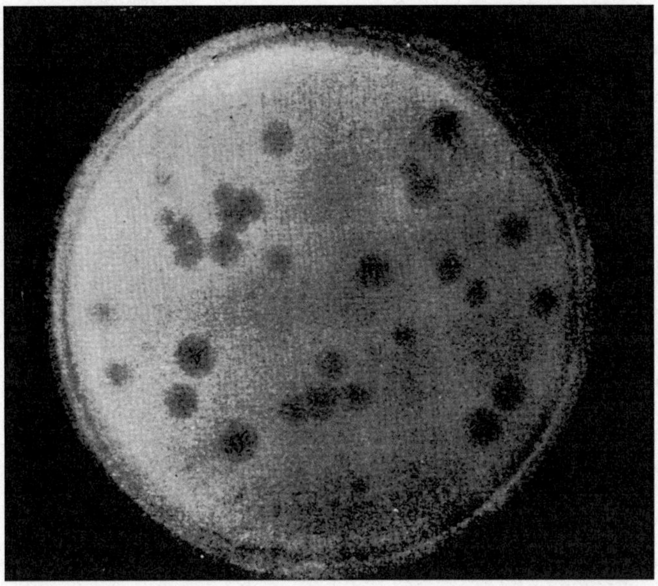

Plate 1. Plaques on the indicators without an R factor or with R factors other than N-1

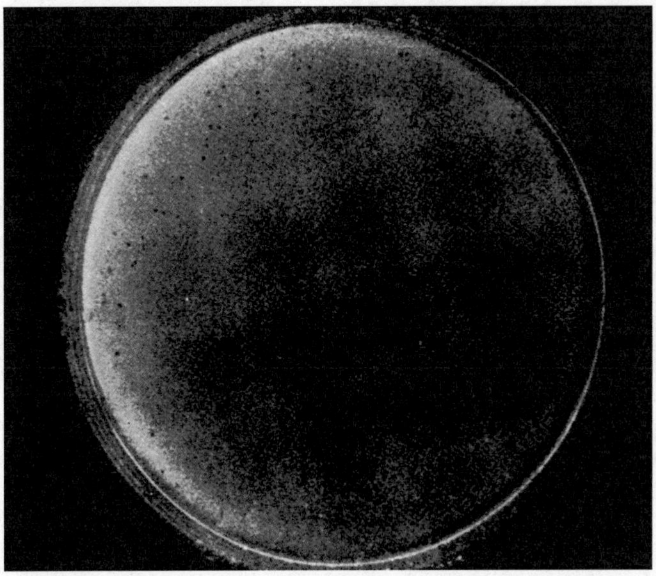

Plate 2. Plaques on the indicators with an R factor N-1

Fig. 1. Plaques of phage T_1 on *Escherichia coli* K-12

the strains carrying an *fi*$^+$ R factor and an *fi*$^-$ R factor are genetically as stable as the strains with single R factors (unpublished data). Furthermore, the *fi*$^-$ and *fi*$^+$ R factors in a cell are not physically associated in view of our findings of their independent transfer both by conjugation and by transduction with phage P1kc (unpublished data). From these unpublished data, it is obvious that *fi*$^+$ and *fi*$^-$ R factors behave quite differently from each other in their superinfection immunity patters. These results, together with those reported in the present paper, suggest that the RTFs (resistance transfer factors) (WATANABE, 1963a) of *fi*$^+$ and *fi*$^-$ R factors are quite different from each other, excluding a possibility that an *fi*$^-$ RTF has developed from an *fi*$^+$ RTF as a result of mutation or deletion.

The immunity to heterologous phages which is conferred by the presence of a prophage has been called prophage interference (BERTANI, 1953) or dysgonia (LWOFF, 1959). It was found that phage T_1 is not only restricted but also modified in P1-lysogenic hosts (LEDERBERG, 1957; CHRISTENSEN, 1961). The results reported in the present paper suggest that they are possibly analogous to prophage interference or dysgonia in their mechanisms. JACOB, SCHAEFFER, and WOLLMAN (1960) mentioned an hypothesis that phages and non-phage episomes may mutate to each other. No experimental evidence has so far been obtained for this hypothesis. Our results may suggest a genetic similarity between *fi*$^-$ RTFs and phages λ and T_1.

Summary

Episomic drug resistance factors (R factors) isolated from natural specimens are divided into *fi*$^+$ and *fi*$^-$ types. The term *fi* means fertility inhibition or the suppression of the functions of F of *Escherichia coli* K-12. *fi*$^-$ R factors were found to restrict phages λ and T_1 in *E. coli* K-12, whereas *fi*$^+$ R factors did not show such an inhibitory effect. Some of the *fi*$^-$ R factors caused host-induced modifications of these phages but an *fi*$^-$ R factor was found not to cause their host induced modifications. Further, this particular R factor caused the requirement of $CaCl_2$ for the progeny formation of phages λ and T_1. *fi*$^-$ R factors obtained from an *fi*$^+$ R factor by transduction with phage P-22 in *Salmonella typhimurium* did not restrict these phages. It is assumed that *fi*$^+$ and *fi*$^-$ R factors isolated from natural specimens have fairly different RTFs (resistance transfer factors), excluding a possibility that an *fi*$^-$ RTF has developed from an *fi*$^+$ RTF as a result of mutation or deletion.

This work was supported in part by Public Health Service Research Grant (E-4740) from the National Institute of Allergy and Infectious Diseases, U. S. A. and also by a research grant from the Ministry of Education of Japan.

Literature cited

ADAMS, M. H., 1950: Methods of study of bacterial viruses. In „Methods in Medical Research" (J. H. COMROE, Jr., ed.), **2**, 1–73.

BERTANI, G., 1953: Lysogenic versus lytic cycle of phage multiplication. Cold Spring Harbor Symp. Quant. Biol. **18**, 65–70.

BERTANI, G., and J. J. WEIGLE, 1953: Host-controlled variation in bacterial viruses. J. Bacteriol. **65**, 113–121.

Christensen, J. R. 1961: On the process of host-controlled modification of bacteriophage. Virology **13**, 40–43.

Jacob, F., P. Schaeffer, and E. L. Wollman, 1960: Episomic elements in bacteria. Symp. Soc. Gen. Microbiol. **10**, 67–91.

Lederberg, S. 1957: Suppression of the multiplication of heterologous bacteriophages in lysogenic bacteria. Virology **3**, 496–513.

Lennox, E. S., 1955: Transduction of linked genetic characters of the host by bacteriophage Pl. Virology **1**, 190–206.

Luria, E. S., 1953: Host-induced modifications of viruses. Cold Spring Harbor Symp. Quant. Biol. **18**, 237–244.

Lwoff, A., 1959: Interrelation between bacteria and bacteriophage. In ,,Symposium on Latency and Masking in Viral and Rickettsial Infections" (D. L. Walker, R. P. Hanson, and H. S. Evans, eds.), pp 8–19, Burgess, Minneapolis, Minnesota.

Morse, M. L., E. M. Lederberg, and J. Lederberg, 1956: Transduction in *E. coli* K-12. Genetics **41**, 142–156.

Watanabe, T., 1963a: Infective heredity of multiple drug resistance in bacteria. Bacteriol. Rev. **27**, 87–115.

Watanabe, T., 1963b: Episomic resistance factors in *Enterobacteriaceae*. XIX. Analysis of transmissible transductant R-factors of *Salmonella typhimurium*. Medicine and Biology (Tokyo) **66**, 34–37 (in Japanese).

Watanabe, T., and T. Fukasawa, 1961: Episome-mediated transfer of drug resistance in *Enterobacteriaceae*. I. Transfer of resistance factors by conjugation. J. Bacteriol. **81**, 669–678.

Watanabe, T., and T. Fukasawa, 1962a: Episome-mediated transfer of trug resistance in *Enterobacteriaceae*. III. Transduction of resistance factors. J. Bacteriol. **82**, 202–209.

Watanabe, T., and T. Fukasawa, 1962b: Episome-mediated transfer of drug resistance in *Enterobacbacteriaceae*. IV. Interactions between resistance transfer factor and F-factor in *Escherichia coli* K-12. J. Bacteriol. **83**, 727–735.

Watanabe, T., T. Fukasawa, and T. Takano, 1962: Conversion of male bacteria of *Escherichia coli* K-12 to resistance to f phages by infection with the episome ,,resistance transfer factor". Virology **17**, 218–219.

Watanabe, T., and K. W. Lyang, 1962: Episome-mediated transfer of drug resistance in *Enterobacteriaceae*. V. Spontaneous segregation and recombination of resistance factors in *Salmonella typhimurium*. J. Bacteriol. **83**, 422–430.

Watanabe, T., and H. Nishida, 1963: Episomic resistance factors in *Enterobacteriaceae*. XXII. Effects of R-factors on multiplication of phage λ in *Escherichia coli* K-12. Medicine and Biology (Tokyo) **67**, 96–99 (in Japanese).

Yoshikawa, M., and T. Akiba, 1962: Studies on transferable drug resistance in bacteria. IV. Suppression of plaque formation of phages by the resistance factor. Jap. J. Microbiol. **6**, 121–132.

The Integration of Episomes into the Bacterial Chromosome

JOHN SCAIFE and JULIAN D. GROSS

MRC Microbial Genetics Research Unit, Hammersmith Hospital, DuCane Road, London, W 12

There is a striking analogy between temperate bacteriophages and sex factors which control the ability to conjugate in various bacterial species. Both types of element, for which the term *Episome* has been proposed, can exist in alternative states, either multiplying autonomously or existing integrated in the bacterial chromosome and being replicated as part of it (JACOB, SCHAEFFER and WOLLMAN, 1960). The general question considered in this communication concerns the mechanism of the transition between the alternative states of episomes, with particular reference to the sex factor of *Escherichia coli* K-12.

Cells of *E. coli* which carry the sex factor (F) in the autonomous state are termed F^+, those in which F is integrated are known as Hfr (LEDERBERG *et al.*, 1952; HAYES, 1953). F^+ cells transfer the sex factor to female (F^-) cells during conjugation and can lose it either spontaneously or after treatment with various acridine dyes (HIROTA, 1960). Hfr cells arise by integration of the sex factor at any one of numerous points on the bacterial chromosome. They transfer the chromosome in an oriented manner the last marker to enter a female cell being the sex factor itself; those recombinants which inherit the sex factor are Hfr, not F^+. The sex factor in the integrated state is insensitive to acridine treatment. There is good evidence that only cells carrying F in the integrated state are able to transfer the chromosome and that the (low) fertility of F^+ populations is due to the presence of a minority of cells of this Hfr type (JACOB and WOLLMAN, 1956).

Hfr cells may revert to the F^+ state and in addition give rise to rare, variant sex factors (F′ factors) which have incorporated a subterminal segment of the Hfr chromosome (ADELBERG and BURNS, 1960; JACOB and ADELBERG, 1959). These factors are transferred with the same efficiency as F and are sensitive to acridine treatment. Strains harbouring an F′ factor transfer the chromosome with the same orientation as the Hfr in which the factor arose and with about 10% of the efficiency.

The difference between the integrated and autonomous states of the F factor is thus reflected primarily in the ability to bring about transfer of the bacterial chromosome and in the response to acridine dyes. The ability to synthesise the specific components required for conjugation (ØRSKOV and ØRSKOV, 1960; SNEATH and LEDERBERG, 1961) appears to be unaffected by the state of the sex factor.

A hypothetical scheme for the relationship between the sex factor, F′ factors and the Hfr chromosome, accounting for most of the differences in their properties is presented in Fig. 1. The formal similarity between the three structures as depicted derives from the supposition that the Hfr chromosome and F′ factors correspond to F factors into which either

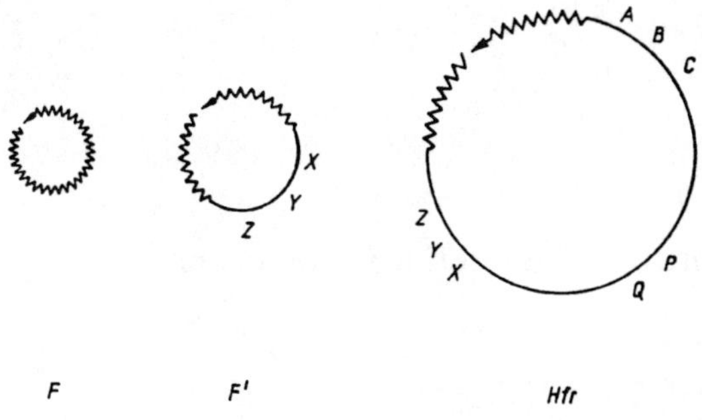

Fig. 1. The relationship between the genetic structures transferred to recipient cells by the three types of donor strains F⁺, F′ and Hfr. The genetic material of the sex factor is represented as a wavy line, that of the bacterial chromosome as a straight line. A, B, C, P, Q, X, Y and Z are genetic markers on the bacterial chromosome. The arrow represents the leading extremity of the structures transferred by the different donor strains. Both distal and proximal moieties of the sex factor must be transferred to an F-cell for the donor property to be inherited.

the whole or a part of the bacterial chromosome has been inserted (CAMPBELL, 1962; GROSS in press.) By making the assumption that transfer of F is itself oriented (as shown by the arrow) the model accounts for the oriented transfer of F′ factors (HIROTA and SNEATH, 1961) and of the Hfr chromosome and for the fact that the donor property in each case is the last to enter the recipient cell. Transfer of the bacterial chromosome by Hfr but not F^+ cells is also explained by this model since it would occur only when the chromosome is inserted into the continuity of the sex factor.

The recent evidence indicating that the chromosome of Hfr cells, like that of F^+ and F^- cells, is circular (TAYLOR and ADELBERG, 1961; CAIRNS, 1963) may be explained in terms of the present model by supposing that the sex factor itself is circular. In that case the arrow would represent the point on the F-factor at which opening and consequent linearization of the structures would occur prior to transfer. This opening may in fact represent a stage in the replication of the chromosome of mated Hfr cells (BOUCK and ADELBERG, 1963; JACOB, BRENNER and CUZIN, 1963).

The proposed structural relationship between the F factor and the Hfr chromosome suggests an obvious mechanism by which the transition from the autonomous to the integrated state could occur, namely by a single reciprocal genetic exchange between a circular sex factor and the circular chromosome. The integration of other episomes could occur by the same mechanism (CAMPBELL, 1962), while reversion of Hfr cells to the F^+ state might take place by reversal of this process. A mechanism of this kind implies the existence of some homology between F and the point on the chromosome where synapsis and exchange occurs and is thus consistent with the observation that F can only become stably integrated at a limited number of positions (MATNEY and GOLDSCHMIDT, 1963; BRODA, pers. comm.).

The validity of this model has not been tested directly in the case of the sex factor itself owing to the absence of adequately marked F factors. However it does lead to a prediction concerning the interaction of F′ factors with the chromosome, which we have tried to verify (SCAIFE and GROSS, 1963). As mentioned previously, cells harbouring an F′ factor transfer their chromosome at a relatively high rate and with the same orientation as the parental Hfr. They thus behave quite differently from populations of F^+ cells. This difference could be explained by supposing that F′ factors, like the F factor, become integrated by a genetic exchange with the chromosome but that the exchange involves the segment of the bacterial chromosome incorporated into the sex factor rather than the genetic material of the sex factor proper. Genetic exchanges between the homologous segments, would be expected to occur more frequently than in the case of pairing between the F factor and the chromosome. The region of homology being greater for the F-prime factor. They would give rise to a structure closely analogous to the Hfr chromosome. The predicted event is shown in Fig. 2 for the case of an F′ factor (F-*lac*) carrying the lactose segment of the chromosome (*lac*) and originating from an Hfr strain which transfers the gene for proline synthesis (*pro*) first and *lac* last.

It may be noted that the resulting structure has two lactose segments, one at each extremity of the transferred chromosome. Consequently, unlike cells of the parental Hfr strain which only transfer *lac* at the distal extremity with *pro* as the leading marker, cells carrying F-*lac* should transfer an entire lactose segment first, followed by the *pro* marker. Moreover in a culture of a strain which has the lac^+ marker on the chromosome and a lac^- mutation in the F-*lac* factor, different types of chromosomal donor would be expected to arise depending on whether the exchange occurs to the left or right of the lac^- mutation. In the former case the resulting structure transfers lac^+ at its leading extremity and lac^- at the distal end (Fig. 2, type 2), while in the latter the position of the markers is reversed (type 1).

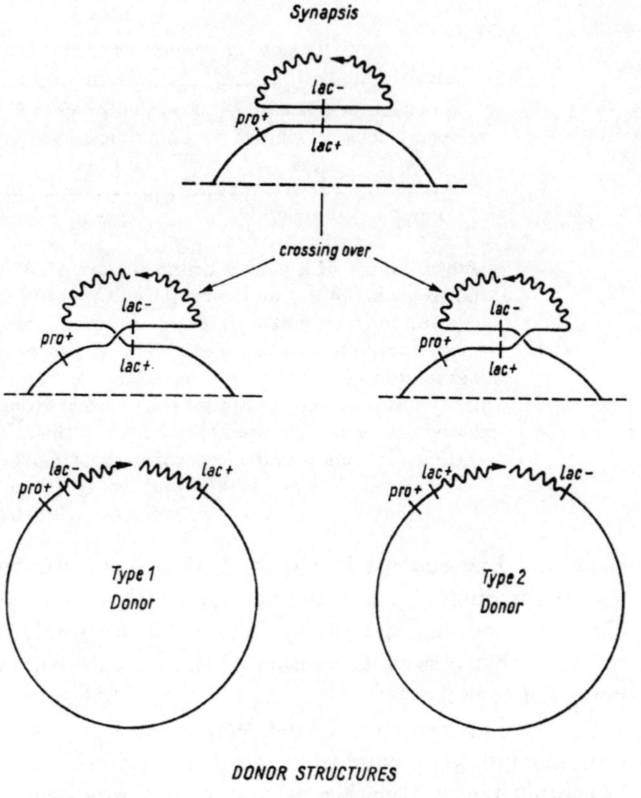

Fig. 2. The mechanism of integration of an F-*lac* factor into the bacterial chromosome. The genetic material of the sex factor is represented as a wavy line, that of the chromosome as a straight line. The arrow represents the leading extremity of the structure transferred during conjugation.

To test this model we have sought evidence for these two types of donor cell. Crosses were performed between a lac^+/F-lac^- donor (see Fig. 2) and a pro^- lac^- recipient, to detect joint transfer of pro^+ and lac^+ and with a pro^+ lac^+ recipient to detect joint transfer of pro^+ and lac^- (type 1 donor). Mixtures of W 1485 $pro^+ lac^+ S^s$ (F-lac^-) and either W 945 $pro^- lac^- S^r F^-$ or a lac^+ derivative of this strain were incubated with gentle aeration and aliquots of a diluted suspension plated on appropriately supplemented minimal agar plates. The $pro^+ S^r$ and $lac^+ S^r$ recombinants obtained in this way were then restreaked to score for inheritance of the lac^+ and pro^+ markers respectively.

The results obtained in a cross of the first kind are given in Table 1 (Scaife and Gross, 1963; see also Pittard and Adelberg, 1963). The yields of pro^+ and lac^+ recombinants are presented as a fraction of the total number of cells taking part in mating, estimated from the yield of $lac^+ S^r$ recombinants in a parallel cross with the same recipient and a F-lac^+ donor. As is to be expected, only a small fraction (2%) of the mated cells become lac^+ since the majority only receive the F-*lac* factor carrying the lac^- mutation. However it may be seen that a considerable proportion (15%) of those cells inheriting the pro^+ marker also inherit lac^+. This result, together with the fact that a large fraction (31%) of the lac^+ recombinants are also pro^+, demonstrates frequent joint transfer of the pro^+ and lac^+ markers. The lac^+ character of the majority of lac^+ pro^+ is in fact stable on subculture in the presence of acridine orange indicating that it is not due to the presence of a F-lac^+ factor but rather to transfer and integration of the lac^+ marker along with the pro^+ marker as part of a chromosomal

Table 1

The donor properties of W 1485 *lac*$^+$ (F-*lac*$^-$)

Fraction of mated recipient cells which are *pro*$^+$	Fraction of mated recipient cells which are *lac*$^+$	Fraction of *pro*$^+$ S^r recombinants which are *lac*$^+$	Fraction of *lac*$^+$ S^r recombinants which are *pro*$^+$
2.5%	2.2%	15%	31%

One millilitre of a young broth culture of W 1485 *pro*$^+$*lac*$^+$$S^s$(F-*lac*$^-$) was mixed with 1 ml. of an overnight culture of W 945 *pro*$^-$*lac*$^-$$S^r$. After gentle aeration for 60 minutes the mixture was diluted, agitated violently to stop further transfer and aliquots were then spread on appropriately supplemented plates to select for *pro*$^+$$S^r$ and *lac*$^+$ S^r recombinants. The recombinants obtained were scored for the unselected character. The total number of mated cells was estimated by measuring the number of recipient cells which became *lac*$^+$ in a parallel experiment mating the same recipient strain with the W 1485 *pro*$^+$ *lac*$^+$ S^s (F-*lac*$^+$) donor.

structure. Experiments in which mating is interrupted at intervals by blending indicate that the fraction of *pro*$^+$ recombinants which are *lac*$^+$ does not increase with increasing time of mating, showing that the *lac*$^+$ marker is invariably transferred before *pro*$^+$. This confirms the view that a sizeable fraction of the recombinants result from chromosome transfer by donors of type 2.

In crosses of the second kind, employing a *pro*$^-$ *lac*$^+$ S^r recipient, about 28% of the *pro*$^+$ recombinants were found to be *lac*$^-$. Once again these recombinants must have received and integrated the *lac*$^-$ marker as part of a chromosomal structure rather than on an F-*lac*$^-$ factor since cells which simply receive F-*lac*$^-$ are heterogenotes and consequently phenotypically *lac*$^+$. It may be noted that in such experiments the transfer of *lac* as a *terminal* marker by either type of donor has a negligible effect on the results owing to the rarity with which the entire chromosome is transferred during conjugation.

These results thus confirm the existence of the two types of donor predicted by the model and indicate that donors of type 1 arise twice as frequently as type 2 donors, since the chromosomal transfer of *lac*$^-$ occurs twice as frequently as that of *lac*$^+$. This difference may be explained by supposing that the *lac*$^-$ mutation lies somewhat towards the right hand end of the F-*lac* factor so that exchanges occur more frequently on its left than on its right. PITTARD and ADELBERG (1963) have, in fact, studied chromosome transfer by a strain harbouring an F-prime factor which differs from the homologous chromosomal segment with respect to several markers and observed that markers near the leading extremity of the F-prime factor are inherited by a greater proportion of chromosomal recombinants than more distal markers. The same workers (PITTARD, LOUTIT and ADELBERG, 1963) have also shown that a marker corresponding to *pro*$^+$ in the F-*lac* system is transferred later by an F′ donor than by the parental Hfr strain and that the length of the delay corresponds to the time required to transfer the segment of chromosome incorporated in the F′ factor. This result provides strong support for the proposed model, as do recent observation of JACOB *et al.*, (1963) who by selective means have isolated derivatives of an F-*lac* strain in which the sex factor is more or less stably integrated; they found that these carry the *lac* region in duplicate, one copy lying at the proximal extremity and another at the distal end.

The present demonstration of the mechanism of insertion of an F-prime factor into the bacterial chromosome, although suggestive, does not in itself constitute proof that the sex factor of an Hfr strain is inserted in the same way. More direct evidence would come from the demonstration that the fragment of the sex factor presumed to be carried by the ♀$_3$ strain of RICHTER (1961) is colinear with the chromosome. Experiments of this type are currently under way in this laboratory.

Literature cited

ADELBERG, E. A., and S. H. BURNS, 1960: Genetic variation in the sex factor of *Escherichia coli.* J. Bact. **79**, 321–330.

BOUCK, N., and E. A. ADELBERG, 1963: The relationship between DNA synthesis and conjugation in *Escherichia coli.* Biochem. biophys. Res. Comm. **11**, 24–27.

CAIRNS, J., 1963: The bacterial chromosome and its manner of replication as seen by autoradiography. J. mol. Biol. **6**, 208–213.

CAMPBELL, A., 1962: Episomes. Advan. Genet. **11**, 101–145.

GROSS, J. D., 1964: Conjugation in bacteria. The Bacteria, Vol V, (I. C. GUNSALUS and R. Y. STANIER, eds.) Academic Press New York, in press.

HAYES, W., 1953: The mechanism of recombination in *E. coli.* Cold Spr. Harb. Symp. quant. Biol. **18**, 75–93.

HIROTA, Y., 1960: The effect of acridine dyes on mating type factors in *Escherichia coli.* Proc Natl. Acad. Sci. U.S. **46**, 57–64.

HIROTA, Y., and P. H. A. SNEATH, 1961: F' and F mediated transduction in *E. coli* K 12. Jap. Journ. Genet. **36**, 307–318.

JACOB, F., and E. A. ADELBERG, 1959: Transfert de charactères génétiques par incorporation au facteur sexual d'*Escherichia coli.* C. R. Acad. Sci. (Paris). **249**, 189–191.

JACOB, F., S. BRENNER, and F. CUZIN, 1963: On the regulation of DNA replication in bacteria. Cold Spr. Harb Symp. quant. Biol. **28**, 329–348.

JACOB, F., P. SCHAEFFER, and E. L. WOLLMAN, 1960: In „Microbial Genetics", p. 67, (HAYES W., and R. C. CLOWES., eds) Cambridge University Press (London).

LEDERBERG, J., L. L. CAVALLI, and E. M. LEDERBERG, 1952: Sex compatibility in *E. coli.* Genetics. **37**, 720–730.

MATNEY, T. S., E. P. GOLDSCHMIDT, and N. S. ERWIN, 1963: The specificity of genomic sites affording registry with the fertility episome in *Escherichia coli* K 12. Biochem. biophys. Res. Comm. **12**, 483–486.

ØRSKOV, I., and F. ØRSKOV, 1960: An antigen termed f$^+$ occurring in F$^+$ *E. coli* strains. Acta. path. microbiol. scand. **48**, 37–46.

PITTARD, J., J. S. LOUTIT, and E. A. ADELBERG, 1963: Gene transfer by F' strains of *E. coli.* K 12. I. Delay in initiation of chromosome transfer. J. Bact., **85**, 1394–1401.

PITTARD, J., and E. A. ADELBERG, 1963: Gene transfer by F' strains of *Escherichia coli.* K 12. II. Interaction between F. merogenote and chromosome during transfer. J. Bact., **85**, 1402–1408.

RICHTER, A., 1961: Attachment of wild-type F factor to a specific chromosomal region in a variant strain of *Escherichia coli.* K 12: the phenomenon of episomic alternation. Genet. Res. Camb., **2**, 333–345.

SCAIFE, J., and J. D. GROSS, 1963: The mechanism of chromosome mobilization by an F-prime factor in *Escherichia coli* K 12. Genet. Res. Camb., **4**, 328–331.

SNEATH, P. H. A., and J. LEDERBERG, 1961: Inhibition by periodate of mating in *Escherichia coli* K 12. Proc. Natl. Acad. Sci. U.S. **47**, 86–90.

TAYLOR, A. L., and E. A. ADELBERG, 1961: Evidence for a closed linkage group in Hfr males of *Escherichia coli* K-12. Biochem. biophys. Res. Comm. **5**, 400–404.

The Environmental Control of the Conjugation in *Escherichia coli* K-12

II. The Effect of Temperature on Effective Pairs Formation and on Chromosomal Transfer

WŁADYSŁAW J. H. KUNICKI-GOLDFINGER and KATARZYNA CZERWIŃSKA

Department of Microbiology, Warsaw University, Warsaw and the Microbiology Department, Wrocław University, Wrocław

Summary

The influence of temperature was studied, separately upon effective pairs formation and chromosomal transfer. It was found that the chromosomal transfer is, in the respect of its temperature dependence, akin to a reversible denaturation process.

Introduction

HAYES (1957) has shown that the rate of chromosome transfer is influenced by temperature, with $Q_{10} = 4.0$. FISHER (1961) has studied kinetics of the conjugation in conditions, which permitted pair formation but prevented chromosome transfer. It appears from his experiments that collision is independent of temperature over the range examined, the effective pairs formation is a temperature dependent process with $Q_{10} = 2.7$.

There is some discrepancy between the results of HAYES and those of FISHER. It seems, therefore, desirable to re-investigate this problem in different experimental conditions, allowing for differentiation between these two phases of conjugation process.

Experimental

Material and Methods

Bacterial strains. $F^- L^- B_1^- M^+ S^r$ strain, derivative of LEDERBERG's 3064 strain, and Hfr $L^+ B_1^+ M^- S^s$, derivative of LEDERBERG's 1895, strain with lowered efficiency of chromosomal transfer, were used. The strains differed also in some other characteristics (phage and azide sensitivity, ability to sugar fermentation), but these markers were not employed in experiments here reported.

Media. Media used were described in previous paper (CZERWIŃSKA, 1964).

Procedure. Technical procedure adopted was identical with described by CZERWIŃSKA (1964), the only difference being as follow. The bacterial suspensions of the strains to be mated were transferred to broth, previously warmed to desired temperature and incubated for appropriate time intervals in an ultrathermostatic bath at different temperatures. At intervals, after mixing, samples were rapidly withdrawn, diluted and plated without washing, on selective media (for recombinants) and on nutrient agar (for total viable count). A final dilution of 10^{-6} for total viable count, and of 10^{-2} for recombinants number were usually used.

The conjugation rate was measured as a number of detectable zygotes in terms of detectable products of zygote formation. As such usually prototrophic recombinants were used, in some experiments other types of recombinants, as described in ,,Results".

Results

Disruption of effective pairs

It is generally assumed that dilution and plating operations disrupt an unknown number of specific pairs, this number, according to current opinion, being very low.

In present research, rapidly made dilutions were rapidly spread on thoroughly dried surface of agar medium. In these conditions the majority of effective pairs were disrupted, the fraction of the undisrupted ones being relatively stable in the range 2–5 per cent. When the number of recombinant colonies is plotted as a function of time a straight line is obtained. The placing of points where the extrapolated lines crossed the abscissa shows that effective pairs were efficiently disrupted (Fig. 1). The linear rise in the number of recombinants is preceded by a lag of different length, dependent of the kind of selective marker used.

The important point is, that the adopted method of effective pairs' disruption, being efficient, at the same time leaves a small fraction of undisrupted pairs. Therefore, if it were possible to assay the ratio of the disrupted to the undisrupted pairs, and to find conditions in which the over-all conjugation rate would be limited only by the rate of effective pairs formation, or only by the velocity of chromosome transfer, then it would be also possible to examine the kinetics of these two phases separately. The number of the undisrupted pairs, which are continuing mating process after plating,

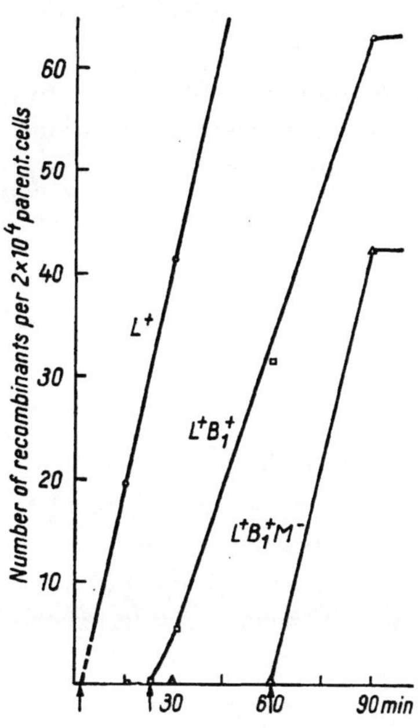

Fig. 1. The variation of recombinant genotype with the period of mating at 44°. Samples were removed at intervals, diluted and plated on selective media + streptomycin. Arrows pointing to the abscissa: the end of the lag phase for L^+, $L^+B_1^+$, and $L^+ B_1^+ M^-$ recombinants, respectively.

may be measured, albeit indirectly. It is also possible to find the conditions in which the over-all conjugation rate is limited either by the rate of effective pairs formation or by the rate of chromosome transfer exclusively. This will be discussed in the next section.

Knowing these conditions and the ratio of disrupted to undisrupted pairs, we should be able to study the kinetics of effective pairs formation (by scoring the number of recombinant colonies arising from undisrupted pairs, when the rate of formation of effective pairs is a limiting factor) and the kinetics of chromosome transfer (by assaying the number of recombinant colonies arising from disrupted pairs, when the velocity of entering of chromosome to F^- cells is a limiting factor).

Effect of temperature

The mȧting mixture was incubated at different temperatures, in the range from 20° to 48°, for one hour, then diluted and plated as discribed previously. The number of $L^+ B_1^+ M^+$ recombinants per 2×10^4 parental cells was plotted against temperature at which mating was carried out (Fig. 2).

Three distinct phases may be distinguished. The first phase, over the range from 20° to 30°, is characterized by a low slope; at higher temperatures it is replaced by the second phase,

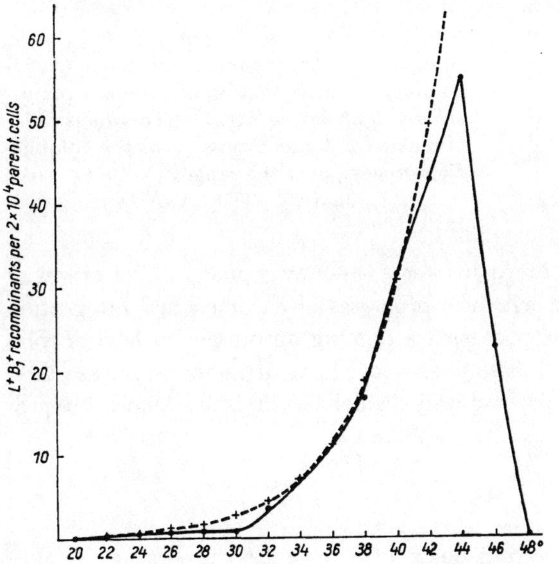

Fig. 2a: Abscissa — temperature of mating; Ordinate-number of prototrophic recombinants per 2×10^4 parental cells (semilogarithmic scale).

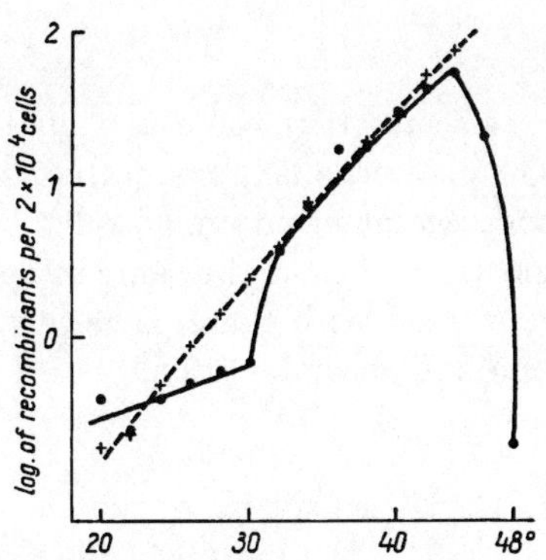

Fig. 2b: Abscissa — temperature of mating; Ordinate — number of recombinants (numerical scale) per 2×10^4 parental cells, full line-observed values, dashed line — calculated (expected) values on the basis of experimental value for 34° and value of μ = 46,800 kcal.

Fig. 2. The effect of temperature on the conjugation rate. The crosses are carried out under usual conditions, but incubated for 1 h at different temperatures, then diluted and plated.

a slope being here very high. The third phase, observed at temperatures 44° and over, is evidently due the thermal inactivation of basic enzymatic processes in the bacterial cells.

When an ARRHENIUT plot of conjugation rate is made, a very characteristic and interesting picture is obtained (Fig. 3).

The critical increments of temperature, μ, of the first phase (20°–30°) amounts to 15.000 kcal, thus being typical for other biological processes. Q_{10} of the first phase is 2.2. The critical increments of temperature, μ, of the second phase (32°–44°) is, on the other hand, exceedingly high, amounting to over 46.000 kcal. The value of Q_{10} of the second phase is also proportionally high: $Q_{10}(32°–40°) = 10$, Q_{10} (34–44°) = 9.6. In this respect the second phase bears striking resemblance to reversible denaturation processes, in which values of μ are of the similar order.

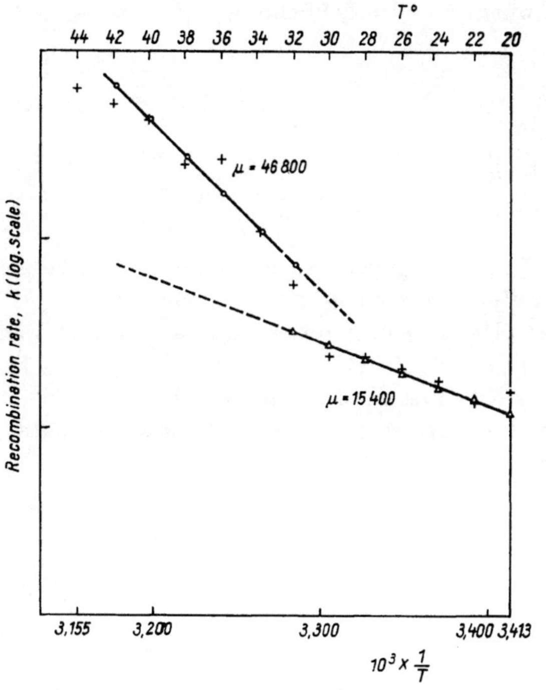

Fig. 3. ARRHENIUS plot of the conjugation rate, assayed by counting prototrophic recombinants after mating at different temperatures for 1 h (see Fig. 2). The values of increments of temperature, μ, of the conjugation process, over the range 32°–40° (–o–o–), and 20°–30° (–Δ–Δ–).

It seems that there is a qualitative difference between these two phases. The origin of this difference is, apparently, not connected with the processes of chromosomal integration and recombination in F^- cells, because these processes are going on on the surface of solid media, always at the same temperature (37°). The observed effects of temperature are then connected with these parts of conjugation process only, which are finished before integration and recombination.

The nature of the first and the second phase of conjugation process

The experimental data obtained over the range 32°–40° have been used for calculation of μ value. Using this value, a theoretical curve was drawn and the numbers of recombinants, which should be found at different temperatures, were calculated and plotted (Fig. 2, dashed line). The theoretical curve at temperatures below 30° deviates from the experimental one in form and in position. The number of observed recombinant colonies is much lower than the number expected. This small fraction of recombinants does not obey the rule, operating at higher temperatures (over 32°). It is clear that at temperatures below 30° the temperature dependent process, affecting the rate of conjugation during the second phase, does not operate. There is then one process common to both phases, and the second one which is limited to the second phase only. This second process has to be consecutive to the first one. The nature of these both processes has now to be explained.

In the small fraction of recombinants, which is found at temperatures below 32°, only the first process is going on during the experiment. The second process is absent in these recombinants, or at least is not completed during incubation in experimental temperatures during mating. It has then to be concluded after dilution and plating operations are carried out. There are two processes, which are finished before integration and recombination: effective pairs formation and chromosome transfer. It may be then inferred that the second process, operating during the second phase and absent in the first one, is chromosome transfer. At lower temperatures there is not enough time for concluding the second process, chromosome transfer, the velocity of which is in these conditions very low. The first process is the effective pairs formation. The first phase (see Fig. 2 and 3) gives the temperature dependence of effective pairs formation, the second one – of chromosome transfer.

The fraction formed by these undisrupted pairs in total effective pairs population may be calculated indirectly by relating the number of their products (e. i. the recombinant colonies from mixtures mating at temperatures below 30°) to the maximal observed number of recombinant colonies at higher temperatures. This has been calculated as 2 to 5 per cent, the calculation being carried out in such a way that the real value is probably much lower.

The first part of the curve (Fig. 2), between 20° and 30°, gives then the effect of temperature on the rate of effective pairs formation. The second part of the same curve, between 32° and 44°, characterizes the temperature dependence of the velocity of chromosome transfer.

The rate of effective pairs formation and of chromosome transfer

The time needed for effective pairs formation and the velocity of chromosome transfer of a given part of a chromosome may be then calculated, albeit indirectly.

In order to do this, the time of appearing of chosen markers (t_m) were measured at various temperatures (see Fig. 1). This time is given approximately by points, at which extrapolated straight lines crossed the abscissa. It is a sum of the time of effective pairs formation (t_e) which is constant at given temperature for all markers, and the time needed for transfer of a part the chromosome (t_{ch}), which depends on the position of a chosen marker.

$$\text{Thus } t_m = t_e + t_{ch}.$$

For a pair markers (a and b) two equations may be formed

$$t_{m'} = t_e + t_{ch}$$
$$t_{m''} = t_e + t_{ch''}$$

where $t_{m'}$ and $t_{m''}$ are the lags of appearance of recombinant colonies of type a and b, t_{ch} and $t_{ch''}$ – the time needed for transfer of a part of chromosome from point 0 to marker a, and from point 0 to marker b, respectively.

Subtracting gives $t_{m''} - t_{m'} = t_{ch''} - t_{ch'}$, thus the time needed for a transfer of a part of chromosome between a and b.

Assuming that the L marker is placed at the extremity or very near the extremity of a chromosome, the values of t_e and subsequently of t_{ch} may be computed, the values of t_m being measured experimentally. This was done for various tested temperatures, and values found were plotted against temperature (Fig. 4).

In Fig. 5 the sum of these both values (e. i. the lag) for each temperature was calculated and plotted in similar manner.

The curve in the Fig. 5 is, to some extent, a mirror picture of the curve from the Fig. 1, which has to be expected if assumptions adopted were correct. From these data the time of the appearance of a marker, which position on the chromosome is known, may be predicted for any temperature in the range examined. That this predicted values are in agreement with the observed ones, shows Fig. 6 for 32°.

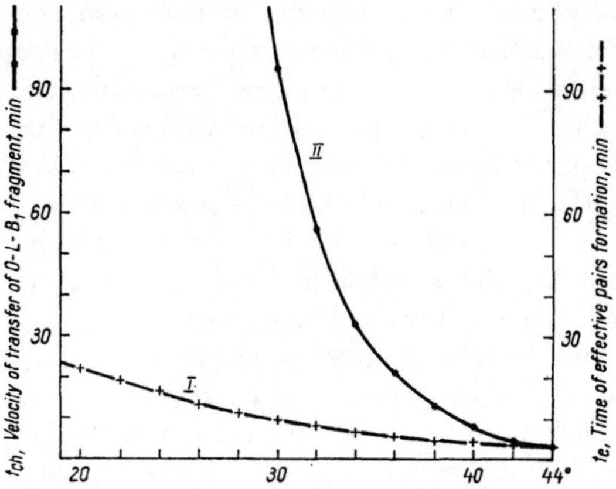

Fig. 4. The kinetics of the conjugation. Effect of temperature on the time needed for effective pairs formation (curve I), and on the velocity of transfer of O-L-B_1 fragment of chromosome (curve II). For further explanations see text.

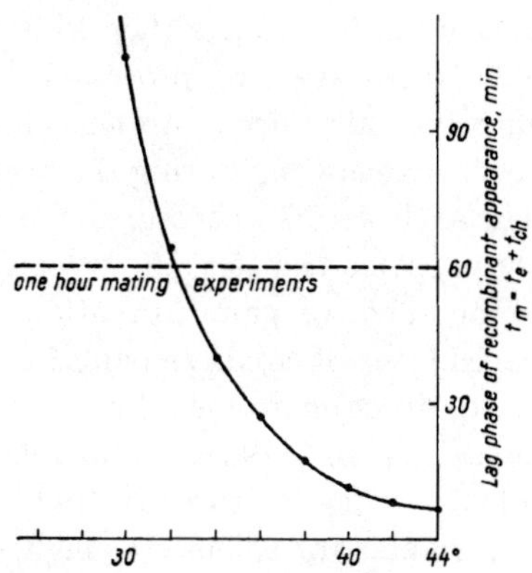

Fig. 5. The kinetics of the conjugation. Effect of temperature on the lag phase (time needed for effective pairs formation + time needed for transfer of O-L-B_1 chromosome fragment) calculated as in Fig. 4. For explanation see text. Circles — observed values.

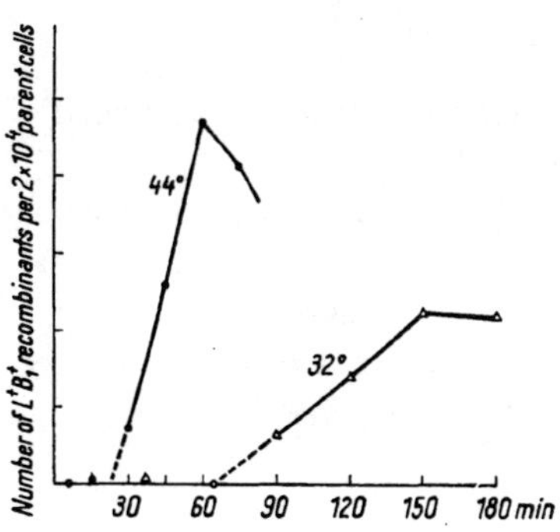

Fig. 6. The observed and expected value of lag phase for $L^+B_1^+$ recombinants at 32°. The open circle marks the expected value point, at which extrapolated straight line based on experimental data crosses the abscissa.

Discussion

The method here adopted of differentiating the two consecutive phases of conjugation process allows for examination of the kinetics of effective pairs formation and of chromosome transfer, separately. This is valid only when certain silent assumptions made previously, are justified. Among these assumptions the most important are: 1. „Production coefficient", by which the number of detectable zygotes is related to the absolute number of zygotes, does not change during the experiment. The validity of this assumption cannot be evaluated directly. Anyhow it is the same as in other researches on the kinetics of conjugation process.

2. The chromosome is transferred from Hfr to F^- cells at an uniform rate, if conditions of the experiment (others than the time of mating) were not changed. This assumption is generally adopted in similar researches. Moreover in the present research the velocities of transfer of the same part of a chromosome were measured at different temperatures, so the conclusions made are rather independent of the correctness of this assumption. 3. The L marker is placed very near the point O, on the extremity of the chromosome entering as the first the F^- cell. The time needed for transfer of the $O - L$ part of the chromosome is negligible small. This seems to be justified by the results reported in the Fig. 1.

The observed dependence on the temperature of the process of effective pairs formation is such as might be expected in any biological, enzymatic process. The exceedingly high value of increments of temperature, μ, which has been found for the process of chromosome transfer, is worth of special consideration and study. In this respect this process resembles a reversible denaturation process.

The so-called bacterial chromosome contains apparently only DNA, at least bonding of DNA with histones or any other proteins is very doubtful (Zubay, Doty, 1959, Bonner, Ru-Chih Huang, 1963). If it were so, the only substances that, with any probability, may suffer denaturation and at the same time be connected with chromosome transfer, are: extrachromosomal, cytoplasmic proteins and/or the DNA itself. These two possibilities are now subjected to further research.

Literature

Bonner, J., Ru-Chih Huang, 1963: Properties of chromosomal nucleohistone. J. Molec. Biol., **6**, 169.

Czerwińska, 1964: The environmental control of the conjugation in *Escherichia coli* K-12. I. The effect of pH, osmotic pressure, surface tension and cations. Acta Microbiol. Polon., **13**, 3.

Fisher, K. W., 1961: Environmental influence on genetic recombination in bacteria and their viruses. Symp. Soc. Gen. Microbiol., **11**, 272.

Hayes, W., 1957: The kinetics of the mating process in *Escherichia coli*. J. gen. Microbiol., **16**, 97.

Zubay, G., P. Doty, 1959: The isolation and properties of deoxyribonucleoprotein particles (DNP) containing single nucleic acid molecule. J. Molec. Biol., **1**, 1.

Competence of Transformable Streptococci

Roman Pakula

Institute of Biochemistry and Biophysics of the Polish Academy of Sciences

Competence can be defined as the physiological state of a bacterial culture that must be developed if the bacteria are to undergo genetic transformation. Transformability of bacteria is limited to a small number of species and only to some strains within these species. The nature of competence remains unexplained and one does not know why some strains are transformable and the others not.

After a careful study of development of competence in streptococcal cultures, we found that appearance of competence resembles in many respects the kinetic of accumulation in cultures of these bacteria of enzymes and toxins as of streptodornase, streptokinase, hyaluronidase and streptolysin O. We assumed, therefore, that streptococci cannot become competent before a substance, capable to convert non-competent cells into competent ones, produced by the germs themselves is accumulated in the culture. This was found true and a factor provoking competence was discovered in sterile supernatants of transformable and competent streptococcal cultures.

Before presenting a characteristic of this factor, it has to be mentioned that, in natural conditions, competence of streptococci develops only in media supplemented with either serum or albumin. In the absence of these substances, transformation does not occur or, if present, it is extremely low. The onset of competency, the period of its duration and the time of its disappearance are strictly dependent on the size of the initial inoculum in the culture. The smaller the inoculum, the later the appearance of competence (Fig. 1).

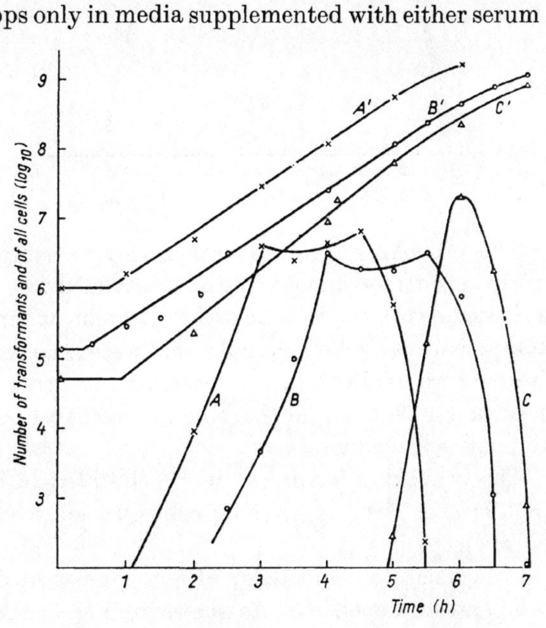

Fig. 1. Time dependence of development of competence in cultures started with inocula of various size.
A-competence, initial density $8{,}9 \cdot 10^5$ cells/ml
B-competence, initial density $1{,}5 \cdot 10^5$ cells/ml
C-competence, initial density $0{,}5 \cdot 10^5$ cells/ml
A′, B′, C′ corresponding growth curves.
Recipient and donor – strain Challis.

Thus conversion to competency of non-competent cultures with the use of provoking factor, can be demonstrated in two different conditions: 1. in cultures grown in the absence of serum or albumin, 2. in cultures grown in media containing serum or albumin. As concerns the second condition, the culture is started with a small initial inoculum and cells are exposed to the action of provoking factor 2 hours before natural competence is expected.

In all experiments, except one to be reported below, the first method of competence provocation was applied. The marker used in the transformation experiments was streptomycin resistance. The recipient and donors were group *H* hemolytic streptococci and strains of *Streptococcus sanguis* of types *I*, *II* and *I*/*II*, regarded to be closely related to group *H* streptococci. Strains of *S. sanguis*, type *I*/*II* share the C polysaccharide characteristic of group *H* streptococci.

With the factor provoking competence in our hands, the following procedure of transformation was developed. Cells were grown in the absence of serum or albumin for 2 hours and then was the provoking factor added. After 30 minutes, the cells were spun down, the supernatant containing the provoking factor discarded, the cells suspended in fresh medium, exposed to the action of DNA for 10 min. and then allowed to grow in the absence of the antibiotic for 110 min. for phenotypic expression. Transformants were scored after 40 hours at 37^0 on blood agar plates containing 250 μg/ml of streptomycin.

Fig. 2 illustrates the time dependence of development of competence and of the production of provoking factor in a culture of strain Challis, a group *H* Streptococcus. Competence disappeared at the end of the logarithmic phase of growth but the competence provoking activities of the sterile supernatant fluids prepared even after 17 hours of growth of the culture did not differ markedly from those prepared at the time of maximum competency.

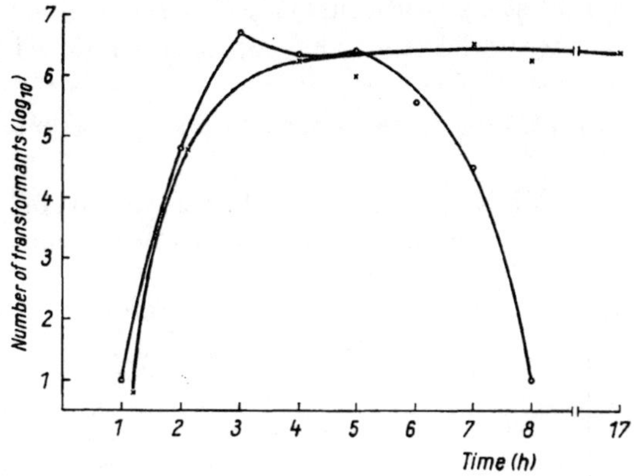

Fig. 2. Development of competence in a culture of strain Challis and competence provoking activity of supernatant fluids prepared at times indicated. The competence-provoking activity was tested on homologous organisms in the absence of serum or albumin.
o — o, — competence
× — ×, — competence provoking activity of the supernatant fluid.

The provoking factor is heat sensitive. Samples of ammonium sulphate concentrates of provoking factor dissolved in nutrient medium, in 0.01 M phosphate buffer or in saline, all adjusted to pH 7.2, were heated for 10 min. at temperatures indicated in Fig. 3 and then their competence provoking activity was tested. Obviously, non-saturating amounts of provoking factor were used in order to observe any decline of activity caused by heating. As can be seen in Fig. 3, the provoking factor seems to be protected by some compounds present in the nutrient medium.

The provoking factor can be precipitated from the supernatant by ammonium sulphate (80–90% of saturation) or by cold ethanol (8 volumes). The first method is more efficient (Fig. 4).

Conversion to competency of non-competent cultures with the use of provoking factor is temperature dependent. As shown in Fig. 5, the provoking factor is not active at 0°, 10°

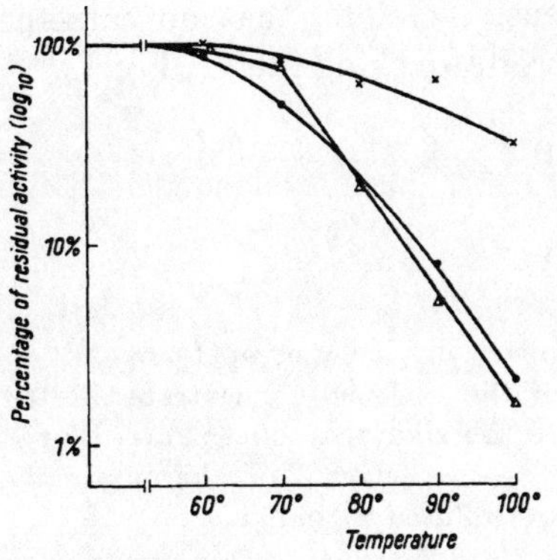

Fig. 3. Heat sensitivity of competence-provoking factor. The activity of the unheated factor is indicated as 100%. × — ×. Concentrate of provoking factor diluted in nutrient medium before heating; · — ·, concentrate diluted in buffer; Δ – Δ, concentrate diluted in saline.

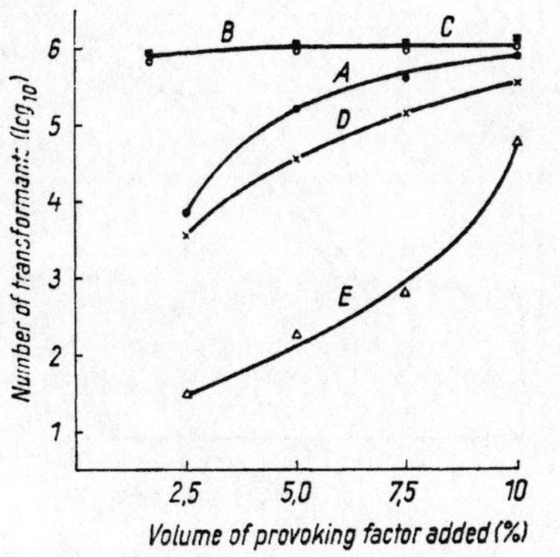

Fig. 4. Competence-provoking activity of a supernatant fluid and of crude concentrates of provoking factor.
A, supernatant fluid; B, ammonium sulphate precipitate dissolved in $^1/_{10}$ of the initial volume; C, ethanol precipitate dissolved in $^1/_{10}$ of initial volume; D, ammonium sulphate precipitate dissolved and diluted to the initial volume of supernatant fluid used for precipitation.

and 20°. Maximum activity was found at 37°. Temperatures higher than 40° could not be tested because they affect growth and viability.

Provocation of competence is also time dependent. The efficiency of transformation was found optimal after 25–35 min. action of provoking factor (Fig. 6).

The provoking factor seems to be rather non-dialysable. Visking dialysis tubings, declared to held back particles of molecular weight greater than 10^4, were filled with crude concentrates of provoking factor and poured into glass vessels containing 20 volumes of 0.01 M phosphate buffer. Some loss of activity was observed but it was not higher than 15–20% of

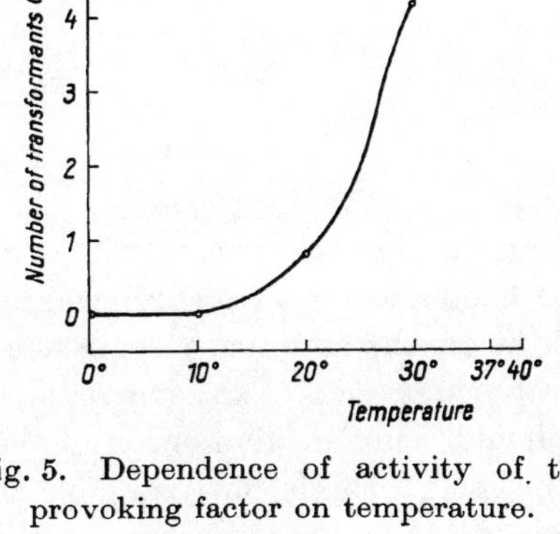

Fig. 5. Dependence of activity of the provoking factor on temperature.

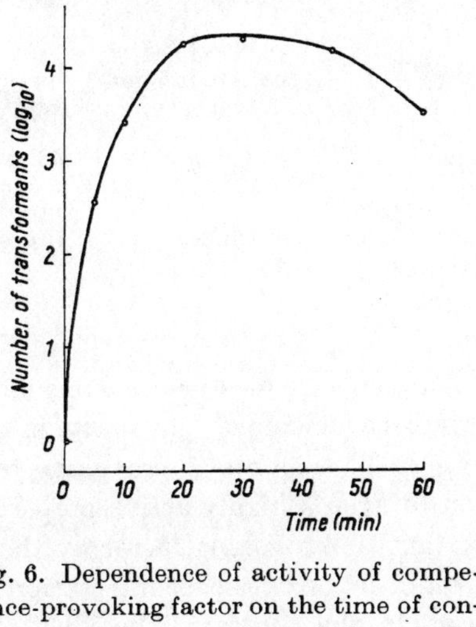

Fig. 6. Dependence of activity of competence-provoking factor on the time of contact with the organisms before DNA addition.

initial activity. It seems, therefore, that no cofactor is necessary for the action of provoking factor (Fig. 7).

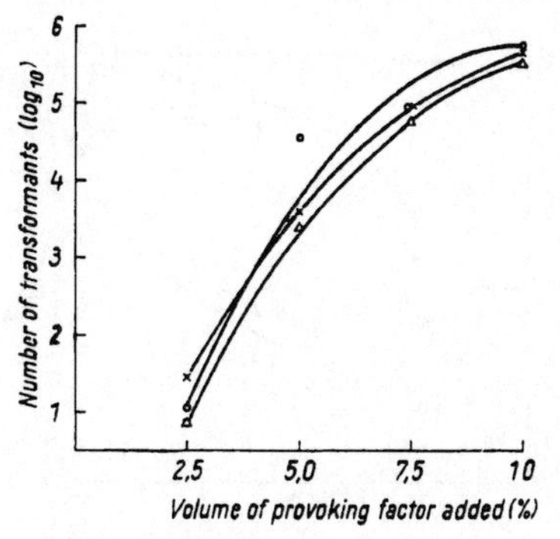

Fig. 7. Effect of dialysis on the activity of competence-provoking factor. × — ×, activity of the dialysed concentrate diluted in buffer; Δ — Δ, activity of the dialysed concentrate diluted in buffer used for dialysis; o — o, activity of the non-dialysed concentrate diluted in buffer.

The efficiency of provoked transformation is dependent on the medium in which the bacteria are suspended for the time of action of provoking factor. This is demonstrated in Table 1. The highest yield was observed when the provoking factor acted on cells in nutrient medium. In saline, containing various amounts of nutrient medium, the efficiency of conversion to competency was as higher as more nutrient medium was added to the saline. Chloramphenicol in a concentration of 7.5–10 μg/ml blocked completely conversion to competency.

Table 1

Conversion to competency in ,,non growth" media

		Media					
		ET 3	saline + 25% of medium ET 3	saline + 15% of medium ET 3	saline + 5% of medium ET 3	saline	ET 3 + 7.5 µg/ml of chlor-amphenicol
Experiments	1	200 × 10^4 transformants ml 100%	61.0%	32.2%	16.1%	7.1%	0
	2	334 × 10^3 transformants ml 100%	55.1%	34.7%	17.4%	6.0%	0
	3	256 × 10^3 transformants ml 100%	49.8%	23.2%	11.9%	5.7%	0
Mean value		100%	55.3%	30.0%	15.1%	6.3%	0
Increase of viable count during 30 minutes action of provoking factor		1.8 times	1.6 times	1.6 times	1.3 times	1.3 times	0.97

A given portion of provoking factor, concentrated or not, can be used several times to provoke competence. Obviously, in this kind of experiments, bacteria were treated repeatedly with small amounts of provoking factor which were much below the saturating concentration of even a highly active preparation. Under such conditions, therefore, any irreversible fixation of provoking factor by the first portion of cells should result in diminution of the effect of action on the second portion of cells. As can be seen in Table 2, this is, however, not the case. On the contrary, the effect of the second application of the factor is superior to the effect of its first use and the results of the third application are, in most instances, as good as of the first one. We have no explanation for the high activity of provoking factor at its second use. We may, however, assume that the first portion of cells absorbs from the crude preparation of provoking factor a substance inhibiting provocation of competence.

Table 2

The effects of repeatable use of provoking factor on conversion to competency

		effects of first use	second use	third use
Experiments carried out with concentrates of provoking factor	1	460×10^2	330×10^3	490×10^2
	2	780×10^3	347×10^4	355×10^3
	3	308×10^2	240×10^3	312×10^2
	4	326×10^3	non tested	322×10^3
Experiment carried out with supernatant of a competent culture as source of provoking factor	5	206×10^2	680×10^2	616×10^2

Competence is a transient state. Streptococcal cells which became competent upon the action of provoking factor lose the ability to be transformed if DNA is not added at proper time. The rate of decline of competency is a function of time and temperature as shown in Fig. 8. In this experiment, bacteria grown for 2 hours were exposed to the action of provoking factor for 30 min., spun down, resuspended in fresh nutrient medium and maintained either at 22° or at 37°. At time intervals, indicated in the figure, aliquots were removed, supplemented with DNA and permitted to grow for phenotypic expression. Transformants were scored in the routine way. The number of viable units was also determined. As can be seen in Fig. 8. at 37° competence disappears completely within 60–90 min. but at 22° it is little affected within 3 hours.

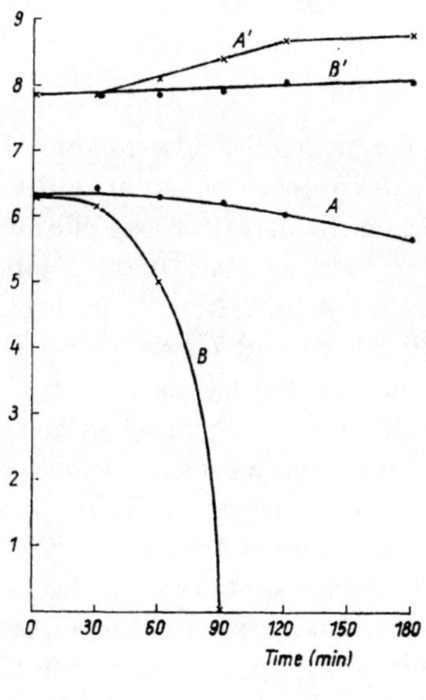

Fig. 8. Loss of competence in nutrient medium at 37° and 22°.
A – loss of competence at 37°
B – loss of competence at 22°
A′ – increase of the number of viable units at 37°
B′ – increase of the number of viable units at 22°

Is the fast loss of transformability at 37° a result of cell division? In order to answer this question, aliquots of competent cells were suspended in nutrient medium which contained 7.5 μg/ml of chloramphenicol or in buffered saline. The bacteria were kept in a 37° water bath and their capacity to undergo transformation tested at times indicated in Fig. 9. Cloramphenicol in a concentration of 7.5 μg/ml does not reduce the viable count but it inhibits multiplication. The rates of drop of competency in buffered saline and in nutrient medium with chloramphenicol are nearly the same as in nutrient medium without chloramphenicol at 37°. In the presence of chloramphenicol, however, there was no increase of the number of cells and in saline it was very insignificant. We conclude, therefore, that not cell division but some metabolic processes, running at 37° but not at 22° result in decline of competency.

Of special interest is the specificity of action of the provoking factor. The kinetic of development of competence was studied in cultures of three transformable streptococcal strains: of two strains of group *H* streptococci Challis and *3437/48* and of one strain *Streptococcus sanguis*, type *I/II*. All these strains share the C polysaccharide common to group *H* beta hemolytic streptococci. The *S. sanguis* strain, however, is alfa hemolytic and differs also with regard to some fermentation reactions from the beta hemolytic group *H* streptococci. All the three strains produce in the presence of serum or albumin exocellular factors capable to provoke competence in conditions in which it naturally never occurs i. e. in the absence of serum or albumin. The specificity of action of the factors was tested on homologous and heterologous, transformable and non-transformable strains. Two different conditions were applied for the test: 1. the provoking factor acted on bacteria grown in the absence of serum or albumin, 2. the factor acted on bacteria grown in the presence of serum. In the latter case cultures started with small initial inocula and the provoking factors were added before natural competence was achieved. Table 3 illustrates the specificity of action of provoking factors tested in the first condition. Strains Wicky, E 91, Channon, Blackborn and H_4 are group *H* streptococci and were received from the Streptococcal Reference Laboratory of the Central Public Health Laboratory, Colindale, London. They all have to be recognized as non-transformable because they could not be transformed when tested by all means in various conditions proper for transformation of other streptococci.

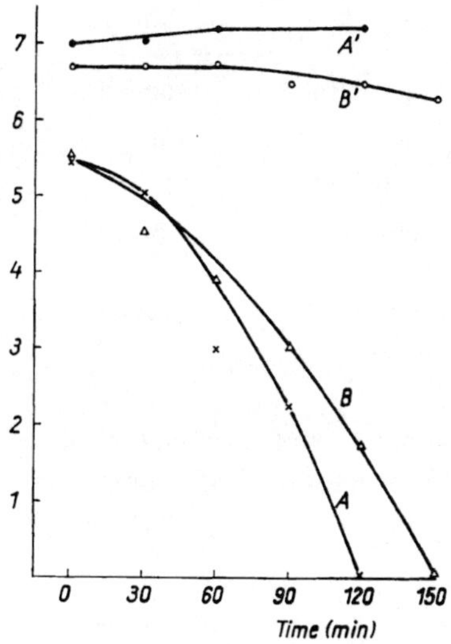

Fig. 9. Loss of competence at 37° in saline (A) and in nutrient medium containing 7,5 μg/ml of chloramphenicol (B). A′ and B′, corresponding curves illustrating viable count.

As can be seen in Table 3, the factor derived from cultures of strain Challis provokes competence in cultures of the homologous strain and of the heterologous strain *3437/48*. The factor produced by strain *3437/48*, vice versa, acts also on bacteria of strain Challis. Both factors provoke transformation in cultures of the naturally non-transformable strain Wicky. The provoking factor of *S. sanguis* acts only on homologous cells.

There is some change of this picture when the test is carried out in the presence of serum (Table 4). In this condition, the factor of strain Challis provokes competence in cultures of *S. sanguis*.

Special attention has to be paid to provocation of competence of the non-transformable strain Wicky. To the best of our knowledge, it is the first example of provoked transformation of naturally non-transformable bacteria achieved as a result of application of a transferable factor produced by a heterologous, related strain. The efficiencies of this transformation are of the same order of magnitude as the efficiencies of provoked, homologous transformations observed with strains: Challis, *3437/48* and *S. sanguis*.

Table 3
Specificity of action of provoking factors tested in media without serum or albumin

Test strains	Control without provoking factor	Transformants in 1 ml of culture — Provoking factors from strains: Challis	*S. sanguis* type *I/II*	*3437/48*
Challis	3×10^0	1×10^6	9×10^1	5×10^4
S. sanguis type *I/II*	1×10^0	2×10^1	17×10^4	0
3437/48	0	21×10^4	0	22×10^4
Wicky	0	52×10^4	7×10^0	20×10^4
E 91/46	0	0	0	0
Channon	0	0	0	0
Blackborn	0	0	0	0
H 4	0	0	0	0
S. sanguis type *I*	0	0	0	0
S. sanguis type *II*	0	0	0	0

In culture supernatants of strain Wicky, no factor provoking competence was found. We assume, therefore, that strain Wicky cannot be transformed because it does not produce the exocellular factor necessary for development of competence.

It is also evident from the above demonstrated data that serum or albumin are not essential for development of competence itself but for the production of provoking factor. After addition of provoking factor, streptococci are converted to competency in the absence of serum or albumin.

Table 4
Specificity of action of provoking factors tested in medium with serum

Test strains	Control without provoking factor	Transformants in 1 ml of culture — Provoking factors from strains: Challis	*S. sanguis* type *I/II*	*3437/48*
Challis	40×10^1	20×10^4	4×10^2	1×10^5
S. sanguis type *I/II*	5×10^1	12×10^4	42×10^4	4×10^1
3437/48	8×10^1	8×10^3	24×10^2	26×10^4
Wicky	0	100×10^4	2×10^1	1×10^5
E 91/46	0	0	0	0
Channon	0	0	0	0
Blackborn	0	0	0	0
H 4	0	0	0	0
S. sanguis type *I*	0	0	0	0
S. sanguis type *II*	0	0	0	0

The kinetic of conversion of non-competent streptococci to competence ones is consistent with an enzymic reaction and the factor itself seems to be a protein of enzymic activity. It is precipitated by ammonium sulphate, it is heat sensitive and does not pass through Visking dialysis tubings. The conversion to competency is time and temperature dependent and very specific. In reciprocal transformations to streptomycin and cathomycin-resistance, strain Challis does not discriminate between homologous DNA and DNA of *S. sanguis*. This is also true for *S. sanguis* which is transformed with the same efficiency by homologous DNA and DNA of strain Challis. The mentioned strains, however, can easyly be distinguished by their provoking factors (Table 3).

The presented findings suggest that development of competence requires the action of an enzyme. The question may, therefore, be asked: what is the substrate of it? This question cannot be answered until the provoking factor has been purified and its action tested on cell constituents. First of all, one has to look after it in the cell wall.

As shown above, chloramphenicol blocks conversion of competence by means of the provoking factor. It has also little effect on cells suspended in „non-growth" media like saline. One may conclude, therefore, that conversion to competency requires cells of non disturbed metabolic activities. Competence, thus, is the result of action of the exocellular provoking factor and of one or more factors produced by fully metabolizing cells. This factor, or factors, is probably a protein, too, because conversion to competency is blocked by chloramphenicol. There is also other evidence that the mechanism of development of competence is rather complicated and that it cannot be explained by the action of a single factor. In Table 3 are mentioned 5 non transformable strains of group *H* streptococci of which only strain Wicky can be converted to competency with the use of provoking factors produced by related strains. Thus, strain Wicky differs in some respects from the other non transformable group *H* streptococci. We could not find the exocellular provoking factor in cultures of strain Wicky but may be that, in contradistinction to the other non transformable group *H* streptococci, it is capable to produce the other component, or components, necessary for development of competence.

Die Induktion lysogener Bakterien durch Halogenderivate des Uracils

E. Geissler

Institut für experimentelle Krebsforschung der Deutschen Akademie der Wissenschaften zu Berlin, Abteilung für Genetik, Berlin-Buch

Eine Infektion mit temperierten Phagen kann in den infizierten Wirtszellen zwei qualitativ verschiedene Reaktionen auslösen (Abb. 1). Die eine, die sog. „lytische Reaktion" ähnelt im Prinzip den Vorgängen nach Infektion mit virulenten Phagen und führt zur Lyse der infizierten Zellen unter gleichzeitiger Freisetzung von Phagennachkommen. Bei der „lysogenen Reaktion" dagegen veranlaßt ein unter der Kontrolle eines Phagengenes produzierter zytoplasmatischer Repressor, daß die Phagengene, die die zur Phagenvermehrung notwendigen Prozesse (z. B. die Synthese „früher Proteine") kontrollieren, reprimiert werden (vgl. Jacob und Wollman 1959; Jacob und Monod 1961). Das reprimierte Phagengenom wird als „Prophage" an einen meist spezifischen Locus des Bakteriengenoms geheftet und mit diesem kontinuierlich repliziert. Auf diese Weise erhalten alle Nachkommen der Zelle, in der eine lysogene Reaktion stattgefunden hat, je einen Prophagen pro Nucleoid und sind damit sämtlich lysogen.

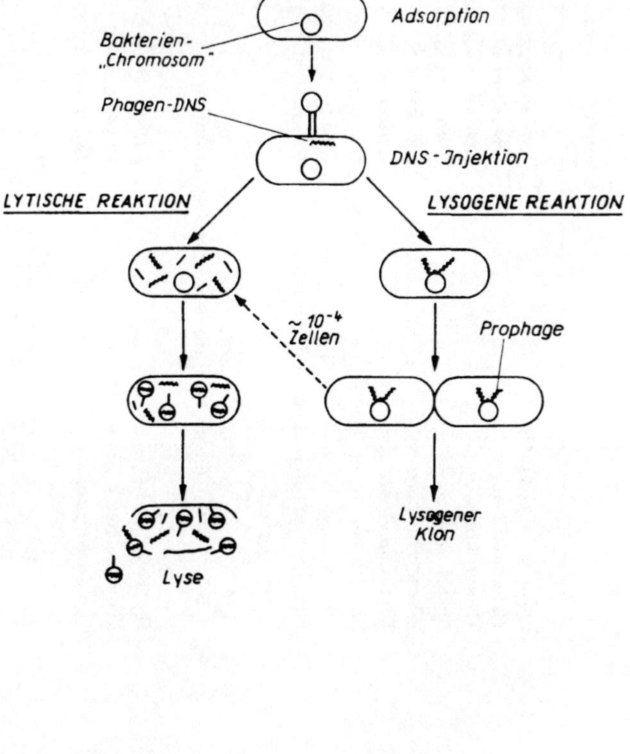

Abb. 1. Folgen einer Infektion mit temperierten Phagen.
Nach der Injektion des Phagengenoms in ein sensibles Bakterium erfolgt meist eine lytische Reaktion, während der innerhalb einer charakteristischen Latenzzeit Phagen-spezifische Enzyme, Phagen-DNS und Phagen-Hüllproteine synthetisiert und reife Phagen produziert werden, die bei Lyse der Zelle ins Medium gelangen. — Gelegentlich erfolgt im infizierten Bakterium eine lysogene Reaktion, wobei das Phagengenom reprimiert, als Prophage an das Bakteriengenom angeheftet und mit diesem vermehrt wird. In einer sehr kleinen Fraktion dieser lysogenen Zellen setzt spontan eine lytische Reaktion ein (Geissler 1963e)

Tabelle 1. Induzierende Noxen

Bezüglich der Literatur bis einschließlich 1961 vgl. GEISSLER 1963e

Noxe	Literatur
reduziertes Glutathion	LWOFF et al. '51
Thiomaleinsäure	LWOFF et al. '52
Thioglykolsäure	LWOFF et al. '52
Ascorbinsäure	LWOFF et al. '52
Wasserstoffperoxyd	LWOFF et al. '52
Tertiobutylperoxyd	LWOFF et al. '52
Phagolessin A 58	HALL-ASHESHOV et al. '56
β-Propiolacton	FIELD et al. '62
4-Nitrochinolin-1-oxyd und -Derivate	ENDO et al. '63
Keine oder nur fragliche Induktion mit:	
Hydroxylamin (mutagen)	LWOFF et al. '52
Äthylmethansulfonat (mut)	LOVELESS '59
Coffein (mutagen)	JACOB et al. '59
Induzierende Noxen, die sicher mit Nukleinsäuren reagieren bzw. mit deren Synthese interferieren	
Ultraviolette Strahlen	LWOFF et al. '50
Ionisierende Strahlen	LATARJET et al. '51
Photodynamischer Effekt von Thiopyronin + Licht	GEISSLER et al. '63
versch. alkylierende Agenzien	versch. Autoren
Mitomycin C	OTSUJI '59
Phleomycin	LEIN et. al. '62
Colicin E 2	ENDO et al. '63
1-Azaserin	GOTS et al. '55
Sulfathiazol	WILLIAMS SMITH '53
UV-bestrahltes Anhydroleucovorin	BOREK et al. '55
Aminopterin	BEN-GURION '62
Amethopterin	GEISSLER et al. '63
5-Fluordesoxyuridin	LEVINE '61
Thymin-Mangel	MELECHEN et al. '60

Der lysogene Regelmechanismus kann zusammenbrechen, was zur Einleitung einer lytischen Reaktion in den betroffenen Zellen führt. Dieser Zusammenbruch – der als Induktion bezeichnet wird – findet in geeigneten Systemen (es gibt auch nichtinduzierbare Prophagen) gelegentlich spontan statt und kann durch eine Reihe physikalischer und chemischer Noxen experimentell ausgelöst werden (vgl. GEISSLER, 1963e). Sehr viele dieser Noxen sind dafür bekannt, daß sie mit den Nukleinsäuren (bevorzugt mit der DNS) reagieren oder mit deren Syntheseprozessen interferieren (Tab. 1). Es liegen aber noch keine konkreten Vorstellungen darüber vor, wie man sich im Einzelnen den Mechanismus der Induktion des Prophagen vorstellen soll.

Wir haben deshalb damit begonnen, den Einfluß von Halogenderivaten des Uracils auf lysogene Zellen zu studieren. Diese Versuche sind noch nicht abgeschlossen. Da sie aber in verschiedener Hinsicht interessant sind, sollen sie im Folgenden kurz zusammengefaßt werden. Über Teilergebnisse wurde gelegentlich bereits kurz berichtet (GEISSLER, 1963a–d).

Material und Methode

Lysogene Bakterien: *Escherichia coli* K 12 (λ) Hfr A' (prot Sm^s)

Indikator-Bakterien: *E. coli* K 12 C 600 (Sm^r)

Medien: *NB*: 10 g Pepton „Grünau", 3 g Bacto beef extract, 5 g NaCl, 1 g Glucose, 1000 ml Aqua dest. *SS*: 30 g Glyzerin, 3 g Bacto vitamin-free Casamino Acids, 0,01 g KH_2PO_4, 0,021 g Na_2HPO_4, 0,3 g $MgSO_4 \cdot 7\ H_2O$, 3,0 g NH_4Cl, 0,3 ml 1 M $CaCl_2$, 1000 ml Aqua dest. *mSS*: wie SS, aber mit Bacto Casamino Acids. *MM*: 5,0 g NH_4Cl,

1,0 g NH_4NO_3, 2,0 g Na_2SO_4, 3,0 g K_2HPO_4, 1,0 g KH_2PO_4, 1,5 g Asparagin, Spuren $CaCl_2$, 0,5 g Glucose, 0,1 g $MgSO_4 \cdot 7\,H_2O$, 1 ml Spurenelemente (20,0 g Bor, 0,4 g $ZnCl_2$, 0,15 g $MnSO_4 \cdot 4\,H_2O$, 0,25 g $(NH_4)\,Mo_7O_{24} \cdot 4\,H_2O$, 0,3 g $CuSO_4 \cdot 5\,H_2O$, 0,5 g $FeSO_4 \cdot 7\,H_2O$, 1000 ml Aqua dest.) 1000 ml Aqua dest.

Nähragar: 8 g Bacto Tryptone, 5 g NaCl, 20 g Agar, 1000 ml Aqua dest.

Weichagar: wie Nähragar, aber nur mit 8 g Agar.

Verdünnungsmedium: 5,85 g NaCl, 1,5 g KH_2PO_4, 4,19 g $Na_2HPO_4 \cdot 2\,H_2O$, 0,02 g $MgSO_4 \cdot 7\,H_2O$, 1000 ml Aqua dest.

Methode

Wenn nicht anders angegeben, wurden lysogene Zellen und (von spontan induzierten Zellen produzierte) freie Phagen aus einer Übernachtkultur 1 : 100 in NB verdünnt, 3 Std. bei 37 °C belüftet und anschließend 1 : 10 in SS verdünnt, das mit den zu prüfenden Substanzen supplementiert worden war. In diesem Medium wurde die lysogene Population 5 Std. bei 37 °C belüftet.

Auswertung

1. Bestimmung der induzierten Zellen

Die Population wurde 20 min mit 1 : 100 verdünntem λ-Antiserum bei 37 °C inkubiert. Nach anschließender Verdünnung wurde ein Teil davon sofort mit Streptomycin (Endkonz. 0,1%) und Indikatorbakterien ausgeplattet, so daß der Titer der nicht-inaktivierten freien Phagen bestimmt werden konnte. Ein anderer Teil der Antiserum-behandelten Population wurde zunächst nur mit Indikatorbakterien ausgeplattet, 2 Std. bei 37 °C bebrütet und dann mit Streptomycin-Lösung (1%ig) besprüht. Auf solchen Platten entstehende Plaques gehen auf nicht-inaktivierte freie Phagen, sowie auf induzierte Zellen zurück. Der Anteil der letzteren kann durch Berücksichtigung der nicht-inaktivierten freien Phagen exakt bestimmt werden. 2. Für viele Zwecke genügte die methodisch einfachere *Q-Methode*: Sofort nach Verdünnung in SS-Medium und im Anschluß an die 5stündige Inkubation wurde die Zahl der

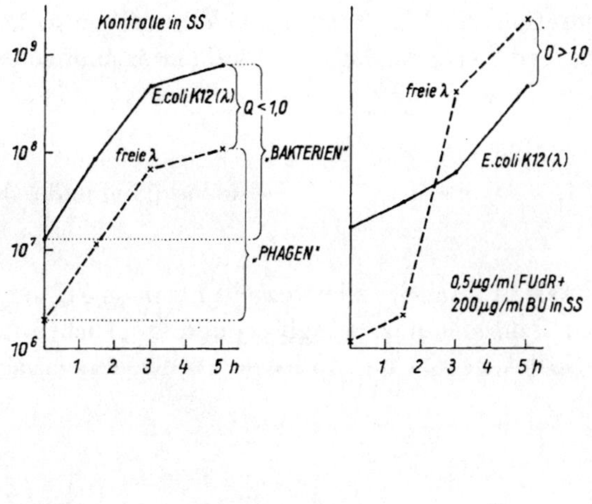

Abb. 2 Auswertung des Einflusses von Substanzen mittels der Q-Methode.
Die in Tab. 2–6 in der Spalte „Bakterien" eingetragenen Werte werden gewonnen durch Division des Bakterien-Titers nach 5 Std. Inkubation durch den Bakterien-Titer zu Beginn der Inkubation. Entsprechend werden auch die in der Spalte „Phagen" eingetragenen Werte ermittelt. Q-Werte werden berechnet durch Division des Phagen-Titers nach 5 Std. durch den Bakterien-Titer nach 5 Std.

Bakterien und freien Phagen ermittelt, so daß man durch Vergleich beider Titer Werte für die Bakterien und Phagenvermehrung erhält (Abb. 2). Außerdem wurde durch Division des Bakterien-Titers nach 5 Std. durch den Phagen-Titer nach 5 Std. ein Quotient Q errechnet, der bei Kontrollkulturen nach 5 Std. Inkubation in SS bei 0,3 liegt und in allen Fällen einer Induktion und Phagen-Produktion den Wert 1 übersteigt (Abb. 2).

Ergebnisse und Diskussion

1. Thymin-Analoga

C 5-substituierte Halogen-Derivate des Uracils werden dann als Thymin-Analoga bezeichnet wenn der van der Waalssche Radius des Substituenten dem der Methylgruppe ähnlich ist (Abb. 3). Dies gilt für die von uns verwendeten Analoga BU und JU, sowie für 5-Chloruracil. Diese Basenanaloga können anstelle von Thymin in die DNS inkorporiert werden (vgl. Handschumacher und Welch, 1960). In der RNS der behandelten Organismen wurden diese Basenanaloga bisher noch nicht nachgewiesen, obwohl in vitro 5-Bromuridintriphosphat anstelle von Uridintriphosphat bei der DNS-gesteuerten RNS-Synthese verwendet und spezifisch eingebaut werden kann (Kahan, 1962). In vivo scheint der Einbau der Thymin-Analoga in die RNS deshalb nicht möglich zu sein, weil für sie – zumindest in *Escherichia coli* – keine Mononucleotidkinase-Aktivität vorhanden ist (Kahan und Hurwitz, 1962).

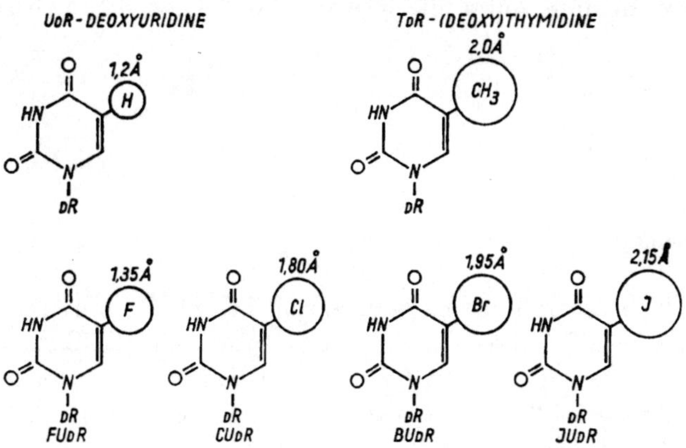

Abb. 3. Chemische Struktur von Desoxyuridin, Thymidin und ihren Analogen.
Die Kreise stellen die van der Waalsschen Radien der Substituenten dar (Szybalski, 1962).

Thymin-Analoga-haltige DNS ist im allgemeinen biologisch voll aktiv (vgl. Handschumacher und Welch, 1960), wenn auch der Einbau dieser Substanzen durch Inkorporations- und Replikationsfehler mutagen wirkt (vgl. Freese, 1959). Außerdem erhöht der Einbau dieser Analoga die Strahlensensibilität der DNS (vgl. Wacker, 1963).

1.1. 5-Joduracil und 5-Joddesoxyuridin

Wie aus Tabelle 2 hervorgeht hemmen JU und JUdR (jeweils 200 µg/ml) die Vermehrung der Bakterien nur geringfügig und im gleichen Ausmaß. Dagegen werden in Gegenwart von JUdR sehr viel mehr Phagen produziert als in Gegenwart der Base, so daß nach JUdR-

Behandlung ein Quotient von 1,1 resultiert. Dies läßt das Vorliegen einer Induktion vermuten. Jedoch zeigt Abbildung 4, daß die Induktionswirkung – wenn sie überhaupt vorhanden sein sollte – außerordentlich schwach ist.

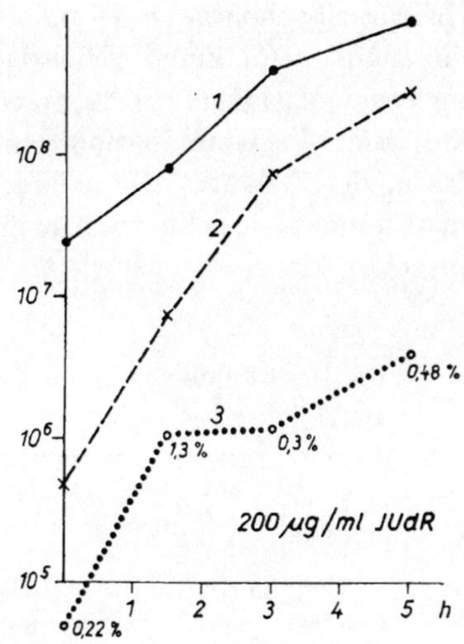

Abb. 4. Bakterienvermehrung, Phagenproduktion und induzierte Zellen in Gegenwart von 200 µg/ml 5-Joddesoxyuridin Mittelwerte aus 4 Versuchen.
1: Bakterien, 2: freie Phagen, 3: induzierte Zellen

1.2. Bromuracil und 5-Bromdesoxyuridin

1.2.1. Wirkung auf den lysogenen Regelmechanismus

Aus Tabelle 2 geht hervor, daß BU (200 oder 20 µg/ml) nicht induziert: Die Q-Werte sind normal bzw. liegen sogar unter dem Normalwert. Das gleiche Resultat erhält man bei der Bestimmung der induzierten Zellen in Gegenwart von 200 µg/ml BU (Abb. 5).

Überraschenderweise findet dagegen durch 200 µg/ml BUdR eine ausgeprägte Induktion statt: Der Quotient liegt bei 17 (Tab. 2), was darauf zurückgeführt werden kann, daß nach 3stündiger Inkubation in Gegenwart von BUdR 12% der Zellen induziert sind (Abb. 5). Das Desoxynucleosid löst also einen qualitativ anderen Effekt aus als die Base – eine Erscheinung, die sich beim JUdR offenbar auch schon andeutet.

Der BUdR-Effekt ist vor allem deshalb so überraschend, weil bekannt ist, daß BU und JU von Bakterien bei Thymin-Mangel zur DNS-Synthese verwendet und anstelle von Thymin in die DNS eingebaut werden können, wozu u. a. ihre Desoxyribosidierung erforderlich ist. Langen und Liss (1962) wiesen nach, daß sogar tierische Zellen (Ascites-Tumorzellen) bei durch

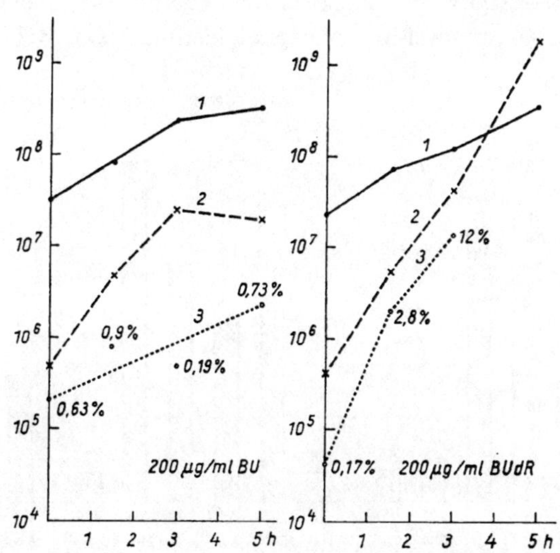

Abb. 5. Bakterienvermehrung, Phagenproduktion und induzierte Zellen in Gegenwart von 200 µg/ml 5-Bromuracil bzw. 5-Bromdesoxyuridin.
Mittelwerte aus je 3 Versuchen

Fluoruracil-gehemmter Thymidylsäure-Synthese BU zur DNS-Synthese verwenden und einbauen, wenn ihnen gleichzeitig Desoxyguanosin oder ein anderes geeignetes Desoxynucleosid als Desoxyribose-Spender angeboten wird. Unter unseren Bedingungen vermag aber auch die Kombination von BU und GdR keine Induktion auszulösen (Tab. 2). Wird das in der Zelle aus BU gebildete BUdR so schnell phosphoryliert, daß es gar nicht erst dazu kommt, den Effekt auszuüben, der von offenbar im Überschuß vorhandenem BUdR ausgelöst wird?

Tabelle 2
Der Einfluß von Thymin-Analoga auf Bakterienvermehrung und Phagenproduktion
Mittelwerte aus N Versuchen

Medium	N	Bakterien	Phagen	Q
Kontrolle (SS)	7	45 ± 8,4	960 ± 240	0,31 ± 0,052
JU (200 µg/ml)	4	32 ± 6,5	420 ± 110	0,19 ± 0,013
JUdR (200)	8	34 ± 4,6	1500 ± 370	1,1 ± 0,34
BU (20)	3	32 ± 5,0	510 ± 180	0,24 ± 0,064
BU (200)	6	5,6 ± 0,54	29 ± 6,3	0,082 ± 0,014
BUdR (20)	4	44 ± 8,0	1500 ± 230	0,68 ± 0,11
BUdR (200)	6	7,4 ± 1,4	10000 ± 1100	17 ± 1,9
BU (200) + GdR(200)	5	5,4 ± 0,49	56 ± 4,9	0,35 ± 0,032

1.2.2. Wirkung auf die Vermehrung von *E. coli* K 12 (λ)

Ferner zeigt Tabelle 2 deutlich, daß BU und BUdR (200 µg/ml) im Gegensatz zu JU und JUdR stark die Vermehrung der Bakterien hemmen. Das ist im Hinblick auf die bereits erwähnten Befunde hinsichtlich des nahezu vollwertigen Ersatzes von T durch BU unerwartet, zumal man unter unseren Bedingungen (nicht-gestörte Thymidylsäure-Synthese) von vornherein keinen ausgeprägten Einbau des BU in die DNS erwarten kann.

Szybalski (1962) nimmt an, daß phosphorylierte BUdR-Derivate – wie Thymidintriphosphat und vor allem Desoxyguanosintriphosphat und Desoxyadenosintriphosphat (Reichard, Canellakis und Canellakis, 1960) – die Reduktion von Cytidindiphosphat zu Desoxycytidindiphosphat hemmen. Die BU-Wirkung kann aber nicht auf einen derartigen Block zurückzuführen sein, da sie sowohl durch 200 µg/ml CdR als auch durch gleiche Mengen von CR und C weitgehend und statistisch signifikant aufgehoben werden kann (Abb. 6). Der gleiche Ef-

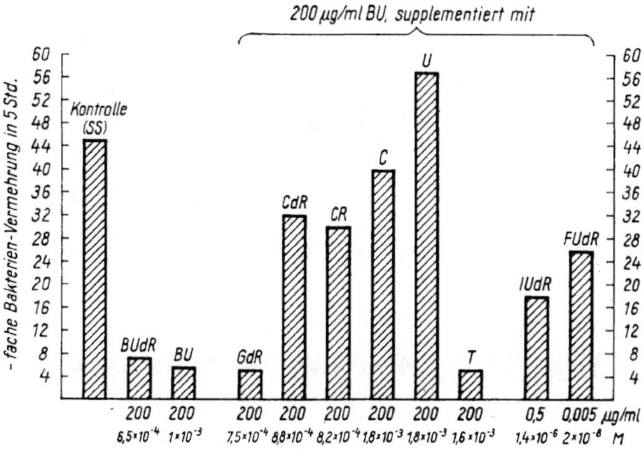

Abb. 6. Der Einfluß verschiedener Substanzen auf die Hemmung der Bakterienvermehrung durch 200 µg/ml 5-Bromuracil
Mittelwerte aus jeweils (von links nach rechts) 7, 9, 6, 5, 5, 9, 6, 4, 7, 7 bzw. 5 Versuchen

fekt wird auch durch U (200 μg/ml) erzielt. Daß GdR den BU-Effekt nicht aufzuheben vermag wäre verständlich, wenn man an irgendeinen Eingriff des BU in den Pyrimidin-Metabolismus glaubt. Dagegen ist der Befund völlig überraschend, daß auch 200 μg/ml T in dieser Hinsicht unwirksam sind. Völlig unübersichtlich wird der ganze Problemkomplex schließlich durch die Tatsache, daß nicht nur 0,5 μg/ml JUdR ($1{,}4 \times 10^{-6}$ M), sondern sogar auch 0,005 μg/ml FUdR (2×10^{-8} M) die BU-Hemmung statistisch signifikant aufheben.

An Hand dieser Daten kann man sich kein Bild über den Mechanismus der BU-Hemmung machen. Lediglich folgende Schlüsse können gezogen werden:

a) BU oder seine Derivate hemmen nicht die Konversion von Cytidindiphosphat zu Desoxycytidindiphosphat.

b) BU oder seine Derivate hemmen nicht – wie Thymidylsäure, Thymidindiphosphat, Thymidintriphosphat (Maley und Maley, 1961) – die Desaminierung von Desoxycytidylsäure zu Desoxyuridylsäure (sonst dürften C, CR, CdR sowie U nicht schützen, während T die BU-Wirkung aufheben müßte).

c) Es ist wenig wahrscheinlich, daß BU oder seine Derivate irgendwie die DNS-Synthese hemmen, da T nicht vor der BU-Wirkung zu schützen vermag, und da 200 μg/ml BUdR eine 10^4-fache Phagenvermehrung (Tab. 2) und 200 μg/ml BU in Gegenwart von 0,05 μg/ml FUdR eine $5{,}4 \times 10^3$fache Phagenvermehrung (Tab. 4) gestatten, wozu DNS-Synthese erforderlich ist. Wir sind augenblicklich dabei, zur weiteren Klärung dieses Problems den Einfluß von BU auf die DNS- und RNS-Synthese zu verfolgen.

2. Uracil-Analoga

5-Fluoruracil ist ein Analogon des Uracils, da der van der Waalssche Radius des F dem eines H-Atoms sehr viel ähnlicher ist als dem der Methylgruppe des Thymins (Abb. 3). Tatsächlich wird FU als Fluoruridintriphosphat in die RNS eingebaut, wobei es zu Störungen der RNS-Synthese selbst (vgl. Handschumacher und Welch, 1960), zur Produktion von Proteinen mit fehlerhafter Aminosäure-Zusammensetzung (Naono und Gros, 1960) und – Sequenz (Bussard, Naono, Gros und Monod, 1960) und damit auch zur phänotypischen Reversion von Mutationen (Champe und Benzer, 1962) kommt.

Außerdem bewirkt eine FU-Applikation Störungen der DNS-Synthese, da FU auch desoxyribosidiert wird und dann als Fluordesoxyuridylsäure die Thymidylsäure-Synthese hemmt (vgl. Handschuhmacher und Welch, 1960). Solche DNS-Effekte (die zum Thymin-Mangeltod führen) resultieren bevorzugt nach Applikation von FUdR, da dies zum größten Teil phosphoryliert und nur in begrenztem Maße hydrolysiert wird und dann als FU RNS-Schäden hervorruft.

2.1. 5-Fluordesoxyuridin

Die Induktionswirkung von FUdR wurde bereits von Levine (1961) sowie von Frey und Melechen (zit. von Melechen und Skaar, 1961) beobachtet. Letztere Autoren verwendeten FUdR in einer Konzentration von 10^{-4} M = 24,6 μg/ml (Melechen, 1963).

Abbildung 7 zeigt, daß FUdR selbst in einer Konzentration von 0,5 μg/ml während einer 5stündigen Inkubation noch 4,6% der Zellen induziert. Die Induktionswirkung dieser FUdR-

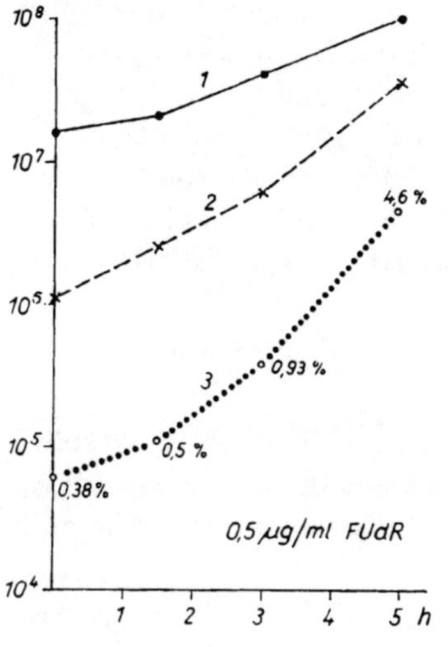

Konzentration ergibt sich auch mit der Q-Methode (Tab. 3), mit der gleichzeitig ersehen werden kann, daß dieser FUdR-Effekt auf die Hemmung der Thymidylsäure-Synthese zurückzuführen sein dürfte. Durch 0,5 μg/ml T kann er aufgehoben werden, nicht aber durch 0,5 μg/ml U oder 25 μg/ml CdR. Warum der Effekt durch 5 μg/ml U aufgehoben wird, müssen weitere Untersuchungen zeigen.

Abb. 7. Bakterienvermehrung, Phagenproduktion und induzierte Zellen in Gegenwart von 0,5 μg/ml 5-Fluordesoxyuridin Mittelwerte aus 2 Versuchen

Interessant ist die Tatsache, daß selbst 5 μg/ml T noch nicht ausreichen, die von 0,5 μg/ml FUdR bewirkte Vermehrungshemmung aufzuheben, während dies durch 5 μg/ml U weitgehend möglich ist. Offenbar ist die Vermehrungshemmung auf RNS-Effekte zurückzuführen, die hydrolytisch entstandenem FU zuzuschreiben sind.

Tabelle 3
Der Einfluß verschiedener Basen und Desoxynucleoside auf die Wirkung von 0,5 μg/ml 5-Fluordesoxyuridin

0,5 μg/ml FUdR +	N	Bakterien	Phagen	Q
–	8	1,6 ± 0,52	54 ± 14	1,8 ± 1,1
T (0,5 μg/ml)	6	4,9 ± 0,87	96 ± 20	0,55 ± 0,067
T (5,0)	6	5,0 ± 0,51	37 ± 4,5	0,24 ± 0,021
TdR (200)	5	33 ± 8,9	95 ± 19	0,045 ± 0,0092
U (0,5)	5	8,8 ± 3,8	470 ± 110	1,4 ± 0,06
U (5,0)	5	32 ± 5,0	900 ± 330	0,42 ± 0,09
CdR (25)	8	19 ± 3,2	620 ± 220	1,3 ± 0,44

Höhere FUdR-Konzentrationen – etwa 5,0 μg/ml – wirken weitaus stärker induzierend (schon nach 90 min Inkubation sind 30% der behandelten Zellen induziert). Bei dieser hohen FUdR-Konzentration erfolgt aber keine Phagenproduktion, so daß hier eine Anwendung der Q-Methode nicht möglich ist.

2.2. 5-Fluordesoxyuridin in Kombination mit 5-Bromuracil

Schon oben war referiert worden, daß BU bei T-Mangel T im allgemeinen weitgehend ersetzen kann und in die DNS eingebaut wird. Tatsächlich ist BU (200 μg/ml) in der Lage, die induzierende Wirkung von 5,0 μg/ml FUdR beträchtlich zu vermindern, so daß nach 90 min Inkubation in Gegenwart beider Substanzen nur noch 2% induzierte Zellen gefunden werden.

Völlig andere Ergebnisse erhält man dagegen, wenn man 200 μg/ml BU mit geringeren FUdR-Konzentrationen kombiniert. Während 200 μg/ml TdR sowohl die Induktion als auch die Vermehrungshemmung durch 0,5 μg/ml FUdR aufheben, hat 200 μg/ml BU auf die hemmende Wirkung dieser FUdR-Konzentration keinen Einfluß – vermutlich weil es selbst hemmt –, während es andererseits die Produktion freier Phagen außerordentlich verstärkt (Tab. 4). Dies ist eindeutig darauf zurückzuführen, daß der Anteil der induzierten Zellen

Tabelle 4

Die kombinierte Wirkung verschiedener Konzentrationen von 5-Fluordesoxyuridin und 5-Bromuracil

FUdR μg/ml	BU μg/ml	N	Bakterien	Phagen	Q
0,5	–	8	1,6 ± 0,52	54 ± 14	1,8 ± 1,1
0,05	–	7	33 ± 6,8	1100 ± 400	0,55 ± 0,1
–	200	6	5,6 ± 0,54	29 ± 6,3	0,082 ± 0,014
–	20	3	32 ± 5,0	510 ± 180	0,24 ± 0,604
0,5	200	7	6,6 ± 3,7	3200 ± 1800	37 ± 18
0,05	200	6	3,8 ± 1,5	5400 ± 1100	63 ± 16
0,005	200	5	26 ± 5,1	290 ± 89	0,38 ± 0,04
0,5	20	9	6,9 ± 2,3	93 ± 35	0,41 ± 0,22
0,05	20	6	40 ± 5,6	3200 ± 130	0,9 ± 0,1

beträchtlich erhöht wird (Abb. 8): Während 0,5 μg/ml FUdR allein innerhalb von 3 Std. lediglich 0,93% der Zellen induziert und damit die spontane Induktionsrate noch nicht einmal verdreifacht, werden im gleichen Zeitraum durch 0,5 μg/ml FUdR + 200 μg/ml BU 68% der Zellen induziert.

Weiter ergibt sich aus Tabelle 4, daß BU auch in Kombination mit 0,05 μg/ml FUdR noch induziert, in Kombination mit einer FUdR-Dosis also, die allein von den Zellen nahezu schädigungslos vertragen wird. Eine weiter verringerte FUdR-Konzentration vermag dann allerdings auch in Kombination mit BU nicht mehr zu induzieren – sie vermag sogar die BU-Hemmung zum Teil auszugleichen, ein Phänomen, das schon weiter oben erwähnt wurde.

Andererseits wird die induzierende Wirkung von 0,5 μg/ml FUdR durch 20 μg/ml BU völlig aufgehoben und die von 0,05 μg/ml FUdR durch 200 μg/ml BU offenbar stark reduziert (der zuletzt genannte Effekt kann erst nach der beabsichtigten Bestimmung der induzierten Zellen präziser dargestellt werden). Somit ist BU also befähigt, in bestimmten Konzentrationen die induzierende Wirkung bestimmter FUdR-Konzentrationen aufzuheben oder zu vermindern und in anderen Konzentrationen die induzierende Wirkung von FUdR außerordentlich zu verstärken. Für

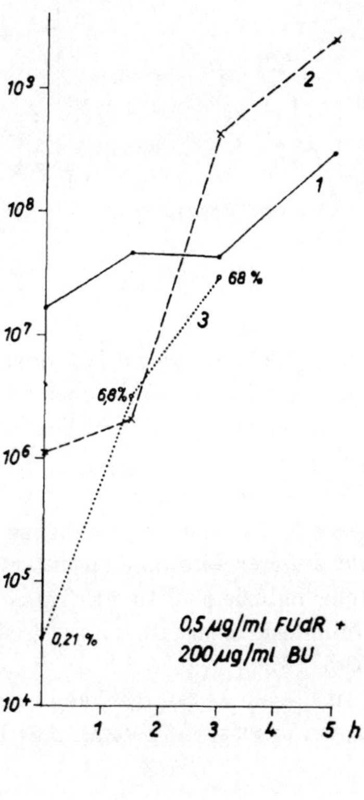

Abb. 8. Bakterienvermehrung, Phagenproduktion und induzierte Zellen in Gegenwart von 0,5 μg/ml 5-Fluordesoxyuridin und 200 μg/ml 5-Bromuracil
Mittelwerte aus 2 Versuchen

dieses widersprüchliche Verhalten haben wir noch keine Erklärung. Sicherlich handelt es sich bei der Verstärkerwirkung durch BU aber nicht darum, daß durch eine Transdesoxyribosidierung BUdR gebildet wird. Aus Tabelle 2 ging hervor, daß GdR in einer sehr wesentlich höheren Konzentration als FUdR nicht befähigt ist, BU (als BUdR) eine Induktionsfähigkeit zu verleihen. Ebenso erwies sich auch CdR (200 μg/ml) dafür als unwirksam.

2.3. 5-Fluoruracil

In Gegenwart von FU (0,5 μg/ml) werden in SS-Medium innerhalb von 90 min 27% der in NB präincubierten Zellen induziert (Abb. 9). FU ist damit wesentlich stärker wirksam als die gleiche Menge FUdR. Wie Tabelle 5 zeigt, kann die induzierende Wirkung von FU aufgehoben werden durch TdR, BU (!!), U und UdR sowie CdR. Somit kann die Induktion durch FU weder auf eine spezifische Hemmung der DNS-Synthese noch spezifisch auf den Einbau des FU in die RNS und/oder auf damit verbundene Folgen zurückgeführt werden.

Auch die inaktivierende Wirkung des FU ist spezifisch weder auf einen DNS- noch auf einen RNS-Effekt zurückzuführen: auch sie kann durch alle eben genannten Substanzen aufgehoben werden. Dagegen gibt sich die Hemmung der Bakterienvermehrung durch FU eindeutig als RNS-Effekt zu erkennen, kann sie doch weder durch 200 μg/ml TdR oder 200 μg/ml BU, dagegen recht gut schon durch 25 μg/ml U aufgehoben werden. Wieso aber 25 μg/ml UdR und sogar CdR besser wirken als 25 μg/ml U ist uns noch völlig unklar (die Differenz U/UdR ist mit $p = 0{,}007$ statistisch einigermaßen gesichert).

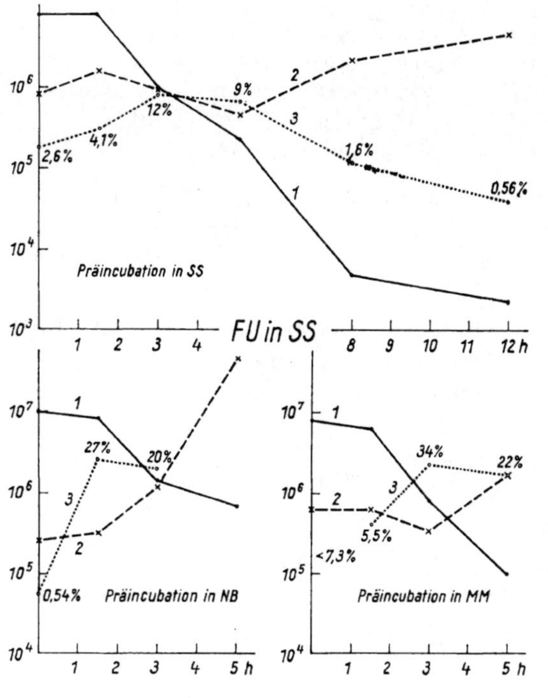

Abb. 9. Bakterienvermehrung, Phagenproduktion und induzierte Zellen in Gegenwart von 0,5 μg/ml 5-Fluoruracil nach Präincubaction in SS-, NB- bzw. MM-Medium Mittelwerte aus je 3 (SS), 2 (NB) bzw. 3 (MM) Versuchen

Ferner ergibt sich aus Tab. 5, daß auch einige Vitamine die induzierende und inaktivierende FU-Wirkung aufheben bzw. vermindern. Wir haben begonnen, den Effekt dieser und anderer Vitamine zu untersuchen, nachdem sich gezeigt hat, daß FU in mSS offenbar nicht induziert (Tab. 6). Tatsächlich konnten wir nachweisen, daß in mSS-Medium nur zumindest innerhalb einer dreistündigen Inkubation gar keine Zellen induziert werden (Abb. 10).

In diesem Zusammenhang erinnerten wir uns daran, daß wir zu Beginn unserer Versuche fanden (Geissler, 1963a), daß FU in NB nicht zu induzieren vermag. Wir prüften deshalb

Tabelle 5

Der Einfluß verschiedener Basen und Desoxynucleoside sowie einiger Vitamine auf die Wirkung von 5-Fluoruracil in SS auf Zellen, die in NB präincubiert worden waren

0,5 µg/ml FU +	N	Bakterien	Phagen	Q
—	13	0,15 ± 0,068	130 ± 51	52 ± 18
U (0,5 µg/ml)	6	1,9 ± 0,61	19 ± 7	0,35 ± 0,11
U (25)	4	28 ± 1,9	330 ± 110	0,32 ± 0,055
UdR (0,5)	6	2,3 ± 0,25	71 ± 14	0,85 ± 0,16
UdR (25)	4	51 ± 5,5	570 ± 47	0,26 ± 0,012
CdR (25)	6	41 ± 6,2	260 ± 31	0,1 ± 0,01
TdR (200)	4	2,4 ± 0,79	6,2 ± 2,8	0,035 ± 0,007
TdR (200) + U (0,5)	4	15,7 ± 0,31	28 ± 9,5	0,035 ± 0,002
BU (200)	4	4,2 ± 1,6	62 ± 30	0,22 ± 0,04
Folsäure (0,01)	7	1,2 ± 0,23	47 ± 5,1	0,69 ± 0,081
Cholin (2)	7	1,1 ± 0,14	42 ± 5,1	0,76 ± 0,15
Nikotinsäure (0,1)	6	0,86 ± 0,1	78 ± 11	1,8 ± 0,56

Tabelle 6

Die Rolle des Mediums und des Präincubationsmediums bei der Induktion durch 0,5 µg/ml 5-Fluoruracil

Präincubation in	0,5 µg/ml Fu in	N	Bakterien	Phagen	Q	Induktion	Phagen Prod.
NB	SS	13	0,15 ± 0,068	130 ± 51	52 ± 18	+	+
mSS	SS	4	0,0035 ± 0,0004	0,22 ± 0,043	—[1]	+	—
SS	SS	6	0,014 ± 0,0048	1,8 ± 0,77	—	+	—
MM	SS	6	0,0037 ± 0,0003	4,1 ± 0,84	—	+	—
NB	mSS	6	0,29 ± 0,072	6,9 ± 1,1	—	(—)[2]	+
NB	MM	8	2,9 ± 0,81	41 ± 7,8	0,59 ± 0,23	(—)[3]	+
NB	NB	5	19 ± 3,1	13 ± 1,7	0,011 ± 0,0017	—	+

[1]) Q wurde nur dann errechnet, wenn im Falle einer Bakterien-Inaktivierung der Phagentiter nach 5 Std. größer als der Bakterientiter zur Zeit 0 min war.

[2]) Maximale Induktion: 1,9% der Zellen nach 5 Std. Inkubation.

[3]) Maximale Induktion: 2,4% der Zellen nach 3 Std. Inkubation.

die Wirkung von FU in verschiedenen Medien und verwendeten dazu auch lysogene Kulturen, die nicht wie üblich 3 Std. in Nb, sondern in anderen Medien angezogen wurden. Die Ergebnisse dieser Versuche sind in Tabelle 6 und in Abbildung 9 zusammengefaßt und zeigen an, daß nicht nur das Behandlungs-, sondern auch das Präincubationsmedium von entscheidender Bedeutung für die FU-Wirkung ist. Ein „Induktions-Quotient" wird praktisch nur bei in

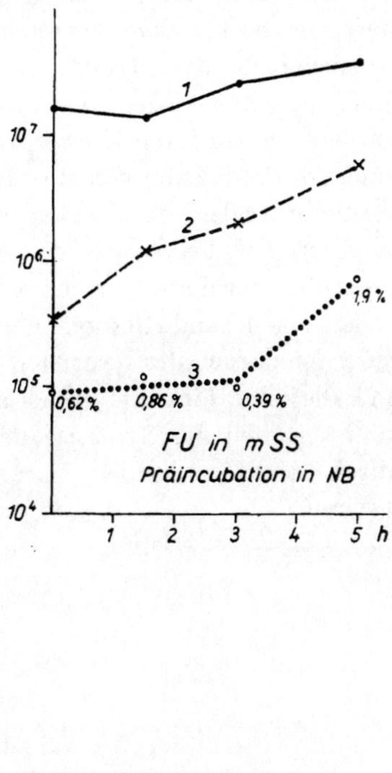

Abb. 10. Bakterienvermehrung, Phagenproduktion und induzierte Zellen in Gegenwart von 0,5 µg/ml 5-Fluoruracil in mSS-Medium nach Präincubation in NB
Mittelwerte aus 4 Versuchen

NB präincubierten Zellen in SS beobachtet. (Dies könnte eine Ursache dafür sein, daß ENDO, ISHIZAWA et al. (1963) mit FU – unbekannter Konzentration – keine Induktion beobachten konnten, da diese Autoren augenscheinlich keinen Mediumwechsel vorgenommen haben.)

Bei diesen Versuchen ergab sich, daß der Q-Methode bei der Analyse von Induktionsversuchen nur ein begrenzter Wert zukommt: Bei der Bestimmung der induzierten Zellen fanden wir, daß FU zwar wie in mSS auch in NB und MM (Präincubation jeweils in NB) keine oder kaum eine Induktion auslöste, während in SS auch solche Zellen durch FU induziert wurden, die in SS, mSS oder MM präincubiert worden waren. In diesen Fällen ergab sich nur deshalb kein „Induktions-Quotient" ($Q > 0,1$), weil keine oder kaum freie Phagen produziert wurden.

Somit gibt es bei Applikation und in Gegenwart von 0,5 µg/ml FU folgende drei Möglichkeiten:

a) Induktion und Phagenproduktion (NB/SS)

b) Induktion, aber kaum Phagenproduktion (SS/SS, MM/SS, mSS/SS)

c) keine signifikante Induktion (NB/mSS, NB/NB, NB/MM).

Demnach findet eine Induktion unabhängig von den – von uns untersuchten – Präincubationsmedien immer in SS, aber in keinem anderen Medium statt. Wir haben dafür noch keine Erklärung, zumal FU in mSS – das sich nur durch den Vitamingehalt von SS unterscheidet – ebenfalls nicht induziert. Andererseits kann der Vitaminmangel allein keine Voraussetzung für die induzierende FU-Wirkung sein, da FU auch in MM – das wie SS keine Vitamine enthält – nicht induzieren kann. Jedenfalls lassen auch diese Befunde in Zusammenhang mit den oben berichteten Ergebnissen vermuten, daß FU möglicherweise an anderer Stelle angreift als in die Synthese der Thymidylsäure oder der RNS.

Während die Induktion unabhängig vom verwendeten Präincubationsmedium stattfindet, ist die Präincubation bzw. ein Mediumwechsel für die Phagenproduktion durch die induzierten Zellen von signifikanter Bedeutung: Eine Phagenproduktion findet in Gegenwart von FU nur in NB (wo das FU auch die Bakterien nicht inaktiviert und nur relativ geringfügig hemmt) oder nur dann statt, wenn ein „shift down" (aus Komplettmedium in Mangelmedium) stattgefunden hat, während kein „shift" (aus SS in SS) oder ein „shift up" (aus MM in SS) den induzierten Zellen keine Phagenproduktion erlaubt. (Ähnliche, aber umgekehrte Verhältnisse beobachtete BEN-GURION (1963): In Trypton präincubierte Zellen produzieren nach lytischer Infektion in Minimalmedium keine Phagen.)

Unter „shift down"-Bedingungen werden weder Ribosomen- noch transfer-RNS synthetisiert, da die im Komplettmedium angezüchteten Zellen Ribosomen und transfer-RNS im Überschuß besitzen (HAYASHI und SPIEGELMAN, 1961, STENT, dieses Symposion). Der von uns beobachtete Effekt wäre nun verständlich, wenn man annehmen würde, daß FU in der von uns verwendeten Konzentration nicht nur induziert, sondern möglicherweise gleichzeitig auch die Produktion von Ribosomen-RNS bzw. von Ribosomen, und/oder von transfer-RNS verhindern oder einschränken würde. Tatsächlich konnte ARONSON (1961) nachweisen, daß 20 µg/ml FU bei *E. coli* die Fertigstellung der 70 s-Ribosomen aus den entsprechenden Vorstufen verhindert. Wenn unsere Vermutung richtig wäre, würden in NB präincubierte Zellen ausreichend Ribosomen und transfer-RNS besitzen, um nach dem durch FU induzierten Zusammenbruch des lysogenen Regelmechanismus Phagen produzieren zu können, während im Falle keines Mediumswechsels oder eines „shift up" deshalb keine Phagen produziert werden könnten, weil die Synthese der dazu benötigten Ribosomen und transfer-RNS-Moleküle durch das FU verhindert würde. Wir versuchen gegenwärtig, diese Probleme näher zu analysieren.

Summary

1. BU (200 µg/ml) inhibits multiplication of the lysogenic cells and does not induce. The inhibitory effect is overcome in presence of either U, or C, CR, CdR, but not in presence of T.
2. BUdR (200) inhibits the multiplication of the bacteria, too, and induces a great fraction of them.
3. IU and IUdR (200) do not inhibit the growth of bacteria significantly.
4. IU does not induce while IUdR seems to induce some cells.
5. FUdR induces in dependence of its concentration. This effect seems to be the result of an inhibition of the enzyme, thymidylate synthetase.
6. BU enhances or reduces the inducing effect of FUdR in dependence of the concentration of these two substances.
7. FU induces in SS medium. This effect is the result of neither an DNA nor of an RNA effect specifically.
8. Cells induced by FU are able to produce phages, if they had been preincubated in NB medium.

Verwendete Abkürzungen

BU: 5-Bromuracil, BUdR: 5-Bromdesoxyuridin, C: Cytosin, CR: Cytidin, CdR: Desoxycytidin, DNS: Desoxyribonucleinsäure, FU: 5-Fluoruracil, FUdR: 5-Fluordesoxyuridin, GdR: Desoxyguanosin, JU: 5-Joduracil, JUdR: 5-Joddesoxyuridin, RNS: Ribonucleinsäure, T: Thymin, TdR: Thymidin, U: Uracil, UR: Uridin, UdR: Desoxyuridin.

Herrn Prof. Dr. A. Graffi bin ich für seine stete Förderung meiner Arbeit und für anregende Diskussionen sehr zu Dank verpflichtet. Frl. A. Schütt und Frl. I. Tetzlaff danke ich für ihre fleißige umsichtige Mitarbeit bei den Versuchen. Herrn Prof. Dr. A. Wacker und Herrn Prof. Dr. F. Kaudewitz danke ich für die Überlassung von Substanzen.

Literatur

Aronson, A. I., 1961: The effect of 5-fluorouracil on bacterial protein and RNA synthesis. Biochim. Biophys. Acta **49**, 98–107.

Ben-Gurion, R., 1962: On the induction of E. coli K 12 (λ) by aminopterin. Biochem. Biophys. Res. Commun. **8**, 456–461.

Ben-Gurion, R., 1963: The production of phage in induced lysogenic and in infected sensitive bacteria. Virol. **20**, 288–291.

Bussard, A., S. Naono, F. Gros et J. Monod, 1960: Effects d'un analogue de l'uracile sur les propriétés d'une protéine enzymatique synthétisée en sa présence. C. R. Acad. Sci. **250**, 4049–4051.

Champe, S. P., and S. Benzer, 1962: Reversal of mutant phenotypes by 5-fluorouracil: An approach to nucleotide sequences in messenger-RNA. Proc. Nat. Acad. Sci. **48**, 532–546.

Endo, H., M. Ishizawa, T. Kamiya, and S. Sonoda, 1963: Relation between tumoricidal and prophage-inducing action. Nature **198**, 258–260.

Endo, H., T. Kamiya, and M. Ishizawa, 1963: λ-phage induction by colicin E_2. Biochem. Biophys. Res. Commun. **11**, 477–482.

Field, A. K., and H. B. Naylor, 1962: Induction of lysogenic Micrococcus lysodeikticus. J. Bact. **84**, 1129–1133.

Freese, E., 1959: The specific mutagenic effect ot base analogues on phage T 4. J. mol. Biol. **1**, 87–105.

Geissler, E., 1963: Untersuchungen über den Mechanismus der Induktion I. Die Wirkung einiger Basen-Analoga auf lysogene Bakterien. Acta biol. med. germ. **10**, 417–421.

— 1963b: Untersuchungen über den Mechanismus der Induktion III. Der Einfluß von Uracil auf die induzierende Wirkung von 5-Fluoruracil und 5-Fluordesoxyuridin. Acta biol. med. germ. **10**, 432–435.

— 1963c: Untersuchungen über den Mechanismus der Induktion IV. Der Einfluß von 5-Bromuracil auf die Induktion durch 5-Fluoruracil und 5-Fluordesoxyuridin. Acta biol. med. germ. **10**, 684–686.

— 1963d: Untersuchungen über den Mechanismus der Induktion V. Versuche zur Analyse der induzierenden Wirkung halogenierter Basen und ihrer Desoxynucleoside. Acta biol. med. germ. **11**, 286–289.

— 1963e: Die Regulation der Lysogenie und ihre Störung. Biol. Rdsch. **1**, 18–31.

Geissler, E., und E. Bender, 1963: Untersuchungen über den Mechanismus der Induktion VII. Die Induktion lysogener Bakterien durch Amethopterin. Arch. Geschwulstforsch. (im Druck)

Geissler, E., und A. Wacker, 1963: Untersuchungen über den Mechanismus der Induktion VI. Die Induktion lysogener Bakterien durch Belichtung in Gegenwart von Thiopyronin. Acta biol. med. germ. (im Druck).

Handschuhmacher, D. E., and A. D. Welch, 1960: Agents which influence nucleic acid metabolism. In: The Nucleic Acids (E. Chargaff und J. N. Davidson, Edts.) **3**, 453–526, Academic Press Inc., New York und London.

Hayashi, M., and S. Spiegelman, 1961: The selective synthesis of informational RNA in bacteria. Proc. Nat. Acad. Sci. **47**, 1564–1580.

Jacob, F., 1952: Effects de la carence glycidique sur l'induction d'un *Pseudomonas pyocyanea* lysogene. Ann. Inst. Pasteur **82**, 433–459.

Jacob, F., and J. Monod, 1961: Genetic regulatory mechanisms in the synthesis of proteins. J. mol. Biol. **3**, 310–356.

Jacob, F., and E. L. Wollman, 1959: Lysogeny. In The Viruses (Burnet, F. M., and W. M. Stanley, Edts.) **2**, 319–351.

Kahan, F. M., 1962: Incorporation of pseudo-UTP, ribo-TTP and unnatural analogues into RNA by RNA-polymerase. Fed. Proc. **21**, 371.

Kahan, M., and J. Hurwitz, 1962: The role of DNA in RNA synthesis. IV. The incorporation of pyrimidine and purine analogues into RNA. J. biol. Chem. **237**, 3778–3785.

Langen, P., und E. Liss, 1962: Die Verwertung von Thymidin, Bromdesoxyuridin und den freien Pyrimidinbasen Thymin, Bromuracil und Joduracil zur Desoxyribonucleinsäure-Synthese durch Ascites-Tumorzellen in vitro. Biochem. Z. **336**, 139–153.

Lein, J., B. Heinemann, and A. Gourevitch, 1962: Induction of lysogenic bacteria as a method of detecting potential antitumour agents. Nature **196**, 783–784.

Levine, M., 1961: Effect of mitomycin C on interactions between temperate phages and bacteria. Virol. **13**, 493–499.

Maley, G. F., and F. Maley, 1962: Nucleotide interconversions. IX. The regulatory influence of deoxycytidine 5'-triphosphate and deoxythymidine 5'-triphosphate on deoxycytidylate deaminase. J. biol. Chem. **237**, PC 331–PC 3312.

Melechen, N. E., 1963: persönl. Mitteilung.

Melechen, N. E., and P. S. Skaar, 1962: The provocation of an early step of induction by thymine deprivation. Virol. **16**, 21–29.

Naono, S., et F. Gros, 1960: Synthese par E. coli d'une phosphatase modifiée en présence d'un analogue pyrimidique. C. R. Acad. Sci. **250**, 3889–3893.

Reichard, P., Z. N. Canellakis, and E. S. Canellakis, 1960: Regulatory mechanisms in the synthesis of deoxyribonucleic acid in vitro. Biochim. Biophys. Acta **41**, 558–559.

Rosenthal, H.-A. und E. Geissler, 1963: Untersuchungen über den Mechanismus der Induktion II. Die UV-Sensibilität 5-Bromuracil-markierter lysogener Bakterien. Acta biol. med. germ. **10**, 422–425.

Szybalski, W., 1962: Properties and applications of halogenated deoxyribonucleic acids. In: The Molecular Basis of Neoplasia, 147–171. University of Texas Press, Austin, Texas.

Wacker, A., 1963: Molecular mechanisms of radiation effects. Progr. in Nucleic Acid Res. **1**, 369–399, Academic Press, Inc., New York und London.

The Initial Events in Transduction of Galactose Fermentation in *Salmonella typhimurium* Cell

J. Hubáček

Department of Microbial Genetics and Variability, Institute of Microbiology, Czechoslovak Academy of Sciences, Praha 6, Na cvičišti 2

The final product of a stable transduction by the P 22 phage is a recombined microbial cell which transfers the new marker obtained by transduction into all its progeny. It is assumed that the first step which leads to such a recombinant, i. e. injection of DNA of the transducing particles into the recipient cell, is analogous to the first stage of any phage infection. The second stage, i. e. the mechanism of the incorporation of the transducing element into the genetic apparatus of the cell and the period during which the integration processes occur, is the main problem of the genetics of transduction. Very little is known about what happens after the penetration of the transducing element into the recipient cell.

The object of this report is to present some experiments which concern the study of this initial period of transduction. We succeeded in reducing the frequency of transduced *Salmonella typhimurium* cells by a transfer of a suspension of cells soon after the adsorption of the transducing phage from a nutrient (tryptone+yeast extract) to a synthetic medium. This method is in its principle similar to the ,,shift-down" method described by Maaløe (1960). The results of one such experiment are shown in Fig. 1.

Using auxotrophic cells the reduction of transductants after a shift is more marked. The reduction of a number of transductants in the synthetic medium is to some extent abolished by supplementing with casein hydrolysate and/or yeast ex-

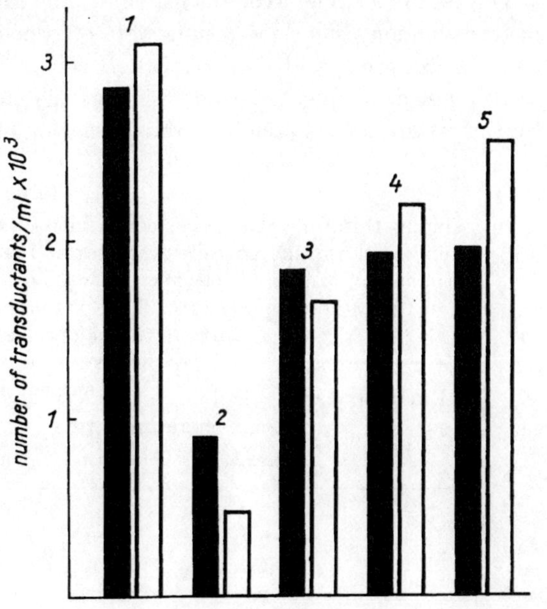

Fig. 1. Column 1 represents the number of transductants in nutrient medium without transfer, column 2 number of transductants after transferring the cells 10 min. after phage adsorption from a nutrient to a synthetic medium and columns 3, 4 and 5 number of transductants in synthetic medium supplemented with casein hydrolysate or yeast extract. The white columns indicate auxotrophic recipient cells used in experiment, the black columns prototrophic back mutant of the auxotrophic strain

tract. The reduced yield of transductants is not paralleled by reduction in the total number of viable recipient bacteria. The columns of transductants are expressed per the same number of cells (3 × 10^9).

The aim of the subsequent experiments was to establish for how long after the phage adsorption the sensitivity of transduced cells to a shift persists. The cell suspensions after 10 min. of phage adsorption were cultivated in nutrient medium and at intervals samples were taken and the cells were transferred to a synthetic medium (Fig. 2).

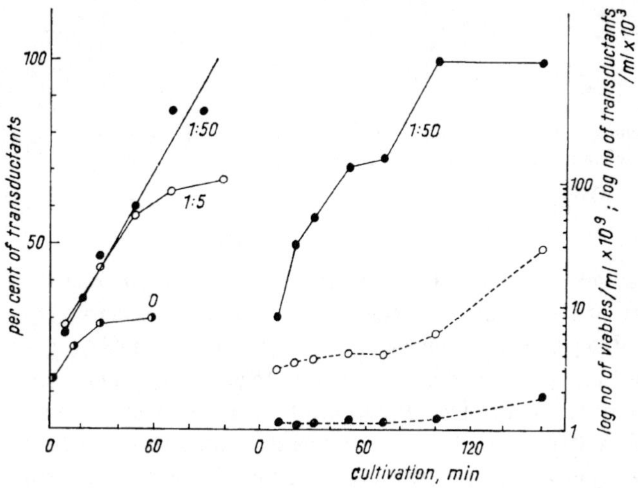

Fig. 2. The ordinate in Fig. 2 indicates the percentage of transductants detectable after shifting the cells to a synthetic medium. This curve (0) demonstrates the sensitivity of potentially transduced cells to a shift in *undiluted* cell suspension after 3, 15, 30 and 60 min. of phage adsorption (number of cells 4,3 × 10^9/ml). It can be seen that sensitivity of transduced cells to a shift is highest at the onset of the transduction process, i. e. 3 min. after phage adsorption. After this time the sensitivity decreases but after 30 min. of adsorption this decrease stops. This phenomenon seems to be due to the high concentration of cells in the adsorption mixture. In the next experiment the cell suspension after 10 min. of phage adsorption was therefore *diluted* 1 : 5 in nutrient medium and cultivated. As indicated by this curve the sensitivity of transductants to a shift at first decreases linearly but after 60 min. of cultivation this decline stops again. Only under conditions which permit growth and multiplication of the cells the sensitivity of transductants to a shift disappears after about 90 min. of cultivation and the frequency of transduced cells is no more influenced. For this purpose the cell suspension after 10 min. of phage adsorption was diluted 1 : 50

The results of these experiments show a 90 min. shift reversible phase in the initial period of transduction. The same results were obtained by Gross who studied the initial period of conjugation process in *Escherichia coli* cells. This shift reversible phase of the potentially transduced or conjugated cells resembles the chloramphenicol reversible phase as described by Ephrussi-Taylor (1958) in transformation of *Pneumococcus*. According to our hypothesis

Table 1

During this time the viable count increases from 5,6 × 10^9 to about 7 × 10^9 but the number of transduced cells decreases at the same time from 4 × 10^3 to about 2 × 10^3. Irradiation of the recipient cells does not increase the effect of acriflavine on the potentially transduced cells. These results show an early flavine reversible phase in more than 50 per cent of transductions

Exposition to acriflavine hrs	Cell suspension with adsorbed phage				
	no. of bacteria/ml × 10^9		no. of gal$^+$ cells/ml × 10^3		elimination
	non-irrad.	irradiated	non-irrad.	irradiated	per cent
0	5,6	5,0	4,0	3,8	0; 0
4	7,2	5,3	2,7	2,3	32,5; 39,3
8	7,0	5,1	2,1	2,0	47,5; 47,7
20	2,5	1,7	0,24	0,2	68,0; 70,0

the 90 min. shift reversible period is the phase during which the transducing element is in the non-integrated state. To verify this idea the elimination of the free transducing element by acriflavine has been followed. First the influence of flavine on the potentially transduced cells, 10 min. after phage adsorption was studied. A suitable concentration used was 10–15 μg of acriflavine/ml and 8 hrs of exposition at 37° (Table 1).

In further experiments the relation between cellular growth and sensitivity of the transducing element to acriflavine was assayed. After 10 min. of phage adsorption the cell suspension (viable count of which was about 2 × 10^9/ml) was diluted 50 × with nutrient medium

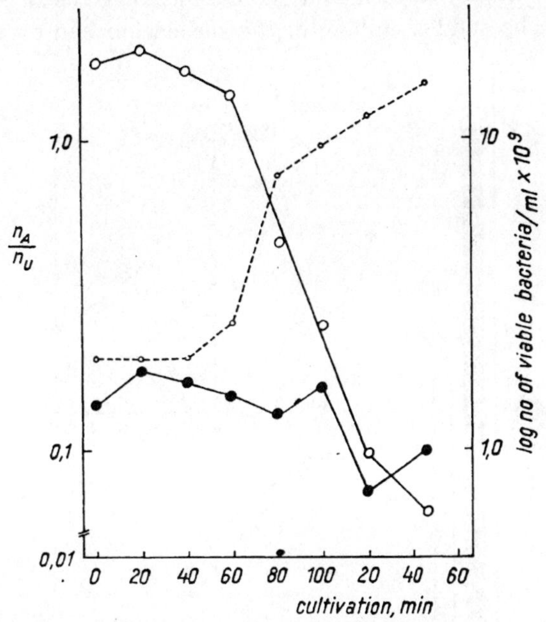

Fig. 3. Figure 3 demonstrates the results of one such experiment. The ordinate shows the ratio between the number of cells after acriflavine treatment and the number of cells in the untreated control sample. The broken line demonstrates the growth curve, the line (—o—) the ratio $\frac{N_a}{N_u}$ for viable count and the line (—●—) the ratio $\frac{N_a}{N_u}$ for the transduced cells. In the early period up to 60 min. of cultivation the number of viable bacteria after acriflavine treatment increases $\left(\text{the ratio } \frac{N_a}{N_u} > 1\right)$ and after this time the cells become sensitive and the viable count is reduced $\left(\text{ratio } \frac{N_a}{N_u} < 1\right)$. The potentially transduced cells are most sensitive to acriflavine in the initial phase of transduction. The number of transductants decreases at about 80 per cent. This early flavine reversible phase lasts during the 60 min. of cultivation. After this time it can hardly be judged when it exactly ends because of the complication of onset of sensitivity to acriflavine of the rest of the culture. Only approximately it can be said that it ends after about 80—120 min. of cultivation.

and incubated at 37°. At intervals samples were taken and divided into 2 parts. One part of each sample served as a control and was not treated by acriflavine at all, the other was treated by acriflavine for 8 hrs at 37° (Fig. 3).

These results suggest a conspicuous relationship between shift reversible and flavine reversible phases. It may be therefore assumed that the 90 min. phase of sensitivity of transductants to a shift is the period in which the transducing element is not integrated into the genome of the recipient cell. In the course of multiplication of the potentially transduced cell in nutrient medium the fragment is apparently stabilized through its integration. This period of cell growth required for incorporation agrees well with the results of the work of Jacob and Wollman (1957) who followed the ability of zygotes to produce recombinants.

What does the effect of the shift-down treatment on the frequency of transduced cells consist in? Our latest experiments show that the frequency of transductants is not influenced by the minimal medium itself. This effect is observed only after shift-down from a nutrient to a synthetic medium but not when the cells after adsorption of the phage in synthetic medium are transferred to synthetic medium again. It may be assumed, therefore, that the reduced frequency of transductants after a shift is not due to deficiency of some elements in the synthetic medium but rather the result of disturbance in the regulation mechanisms in the cell. According to our interpretation the reduced frequency of transduced cells is not due to the death of the cells but rather results from the curing of the cells from the transducing element. The nature of this event was therefore studied in further experiments.

First the influence of a lower temperature on the frequency of transduced cells was studied. After 10 min. of phage adsorption one part of the cell suspension in nutrient medium was transferred to a synthetic medium, quickly chilled to 0° and cultivated for 90 min. at 0°. The cells in the other part were transferred to synthetic medium and exposed for 90 min. at 37° (Fig. 4).

It can be seen that the number of transduced cells is reduced both at 0° as well as 37°. The sudden chilling of the suspension had even a stimulating effect and the reduction of the number of transductants soon after chilling is more marked. A very close relationship was shown between the more conspicuous reduction of the number of transductants in the early period after transfer and chilling the cells to 0° and the loss of some fraction of amino acids from amino acid pool of the cells.

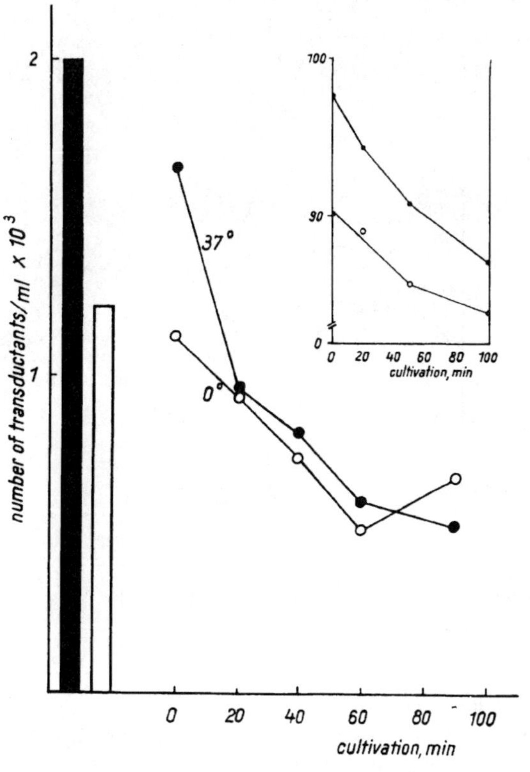

Fig. 4. The black column demonstrates the control number of transductants in the nutrient medium, the white column the number of transductants in nutrient medium suddenly chilled to 0°. It can be seen that the sudden chilling reduced the number of transductants also in nutrient medium without shift to synthetic medium. The curve —●— represents the number of transductants in synthetic medium after shift and cultivation at 37°, —○— the number of transductants after shift and cultivation at 0°.
The inset in the corner (Fig. 4) demonstrates the relationship between time of exposition of the cells in the synthetic medium and fraction of amino acid pool detectable after certain intervals of such exposition. The curve —● - represents the unchilled suspension, the curve —○— the sudden chilled suspension

It can be seen that after sudden chilling of the cells to 0° the higher amount of free amino acids is extracted to the external medium with regard to unchilled suspension. Some amino acids (as glycine, alanine, phenylalanine, leucine and valine) are extracted even from more than 50 per cent (Table 2).

But regardless of this relationship it is probable that the change in the pool by itself does not cause the curing of the cell from the transducing element. When bacteria are starved the assumption is not justified that the only effect is upon the free amino acid pool. Under these conditions the ribosomes in the cell disintegrate, either because of the fall in the concentration of intracellular Mg^{2+} or for some other reason, the RNA becomes exposed to attack and at the same time the degrading enzymes are liberated. In further experiments we have studied the possibility of the stabilization of the transducing element in the cell after shift to a synthetic medium. Various substances (chloramphenicol, streptomycine, 2,4-dinitrophenol, citrate, Mg, Ca, Mn, cadaverine, and putrescine) were used. Only the effect of Mg, Ca, Mn, cadaverine, or putrescine proved to be interesting. It was shown that these substances reverse the influence of a shift-down treatment on the frequency of transduced cells. If added to a synthetic medium the number of transductants after shift remains unchanged. Mg and these amines are known to stabilize ribosomes in the starved cells. In Fig. 5 the reversible effect of Mg on the frequency of transduced cells after a shift from a rich to a poor medium is shown.

Table 2

amino acid	amino acid pool in cell µg/100 mg d. wt.	extracted µg/100 mg d. wt.	per cent
glutamic	306,0	49,8	14,0
aspartic	11,9	1,5	11,4
glycine	1,8	3,0	62,5
alanine	7,8	15,6	66,6
CH_3glutamic	18,3	1,0	4,8
phenylalanine	7,6	5,5	41,8
leucine	20,8	30,5	59,5
valine	7,9	13,1	62,3

The reversible effect of Mg depends on temperature at which the cells are exposed in the synthetic medium. The presence of Mg in the synthetic medium at 0° (column 3) has no protective effect and in order to obtain the same number of transductants as in control sample, Mg is to be added only after transferring the cells to higher temperature (30 min. at 37° – columns 4 and 5). On the other hand when the cells are exposed to the synthetic medium at higher temperature (22° or 37°), in order to obtain the same number of transductants as in the control, it is necessary to add Mg into the synthetic medium already during this period of exposition (column 3). If this is not carried out some irreversible processes occur and the addition of Mg in the course of the following exposure at higher temperature (37°) has no effect (column 4). The optimal concentration of Mg was found to be 0,01 M and a similar effect was obtained by using Ca, Mn, cadaverine, and putrescine.

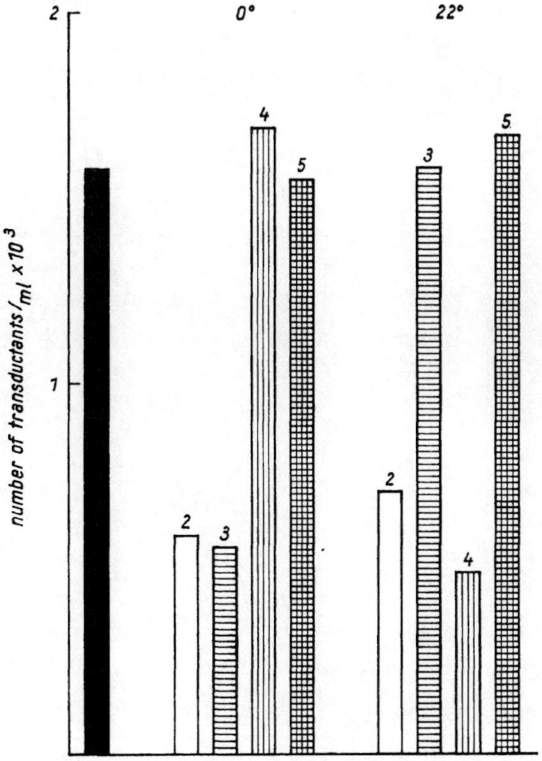

Fig. 5. The number of transductants is expressed in all columns per the same number of cells (about 5×10^9). Column 1 represents the number of transductants in control sample in nutrient medium without transfer, column 2 the number of transductants after transfer to a synthetic medium and 60 min. exposition at 0° or 22° and column 3 the number of transductants after transfer to a synthetic medium with Mg^{2+} (0,1 M) and 60 min. exposition at 0° or 22°; column 4 – experimental conditions are same as column 2 but after 60 min. exposition at 0° or 22° the cells were further exposed 30 min. with Mg^{2+} at 37°; column 5 – experimental conditions are the same as columns 3 but after 60 min. exposition at 0° or 22° the cells were further exposed 30 min. with Mg^{2+} at 37°.

According to these results it might be speculated that the curing process by itself consists at least of two parts. The first can be carried out at 0° and this temperature has even a stimulating effect on the reduction of transductants after shift. The changes in amino acid pool could play some role in this initial period. Transducing element in the cell need not be destroyed (eliminated) during this phase. The second part of the curing process occurs only at a higher temperature and may be inhibited by divalent cations. The nature of this event is being the object of further experiments.

References

Ephrussi-Taylor, H., 1958: Recent Progress in Microbiology. Symposia held at the VII Intern. Congr. for Microbiology, Stockholm, p. 51, Blackwell Scientific Publications 1959.

Gross, J. D.: Ph. D. thesis, London 1963.

Jacob, F., and E. J. Wollman, 1957: Symp. Soc. exp. Biol. 12, 75.

Maaløe, O., 1960: In: Hayes, W., and R. C. Cloves, ed Microbial Genetics. Tenth Symposium of the Society for General Microbiology, London, p. 272, Univ. Press, Cambridge.

Über den Einfluß von Mutationen im Genom des Donor-Stammes auf die Transduktionsfähigkeit des *Proteus*-Phagen π 1

H. Böhme

Institut für Kulturpflanzenforschung Gatersleben, Kr. Aschersleben, der Deutschen Akademie der Wissenschaften

Unter Transduktion verstehen wir die Übertragung von Fragmenten des genetischen Materials eines Donor-Stammes in eine Rezipientenzelle durch einen Bakteriophagen (Hartman, 1957). Bei der unspezifischen Transduktion können theoretisch alle Marker eines Donor-Stammes durch die Phagen eines Lysates übertragen werden. In der Rezipientenzelle werden die transduzierten Fragmente des Donor-Genoms im Laufe eines rekombinativen Prozesses in das Genom der Rezipientenzelle eingebaut. Die Einzelheiten dieses Vorgangs sind bis heute noch nicht völlig klar zu übersehen.

Der Phage π 1 von *Proteus mirabilis* ist zur Transduktion der verschiedensten Marker fähig (Böhme, 1963). Es handelt sich um eine unspezifische Transduktion, die in allen ihren Eigenschaften dem Transduktionssystem bei *Salmonella typhimurium* mit dem Phagen P 22 sehr ähnlich ist (Demerec, 1956). So können auxotrophe Mutanten mit Phagen aus dem Wildtyp oder aus nicht identischen Mutanten zur Prototrophie transduziert werden. Die Häufigkeit der Transduktion liegt zwischen $10^{-5} - 10^{-7}$/Phagenpartikel. Die Methodik ist die gleiche, wie sie bei der Transduktion von *S. typhimurium* mit dem Phagen P 22 angewandt wird (Tab. 1).

Tabelle 1

Rezipient	Donor	Transduktanten	
		Genotyp	Anzahl/10^8 Überlebende
lys$^-$	Wildtyp	*lys*$^+$	901,3
met-49$^-$	Wildtyp	*met*$^+$	1391,0
tyr$^-$	Wildtyp	*tyr*$^+$	312,5
str-d	Wildtyp	*str*-s	332,0
his$^-$*lys*$^-$	Wildtyp	*his*$^+$*lys*$^-$	365,4
		his$^-$*lys*$^+$	958,5
met-29$^-$*lys*$^-$	Wildtyp	*met*$^+$*lys*$^-$	1144,0
arg$^-$*lys*$^-$	Wildtyp	*arg*$^+$*lys*$^-$	1118,0
met-49$^-$*lys*$^+$	*met*-49$^+$*lys*$^-$	*met*$^+$*lys*$^+$	380,0
tyr$^-$*lys*$^+$	*tyr*$^+$*lys*$^-$	*tyr*$^+$*lys*$^+$	383,3

Wir interessierten uns in der letzten Zeit besonders für eine Region des *Proteus*-Chromosoms, die 1 *met*-Locus und mindestens 3 *arg*-Loci enthält. Alle 4 Loci sind eng gekoppelt, so daß sie in einem Phagenteilchen gemeinsam transduziert werden. Bei der Durchführung einer Reihe von Kreuzungen fanden wir, daß der Phage π 1 nach Vermehrung in dem Mutanten-Stamm *met*-43 nicht mehr in der Lage ist, irgendeinen Marker des Donor-Stammes zu transduzieren. Der Stamm *met*-43 kann daher nicht als Donor-Stamm verwendet werden (Tab. 2). Die Mutation *met*-43 wurde durch Äthyl-Methansulfonat im Wildtyp induziert (Böhme, 1962). Anstelle von Methionin kann der Stamm auch auf Cystein wachsen.

Tabelle 2

	Anzahl von Kolonien auf 4 Platten *)
str-d-3; *met*⁺ (x) *str*-s; *met*⁺	781
str-d-3; *met*⁺ (x) *str*-s; *met*-43	0
(Selektion auf Streptomycin-Unabhängigkeit)	
phen-99; *met*-43 (x) *phen*⁺; *met*⁺	311
phen-99; *met*-43 (x) *phen*⁺; *met*-43	1
(Selektion auf Phenylalanin-Unabhängigkeit)	

*) Werte nach Korrektur entspr. der Anzahl spontaner Revertanten

Der Test auf die Transduktionsfähigkeit des Phagen wurde an zwei Transduktionssystemen durchgeführt: 1. Transduktion des Streptomycin-abhängigen Stammes *str-d*-3 zur Streptomycin-Unabhängigkeit und 2. Transduktion der Doppelmutante *phen*-99; *met*-43 zur Phenylalanin-Prototrophie. Im Gegensatz zu dem Verhalten des Donor-Stammes ist das Verhalten des Stammes *met*-43 als Rezipient völlig normal (Tab. 3).

Tabelle 3

	Anzahl der Kolonien auf Platten *)
str-s; *met*-43 (×) *str*-r; *met*⁺	290
(Selektion auf Methionin-Unabhängigkeit)	

*) Werte nach Korrektur entspr. der Anzahl spontaner Revertanten

Auch die Tatsache, daß *met*-43 mit relativ großer Häufigkeit zu *met*⁺ zurückmutiert, schließt die Möglichkeit aus, daß es sich bei der Mutation zur Methionin-Auxotrophie um eine größere Deletion handelt. Wir finden also, daß eine Mutation im Genom des Donor-Stammes zum Verlust der Transduktionsfähigkeit des Phagen π 1 führt.

Tabelle 4

	Anzahl der Kolonien auf 4 Platten *)
str-d-3; *met*⁺; *arg*⁺ (×) *str*-s; *met*-43; *arg*⁺	0
str-d-3; *met*⁺; *arg*⁺ (×) *str*-s; *met*-43; *arg*A-89	308
str-d-3; *met*⁺; *arg*⁺ (×) *str*-s; *met*-43; *arg*F-143	145
str-d-3; *met*⁺; *arg*⁺ (×) *str*-*s*; *met*⁺; *arg*F-72	223
(Selektion auf Streptomycin-Unabhängigkeit)	

*) Werte nach Korrektur entspr. der Anzahl spontaner Revertanten

Tabelle 5

	Anzahl der Kolonien auf 4 Platten *)
phen-99; *met*-43; arg^+ (×) $phen^+$; *met*-43; arg^+	1
phen-99; *met*-43; arg^+ (×) $phen^+$; *met*-43; *arg*A-89	292
phen-99; *met*-43; arg^+ (×) $phen^+$; *met*-43; *arg*F-104	289
(Selektion auf Phenylalanin-Unabhängigkeit)	

*) Werte nach Korrektur entspr. der Anzahl spontaner Revertanten

Dieser Einfluß der Mutation *met*-43 auf die Transduktionsfähigkeit des Phagen kann jedoch aufgehoben werden, wenn im Genom dieser Mutante eine zweite Mutation induziert wird (Tab. 4 und 5).

Aus Tab. 4 ist zu ersehen, daß der Stamm *met*-43 nach Induktion zweier verschiedener *arg*-Mutationen wieder als Donor-Stamm verwendet werden kann. Aus der in dieser Tabelle zuletzt angeführten Kreuzung geht hervor, daß die *arg*-Mutationen allein keinen Einfluß auf die Transduktionsfähigkeit des Phagen haben. Nicht jede zusätzliche Mutation ist in der Lage, den Einfluß der Mutation *met*-43 auf die Transduktionsfähigkeit aufzuheben. Die folgenden Stämme wurden bisher in dieser Hinsicht geprüft, wobei die unter + aufgeführten Stämme transduktionsfähige Phagen produzieren, während die unter – angegebenen Mutanten transduktionsunfähige Phagen erzeugen:

+	–
met-43; *arg*A-89	*met*-43; *arg*G-136
met-43; *arg*F-104	*met*-43; *phen*-99
met-43; *arg*F-143	*met*-43; *phen*-96
met-43; *arg*F-127	*met*-43; *ilva*-95
met-43; *tyr*-123	*met*-43; *phen*-99; *arg*A-145
met-43; *his*-109	*met*-43; *phen*-99; *arg*F-164
met-43; *phen*-99; *arg*A-159	
met-43; *phen*-99; *arg*F-161	
met-43; *phen*-99; *arg*A-162	
met-43; *phen*-99; *arg*A-163	
met-43; *phen*-99; *arg*E-168	

Es ist eine Tendenz vorhanden, daß vor allem Mutationen in *met*-43 benachbarten Regionen zur Wiederherstellung der Transduktionsfähigkeit führen. Es gibt jedoch hiervon auch Ausnahmen; so sind *tyr*-123 und *his*-109, die beide die Transduktionsfähigkeit wiederherstellen können, nicht mit *met*-43 gekoppelt, während *arg*A-145 mit *met*-43 gekoppelt ist, jedoch keinen Einfluß auf die Transduktionsfähigkeit ausübt.

Tabelle 6

	Anzahl der Kolonien auf 4 Platten *)
str-d-3; met^+; arg^+ (×) *str*-s; *met*-43; arg^+	0
str-d-3; met^+; arg^+ (×) *str*-s; $met^{+(43)}$; arg^+	496
str-d-3; met^+; arg^+ (×) *str*-s; *met*-43; *arg*A-89	736
str-d-3; met^+; arg^+ (×) *str*-s; $met^{+(43)}$; *arg*A-89	0
str-d-3; met^+; arg^+ (×) *str*-s; *met*-43; $arg^{+(A\text{-}89)}$	659
(Selektion auf Streptomycin-Unabhängigkeit)	

*) Werte nach Korrektur entspr. der Anzahl spontaner Revertanten

Es war nun von Interesse, das Verhalten verschiedener Reversionstypen zu prüfen. Zunächst fanden wir, daß eine Rückmutation von *met*-43 zu *met*+ die Transduktionsfähigkeit wiederherstellt. Erfolgt diese Rückmutation jedoch in der Doppelmutante *met*-43; *arg*A-89, dann sind die in diesem Stamm produzierten Phagen nicht transduktionsfähig. Eine Reversion zur Arginin-Prototrophie in der Doppelmutante *met*-43; *arg*A-89 führt nicht zum Verlust der Transduktionsfähigkeit (Tab. 6).

Eine echte Deutung der hier beschriebenen Fakten ist nach unserer Ansicht bei dem bisher vorliegenden Versuchsmaterial noch nicht möglich. Folgende Überlegungen können jedoch zu der Frage, in welcher Phase des Transduktionsprozesses die Transduktionsfähigkeit des Phagens durch die Mutation *met*-43 unterdrückt wird, angestellt werden. Wir sehen drei mögliche Antworten auf diese Frage:

1. Es erfolgt keine Inkorporation von genetischem Material des Donor-Stammes in die Phagen während der Phagenvermehrung im Stamm *met*-43.
2. Es erfolgt ein Einbau von Fragmenten des Donor-Chromosoms, die Phagen sind jedoch so stark defekt, daß sie nicht in die Rezipientenzelle eindringen.
3. Die Integration des transduzierten genetischen Materials in das Genom der Rezipientenzelle wird verhindert.

Mir scheint, daß die letzte Möglichkeit ausscheidet, da nicht einzusehen ist, warum auch die Fragmente, die *met*-43 nicht enthalten, nicht inkorporiert werden sollen. Die zweite Möglichkeit erscheint ebenfalls unwahrscheinlich, da in diesem Fall der Zusatz von Hilfsphagen eine Transduktion ermöglichen sollte. Eine Reihe von Versuchen, in denen den im Stamm *met*-43 vermehrten Phagen Hilfsphagen zugesetzt wurden, verliefen negativ. Wir gehen bei der weiteren Planung von Experimenten von der Arbeitshypothese aus, daß bei der Phagenvermehrung im Stamm *met*-43 der Einbau von genetischem Material des Donor-Genoms in die Phagen unterbleibt. Es ist jedoch noch zu früh, über den möglichen Mechanismus dieses Vorgangs zu spekulieren. Der hier beschriebene Einfluß von Mutationen im Donor-Genom auf die Transduktionsfähigkeit der Phagen weist jedoch darauf hin, daß bei *Proteus* der Einbau von genetischem Material der Bakterienzelle in die Phagenteilchen unter einer gewissen Kontrolle durch das Donor-Genom steht.

Summary

The temperate phage π 1 of *Proteus mirabilis* is able to transduce various bacterial markers from donor cells into recipients. Auxotrophic mutants can be transduced to prototrophy by phages grown either in the wildtype or in nonidentical auxotrophic mutants. The following results pointing out influences on the transducing ability of the phage by mutations within the genome of the donor strain have been found in the course of studies on the genetic fine structure of some *met*- and *arg*-loci.

1. Loss of transducing ability of phages following the mutation from *met*+ to *met*-43 in the donor cell

Complete loss of transducing ability of the phage has been found to be the consequence of his being grown in mutant strain *met*-43. The phages produced are unable to transduce any allele of the donor strain. All other phage characters studied (f. i. lysogenisation) remained unchanged.

2. Restoration of transducing ability following the induction of a second mutation within the genome of the donor strain

Double mutants originating by a second independent auxotrophic mutation in strain *met*-43 may again function as donor strain. These double mutants are producing phages with normal transducing ability. The restoration of transducing ability following growth in the double mutant strain is dependent on the locus of the second mutation.

3. The transducing ability of phages grown in different reversion types

Phages with normal transducing ability are produced after the reversion of

met-43 to met^+

in the donor strain. This reversion, however, occuring in the double mutant

met-43; *arg*A-89 to met^+; *arg*A-89

causes the loss of transducing ability of phages grown in this revertant strain. A reversion to arginine prototrophy in the double mutant is without influence on the transducing ability.

Literatur

Böhme, H., 1962: Die Beeinflussung der inaktivierenden und mutagenen Wirkung von Äthyl-Methansulfonat durch Mangan- und Magnesiumchlorid. Biol. Zbl. **81**, 267–275.

– 1963: Transduction of prototrophy to auxotrophic mutants of *Proteus mirabilis*. Biochem. Biophys. Res. Comm. **10**, 60–62.

Demerec, M., 1956: A comparative study of certain gene loci in *Salmonella*. Cold Spring Harbor Symposia Quant. Biol. **21**, 113–120.

Hartman, Ph. E., 1957: Transduction: A comparative Review. In: W. D. McElroy and B. Glass, The Chemical Basis of Heredity. The John Hopkins Press, 408–462.

Regulation of RNA Synthesis in Bacteria[1])

GUNTHER S. STENT

Virus Laboratory, University of California, Berkeley, California, U.S.A.

More than 80 percent of the ribonucleic acid (RNA) of *Escherichia coli* is represented by ribosomal RNA molecules, the nucleic acid moiety of the ribosomes that are the site of protein synthesis in the cell, and most of the remainder of the RNA is accounted for by the transfer RNA molecules that function as amico acid „adaptors" in protein synthesis. Finally, a quantitatively minor, albeit qualitatively most important, fraction of the RNA is represented by the ephemeral *messenger* RNA molecules that harbor the sequence information for the ordered copolymerization of amino acids into specific polypeptides (JACOB and MONOD, 1961). In this discussion, I should like to summarize briefly some recent ideas that lead to the notion that, besides being the amino acid adaptor, and thus the agency that „knows" the genetic code, the transfer RNA may also play a role in the regulation of bacterial biosynthesis, in particular that the transfer RNA may intervene in the general regulation of the synthesis of RNA.

Amino Acid Control of RNA Synthesis

There exist numerous observations that indicate that the availability to the bacterium of amino acids governs its differential rate of RNA synthesis. Since most of the experiments relevant to this regulation of RNA synthesis were concerned with measurements of *total* RNA, I shall not attempt to distinguish here between the possibly separate control of synthesis of ribosomal, transfer and messenger RNA. One set of such observations pertains to the *upshift* and *downshift* experiments (KJELDGAARD, MAALØE and SCHAECHTER, 1958; SCHAECHTER, MAALØE and KJELDGAARD, 1958; NEIDHARDT and MAGASANIK, 1960). These experiments show that there ensues an immediate acceleration in the synthesis of RNA upon transfer of a bacterial culture from a minimal to an amino acid-supplemented medium (upshift); this increase in the rate of RNA synthesis occurs well before any later acceleration of other biosynthetic functions becomes manifest (reflected in such properties of the culture as its turbidity, viable cell count, or DNA content). The time lag between the accelerations of the syntheses of RNA and of other cell constituents accounts for the higher relative

[1]) This investigation was supported by Public Health Service Research Grant CA 02129, from the National Cancer Institute.

RNA content of bacteria in an amino acid-supplemented than in a minimal medium (MAALØE, 1960). Conversely, there ensues an immediate halt of RNA synthesis upon transfer of a culture from an amino acid supplemented to a minimal medium (downshift). The complete halt in RNA synthesis persists after other biosynthetic functions again proceed at the lower rate characteristic of the minimal medium and RNA synthesis finally resumes only after the specific RNA content of the post-downshift culture has fallen to the pre-upshift level.

A second set of experiments pertains to RNA synthesis in amino acid-requiring bacterial auxotrophs. Such auxotrophs stop synthesizing not only protein but also RNA as soon as they are deprived of an exogenous source of the required amino acid. However, if synthesis of protein is inhibited, e. g., by addition of the antibiotic chloramphenicol to the culture, then a very small concentration of the required amino acid – far below that otherwise necessary for optimal growth – suffices to promote RNA synthesis at a nearly maximal rate (GROS and GROS, 1956; 1958; PARDEE and PRESTIDGE, 1956; ARONSON and SPIEGELMAN, 1958). That is, the requirement for amino acids in RNA synthesis appears to be *catalytic*, rather than stoichometric. This catalytic role of amino acids is suggested also by the finding that addition of chloramphenicol to a culture of non-auxotrophic bacteria growing in a minimal medium engenders a temporary acceleration of RNA synthesis. Here the antibiotic appears to prevent the neutralization of free amino acids liberated by the spontaneous breakdown of bacterial proteins and thus to allow the build-up of an intracellular amino acid pool, mimicking the conditions of „upshift" (KURLAND and MAALØE, 1962).

The catalytic intervention of amino acids in the control of bacterial RNA synthesis allows the bacterium to adjust its steady state level of RNA in accordance with the nutritional limitations imposed on the overall rate of protein synthesis: as long as all of the 20 standard amino acids are in abundant supply, the cell can utilize the maximum amount of ribosomal and messenger RNA molecules in order to effect protein synthesis at the maximum rate; as soon as the supply of any one amino acid falls to a suboptimal level, protein synthesis must necessarily decelerate and render supernumerary some of the cellular RNA. It is possible to understand the nature of this regulatory process by supposing that there exists within the bacterium a set of 20 *inhibitors* of RNA synthesis, each inhibitor species subject to neutralization by one particular kind of amino acid. Hence, the lower the intracellular concentration of amino acids, the higher the effective inhibitor concentration, and hence, the smaller the rate of RNA synthesis. Furthermore, as soon as the concentration of any one amino acid falls to the very low level that obtains in an auxotroph starved for its growth factor, the effective concentration of the inhibitor homologous to that amino acid rises high enough to cut off RNA synthesis altogether.

The set of 20 or more transfer RNA species, each of which is known to enter into combination with only one cognate amino acid (BERG and OFENGAND, 1958) commended itself as a likely possibility for the postulated inhibitors of RNA synthesis (STENT and BRENNER, 1961; KURLAND and MAALØE, 1962). Thus, amino acid-free transfer RNA molecules would inhibit RNA synthesis, whereas enzymatic transfer of the cognate amino acid to the ribose moiety of the terminal adenine nucleotide of the homologous transfer RNA molecule would abolish the inhibitory effect. The hypothesis of the transfer RNA molecules as regulators of RNA synthesis subsequently derived support from the finding (TISSIÈRES, BOURGEOIS and GROS, 1963) that the *in vitro* action of the DNA-dependent RNA polymerase – the enzyme presumed to be responsible for the *in vivo* synthesis of bacterial messenger RNS – is inhibited by amino acid-free transfer RNA and that this inhibition can be relieved by charging the transfer RNA molecules with amino acids. Thus if the DNA-dependent RNA polymerase is responsible not only for the synthesis of messenger but also for the synthesis of the total bacterial RNA, as would be the case if the bacterial DNA really provides the template for all species of RNA polynucleotides – then the amino acid control of RNA synthesis could be understood in terms of the inhibition of RNA polymerase function by amino acid-free transfer RNA molecules.

Relaxed Control and the Catholic Inducer

There exists, however, an exception to this general finding of *stringent* amino acid control of bacterial RNA synthesis, namely the behavior of the methionine-requiring mutant 58–161 of *E. coli*, K 12 (Borek, Rockenbach and Ryan, 1955; Borek, Ryan and Rockenbach, 1955). Cultures of this mutant strain continue to synthesize RNA even after having been deprived of all exogenous methionine. During methionine starvation, the bacteria more than double their relative content of both ribosomal as well as transfer RNA (Mandel and Borek, 1962; Neidhardt, 1963) and, without having lost the ability to give rise to colonies on nutrient agar, undergo a progressive physiological deterioration that delays the resumption of normal anabolic activities after restoration of methionine to the growth medium. The reason for the methionine-independent RNA synthesis in this strain is not that methionine, unlike other amino acids, does not happen to participate in the control of RNA synthesis, since methionine-auxotrophs of *E. coli* other than strain 58–161 do cease net synthesis of RNA as soon as methionine is removed from their growth medium. Subsequent experiments with auxotrophic derivatives of this strain requiring various amino acids, such as leucine, isoleucine, valine, threonine, arginine, histidine, lysine or tryptophan showed that in this exceptional strain RNA synthesis can proceed in the absence of not only methionine but also of other amino acids necessary for growth. That is, in strain 58–161 the normally stringent amino acid control of RNA synthesis is *relaxed*.

Genetic crosses involving conjugation between Hfr donor bacteria derived from strain 58–161 and F^- recipient bacteria derived from other lines of *E. coli*, K 12 that manifest the normal, stringent control of RNA synthesis, showed that the property of relaxed amino acid control of RNA synthesis can be transferred from donor to recipient cell, and that it segregates among the recombinant bacteria produced. Hence there appears to exist an RNA control, or *RC*, genetic locus in *E. coli* which is involved in the regulation by amino acids of RNA synthesis, and which can exist in two allelic states, *stringent*, or RC^{st}, and *relaxed*, or RC^{rel} (Stent and Brenner, 1961). Amino acid auxotrophs carrying the RC^{st} allele stop synthesizing not only protein but also RNA as soon as they are deprived of an exogenous source of their amino acid growth requirement, whereas auxotrophs carrying the RC^{rel} allele continue to synthesize RNA at a nearly normal rate for a considerable period after removal of the required amino acids from the growth medium. More detailed study of the segregation pattern of complementary *RC* genotypes among the recombinant progeny of such crosses showed that the *RC* gene is situated on the *E. coli* chromosome between the loci responsible for resistance to streptomycin (Str) and for synthesis of serine (*Ser/Gly*) (Alföldi, Stent and Clowes, 1962).

Study of the physiology of growth of RC^{rel} bacteria showed that their synthesis of RNA appears to be under normal control under most conditions of balanced or unbalanced growth. Thus, it is true for RC^{rel} strains, as it is for the normal RC^{st} strains, that the richer the growth medium, and hence the faster the rate of bacterial growth, the greater the differential rate of RNA synthesis, and hence the greater the relative cellular content of RNA. Furthermore, it is true for RC^{rel} strains, as it is for RC^{st} strains, that upon downshift of growing cultures into media of nutritionally inferior carbon and energy or nitrogen sources, there ensues an immediate reduction in the differential rate of RNA synthesis (Neidhardt and Eidlic, 1963). However, a striking difference in the behavior of RC^{rel} bacteria is evident upon downshift from amino-acid supplemented to minimal media. Under these conditions, RC^{rel} bacteria *continue* rather than cease their synthesis of RNA and enter a long lag, lasting for many hours, before resuming growth in the minimal medium. Apparently, the unbalanced, post-downshift accumulation of RNA drives the RC^{rel} bacteria into a physiological impasse in which the synthesis of previously repressed enzymes necessary for the resumption of growth has become very difficult. Indeed, colony assay on minimal glucose agar of RC^{rel} bacteria growing rapidly in amino acid supplemented medium reveals that only about 20% of the cells thus subjected to downshift are ultimately able to escape from this impasse. *Leucine* greatly aggravates the deleterious effects of downshift transfer for RC^{rel} genotypes, since the presence of leucine in the minimal glucose agar reduces to 0.1% the fraction of cells capable of ever resuming growth, i. e., of forming a colony on the minimal agar (Alföldi, *et al.*, 1963). Thus the regulatory aberration of RC^{rel} bacteria becomes manifest only upon starvation of the bacteria for *one or a few required amino acids.* It is under this special metabolic restriction that the normal control of RNA synthesis shown by RC^{st} genotypes breaks down in RC^{rel} genotypes.

Since the behavior of RC^{rel} bacteria is quite normal under most conditions of balanced and unbalanced growth, it follows that their RNA synthesis is not to be considered amino acid-independent, or ,,constitutive". Rather, their behavior suggests that the regulatory aberration of RC^{rel} bacteria derives from a *breakdown of the specificity* of the neutralization reaction between the amino acids and the postulated inhibitors of RNA synthesis. That is, one may suppose that, in contrast to normal RC^{st} genotypes, in which each inhibitor species can be neutralized by only one of the standard amino acids, in RC^{rel} bacteria each inhibitor species can be neutralized not only by its cognate amino acid but also by a *catholic inducer.* This catholic inducer might be a metabolite that bears some structural or metabolic relation to amino acids, or might in fact, *be itself* an amino acid. In RC^{rel} bacteria, just as in RC^{st} bacteria, RNA synthesis would then proceed at a reduced rate as long as nutritional limitations of the growth medium render many amino acids in short intracellular supply. These same nutritional limitations would cause the postulated catholic inducer also to be in short supply, and its intracellular concentration to be insufficient for the neutralization of an appreciable fraction of the amino acid free-inhibitor molecules. However, if RC^{rel} bacteria are starved for only one, or a very few required amino acids, then the intracellular concentration of the catholic inducer would suffice to neutralize enough inhibitor molecules cognate to the few missing amino acids to allow maintenance of RNA synthesis. Leucine would be thought to bear a metabolic relation to the catholic inducer, so that its toxic effect during downshift tranfer from amino acid-supplemented to minimal medium would be explained by an increase in the internal concentration of the inducer and hence by an overstimulation of the pernicious, post-downshift RNA synthesis.

Three alternative roles can now be envisaged for the *RC* locus. (1) *RC* might govern the structure of the inhibitor molecules; here, the RC^{rel} allele would produce a structural modification of all inhibitor species, so that they would accept the catholic inducer. (2) *RC* might govern the synthesis of one or more enzymes that catalyze the combination of the amino acids with the cognate inhibitor; here, the RC^{rel} allele would produce a modified enzymatic ensemble that could combine the catholic inducer with all inhibitor species. (3) *RC* might govern the synthesis of the catholic inducer; here the RC^{rel} allele would produce an increase in the intracellular concentration of the catholic inducer. At present I favor the last of these three hypotheses.

Experiments have been carried out to test directly whether, provided that the transfer RNA molecules are really the inhibitors of RNA synthesis, one of the 20 standard amino acids is the postulated catholic inducer (MARTIN, YEGIAN and STENT, 1963). For this purpose, transfer RNA molecules extracted from RC^{rel} bacteria were charged with one or more of the 20 standard amino acids by use of amino acid activating enzymes isolated from the same bacteria. The charged transfer RNA was oxydized with periodate, and then reisolated and retested for its residual capacity to accept an amino acid that was absent from the preliminary charging mixture. If preliminary charging transferred an amino acid to a non-cognate transfer RNA species belonging to an absent amino acid, then the acceptor capacity for the missing amino acid would survive periodate oxidation and reveal its presence on recharging with that amino acid after post-periodate reisolation of the transfer RNA (BERG, LAGERKVIST and DIECKMANN, 1962). The results of these experiments showed that there does *not* appear to exist any major breakdown in amino acid transfer specificity in RC^{rel} bacteria: preliminary charging of the transfer RNA from RC^{rel} bacteria with 19 of the 20 standard amino acids does not afford protection against periodate oxydation for any appreciable fraction of the transfer RNA molecules cognate to the absent 20th amino acid. It is unlikely, therefore, that the catholic inducer is one of the 20 standard amino acids. If, as is of course possible despite the suggestive evidence, transfer RNA is not, after all, the inhibitor of RNA synthesis, and amino acids exert their regulatory role by combining with and neutralizing an entirely different class of inhibitor molecules, then the present experiments are not relevant to the nature of the catholic inducer. But if one wishes to retain both notions of the regulatory role of transfer RNA and of the presence of a catholic inducer in RC^{rel} strains, one is led to infer that the catholic inducer may be a non-standard amino acid, or simply an organic acid, that combines aspecifically with the terminal adenosine residues of amino acid-free transfer RNA molecules and thus neutralizes their inhibitory effect on the RNA polymerase. Accordingly, we are now attempting to ascertain whether, as predicted by this idea, transfer RNA molecules extracted from amino acid-starved RC^{rel} bacteria are, in fact, combined with a substance that is not their cognate amino acid.

It should be evident from this discussion that none of the main hypotheses presented here concerning the mechanism of amino acid control of RNA synthesis, plausible as they may appear, can as yet lay claim to very much *direct* experimental support. In that respect, however, they may not be at a very serious disadvantage *vis a vis* some other theories designed to render account of various regulatory phenomena. Furthermore, these hypotheses would seem to have at least the virtue of suggesting further experiments that should be capable of testing their validity, experiments that we are presently endeavoring to carry out.

References

ALFÖLDI, L., G. S. STENT, and R. C. CLOWES, 1962: J. Mol. Biol. **5**, 348.
ALFÖLDI, L., G. S. STENT, M. HOOGS, and R. HILL, 1963: Z. Vererbungsl. **94**, 285.
ARONSON, A. I., and S. SPIEGELMAN, 1958: Biochim. Biophys. Acta **29**, 214.
BERG, P., V. LAGERKVIST, and M. DIECKMANN, 1962: J. Mol. Biol. **5**, 159.
BERG, P., and E. J. OFENGAND, 1958: Proc. Natl. Acad. Sci. Wash. **44**, 78.
BOREK, E., J. ROCKENBACH, and A. RYAN, 1955: J. Bacteriol. **71**, 318.
BOREK, E., A. RYAN, and J. ROCKENBACH, 1955: J. Bacteriol. **69**, 460.

GROS, F., and F. GROS, 1956: Biochim. Biophys. Acta **22**, 200.
GROS, F., and F. GROS, 1958: Exptl. Cell Research **14**, 104.
KJELDGAARD, N. O., O. MAALØE, and M. SCHAECHTER, 1958: J. Gen. Microbiol. **19**, 607.
KURLAND, C. G., and O. MAALØE, 1962: J. Mol. Biol. **4**, 193.
JACOB, F., and J. MONOD, 1961: J. Mol. Biol. **3**, 318.
MAALØE, O., 1960: Symposium Soc. Gen. Microbiol. **10**, 272.
MANDEL, L. R., and E. BOREK, 1962: Biochem. Biophys. Res. Comm. **9**, 11.
MARTIN, E. M., C. YEGIAN, and G. S. STENT, 1963: Z. Vererbungsl. **94**, 303.
NEIDHARDT, F. C., 1963: Biochim. Biophys. Acta **68**, 365.
NEIDHARDT, F. C., and L. EIDLIC, 1963: Biochim. Biophys. Acta **68**, 380.
NEIDHARDT, F. C., and B. MAGASANIK, 1960: Biochim. Biophys. Acta **42**, 99.
PARDEE, A. B., and L. PRESTIDGE, 1956: J. Bacteriol. **71**, 677.
SCHAECHTER, M. O., O. MAAØLE, and N. O. KJELDGAARD, 1958: J. Gen. Microbiol. **19**, 529.
STENT, G. S., and S. BRENNER, 1961: Proc. Natl. Acad. Sci. Wash. **47**, 2005
TISSIÈRES, A., S. BOURGEOIS, and F. GROS, 1963: J. Mol. Biol. **7**, 100.

Restoration of Operon Activity by Suppressors

Jonathan R. Beckwith [1])

MRC Microbial Genetics Research Unit, Hammersmith Hospital, Du Cane Road, London, W. 12, England

The sequence of nucleotide bases which make up a structural gene must contain several sorts of information. (1) The sequence of bases provides information for the coding of amino acids in the ultimate gene product, the protein. (2) There is evidence that at least some structural genes also carry sites which determine the sensitivity to regulation of the synthesis of their proteins (Jacob and Monod, 1961). (3) The individual gene must contain information which determines the maximum rate at which its protein can be produced. It is evident that not all proteins are produced at the same rate even when fully induced (Pardee and Beckwith, 1962a). (4) There must be sites at the beginning of individual genes which result in separate proteins being produced from each unit of structure even in linked groups of genes. Although all this information must be present, in many cases we do not know how or at what level it is expressed.

Much of our knowledge concerning the expression of gene functions comes from studies on the enzymes involved in lactose metabolism in *E. coli* (Jacob and Monod, 1961). The genes for three enzymes, β-galactosidase (z), galactoside permease (y) and galactoside transacetylase, are closely linked on the chromosome. In the absence of an inducer, the synthesis of these enzymes is inhibited by a cytoplasmic repressor produced by a fourth gene (i). The operator (O), a region at the end of the z gene, determines the sensitivity of all three enzymatic activities to control by the repressor. A group of genes whose activity is regulated in this way is known as an operon. Two classes of mutants have been detected in the operator region. O^c (operator-constitutive) mutants produce the enzymes of the operon constitutively in the presence of repressor. The mutation has resulted in a loss of sensitivity of the operator to the repressor. In O^o (operator-negative) mutants, the synthesis of all three enzymatic activities is abolished.

It has been established that the primary products of the lactose operon genes are complementary RNA molecules (messenger-RNA) which are probably the direct template for protein synthesis (Attardi, Naono, Gros, Brenner and Jacob, 1962; Hayashi, Spiegelman, Franklin and Luria, 1963). However, this specific operon messenger-RNA can only be detected in cells which have been exposed to a β-galactosidase inducer. In the absence of inducer, the repressor apparently acts at the operator site to prevent transcription of messenger-RNA from the operon genes. The same techniques used with induced cells have been used to measure operon messenger-RNA production in O^o mutants (Attardi, Naono, Gros and

[1]) United States Public Health Service Postdoctoral Fellow.

JACOB, personal communication). In O^o mutants, no specific operon messenger-RNA could be detected, even in the presence of inducer. As a result, it has been proposed that the operator region serves both as an initiation site for the transcription of messenger-RNA from the operon and as a repressor-sensitive site.

Another function of the operator site has been suggested by experiments with revertants of an O^o mutant (PARDEE and BECKWITH, 1962b). According to this model, the structure of the operator site determines the maximum rate of messenger synthesis and consequently the maximum rate of protein synthesis of which a gene is capable. Thus, the several sorts of information contained within the operator region are thought to be expressed directly at the DNA level rather than at the messenger-RNA level.

The work described here was initiated to determine more precisely the nature of the operator site and of O^o mutations by characterizing revertants of an O^o mutant. In contrast to the experiments mentioned above, the results suggest that O^o mutants are not blocked at the level of messenger-RNA synthesis. In addition, the results provide more information on the genetic sites involved in various gene functions. A preliminary report of this work has appeared (BECKWITH, 1963).

Results

We have described the isolation of *lac*$^+$ (z^+y^+) revertants of an O^o mutant for the lactose operon (PARDEE and BECKWITH, 1962b). It was possible to isolate a new type of revertant (z^-y^+) of this same mutant by using as a selective agent, melibiose, an α-galactoside which requires galactoside permease but not β-galactosidase for its metabolism (PARDEE, 1957). Using this compound, one can select for revertants in which the reading process affected by the O^o mutation, but not necessarily β-galactosidase activity, is restored. An $F^-i^-O^o$ strain, 2320 (obtained from Dr. F. JACOB), gave rise to a large number of revertants when incubated on melibiose-minimal agar for 2 to 3 days. About half of these revertants were phenotypically z^-y^+. These permease-positive revertants are not the result of a mutation at another structural gene producing a new type of permease, since mutants deleted in the *lac* region do not revert in this manner. The permease activity in these revertants ranged from close to 0% to 90% of the level in a fully constitutive strain.

Outside suppressors

Recombinational studies were carried out to determine whether any of the reversions in both z^-y^+ and z^+y^+ strains were due to mutations at suppressor loci outside the *lac* region. At least three distinct suppressor loci were defined by these mapping studies (Figure 1). The reversions in 4 of the „z^-y^+“ strains are a result of mutations at a locus or loci, su_A, which is closely linked to one of the methionine markers. The 4 were distinguishable from each other both by the level of permease restored and by the effect of the mutation on the generation time on other media. A second suppressor locus, su_B, is very closely linked to the *gal* genes. Mutations in this locus restore both β-galactosidase and permease and also lower the growth rate on other media. In two other suppressed „z^+y^+“ strains, a third suppressor locus, su_C, could be defined, mapping near the tryptophan operon. This suppressor does not affect the growth of the mutants on other media in contrast to su_A and su_B.

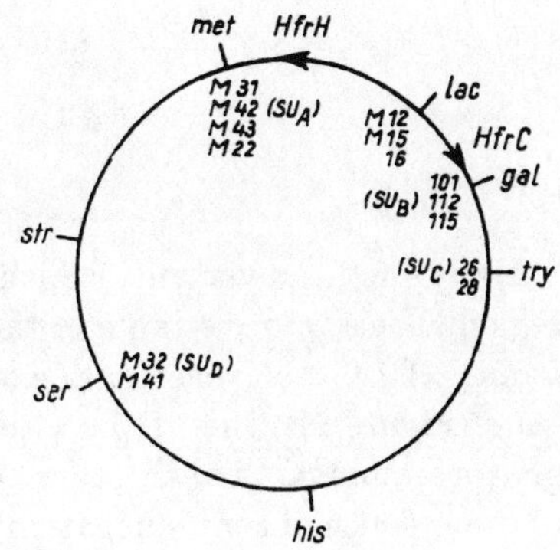

Fig. 1. The chromosomal location of O^0 suppressors
The four suppressor loci are described in the text. The M prefixed to some numbers indicates z^-y^+ mutants. Numbers at the *lac* region are for reversions which have occurred within the operon. The abbreviated markers are as follows: *lac*- lactose, *gal*- galactose, *try*- tryptophan, *his*- histidine, *ser*- serine, *str*- streptomycin and *met*- methionine. The origins and polarities of transfer of 2 of the Hfr's used for mapping the suppressors, HfrCavalli and HfrHayes, are shown

The technique of mapping used pointed to the existence in 2 z^-y^+ revertants of a fourth suppressor locus, su_D, lying near the serine marker. However, further studies with one of these, M 41, have shown that the reversion is at least partially due to a mutation within the *lac* region. This revertant displays other unusual properties which suggest that the events responsible for the restoration of permease activity may be quite complex. Several revertants were shown to be the result of mutational events within the *lac* region. These will be discussed in the section on „internal reversion".

Ames, Hartman and Jacob (1963) have shown that some revertants of an O^0-type mutant for the histidine operon in *Salmonella typhimurium* are due to a duplication of the operon outside the histidine region. The possibility was considered that the suppressors described here were actually translocated *lac* operons under the control of a new operator. If this were the case, one would expect that these loci would produce active enzyme by themselves in the absence of the *lac* region containing the O^0 mutation. This hypothesis was tested by mating lac^- (not O^0) Hfr's with representative strains of the three established suppressor loci. It was found that in interrupted mating experiments lac^- (or $melibiose^-$) recombinants appeared immediately the *lac* region of the Hfr donor chromosome entered the recipients. The activity of the original suppressed strains could be restored by recombining the original O^0 mutation into these lac^- (or $melibiose^-$) recombinants still carrying the active suppressor loci. Thus, although the suppressor mutation was still present in these recombinants, their phenotype was not expressed unless the O^0 mutation was also present. These experiments show that the suppressor loci are not reactivated translocations of the defective operon.

The natur of these suppressors has become clearer as a result of experiments carried out in collaboration with Dr. Sidney Brenner. The results provide strong evidence that su_B, and, by inference, all the O^0 suppressors, act on the translation of messenger-RNA information into protein. It has been shown that su_B restores activity to several rII mutants of the *E. coli* bacteriophage, T 4. Many of these mutants are also suppressed by the „nonsense" suppressor studied by Benzer and Champe (1962). These suppressors are thought to act by coding in the translation process for a previously untranslatable („nonsense") coding unit in the messenger-RNA. The finding that all of the rII mutants suppressed by su_B can be partially reverted by adding 5-fluorouracil to the medium is further evidence that the suppressed mutants are blocked in the translation process. It is difficult to explain this action of 5-fluorouracil other than by its incorporation into the messenger-RNA produced by the mutated gene.

Internal reversions

Many of the revertants which were isolated result from events occurring within the *lac* region. The z^-y^+ revertants of this type were further characterized in fine structure mapping studies. Of 6 z^-y^+ revertants examined, 5 were definitely shown to carry deletions in the z gene (Figure 2). One of these deletions, M 12, extends over most of the z region, but still gives recombinants with other O^o mutants. The deletion includes the original O^o mutation (JACOB, personal communication). The other 4 deletions, although beginning at different sites within the z gene, extend beyond the furthest known marker in the operator region. It has not yet been established whether these deletions actually extend out of the z region.

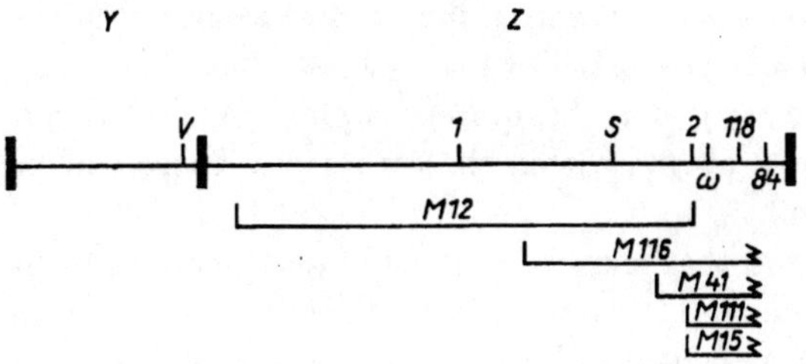

Fig. 2. The extent of deletions in the *lac* region. The deletions were mapped using the z^- and y^- markers indicated on the map. All the deletions except M 12 gave no recombinants with ω, 118, and 84, which are O^o mutants. 2320, the O^omutant used in these studies, is represented on the map by the number 2

Since the repressor-sensitive site is thought to be defined by the operator region, two of the deletion mutants were examined for their sensitivity to repressor. In order to test the repressibility of these i^- strains, it was necessary to introduce an i^+ gene by means of an episomal F-*lac* factor. Diploids with the genetic constitution, F-$i^+ z_S^- y^+/i^- z^- y^+$, were created with two of the deletion mutants, M 12 and M 116, and assayed for permease. The permease of M 12 is strongly repressed by the i^+ product while M 116 is not affected. These results are consistent with the picture of a repressor-sensitive site limited to the operator region. Since M 12 is deleted over all of the z region except the operator, yet is still repressed, there can be little or no information in the deleted segment which is required for repression.

Discussion

The results presented here provide substantial evidence that O^o mutants do produce an operon messenger-RNA. First, the correlation between the activity of one of the O^o suppressors, su_B, and that of the „nonsense" suppressor of BENZER and CHAMPE (1962) indicates that they are acting on the same process, the translation of messenger-RNA coding units into protein. The response of the suppressible rII mutants to 5-fluorouracil also suggests that the suppressors act at this level. Thus, in order for the O^o suppressors to work, there must be a messenger-RNA to work on. That O^o mutants do produce messenger-RNA from the operon is also indicated by the existence of 2 classes of suppressed mutants, „z^- y^+" and „z^+ y^+". These are best explained if one assumes that the O^o mutation, in addition to shutting off the operon activity, is also a structural mutation for β-galactosidase. The suppressors, then, provide some new coding information which acts at the O^o site on the messenger either to code for an amino acid which restores β-galactosidase activity („$z^+ y^+$"), or for an amino acid which results in an inactive z protein being produced („$z^- y^+$"). In both cases, the reading process and consequently permease activity are restored. Finally, the existence of three suppressor loci, in itself, is difficult to explain without assuming an operon messenger, unless the gene transcription process is infinitely more complex than has been supposed.

However, the conclusion that messenger-RNA from the operon must be present in O^o mutants is inconsistent with the finding of ATTARDI *et al.* (personal communication) that no messenger from the operon can be detected in these mutants. This paradox is best resolved by assuming that the messenger-RNA transcribed from the lactose region is particularly unstable in these mutants. An alternative explanation, that O^o messenger represses its own synthesis, appears ruled out since the O^o mutation is not dominant over the wild-type in diploids (JACOB and MONOD, 1961).

If O^o mutants produce messenger-RNA from the operon, this RNA must be of one piece and can not be made up of separate messenger for each gene. Otherwise, O^o mutations located in the z gene should have no effect on permease levels. The existence of a single messenger-RNA for the whole operon has been proposed by AMES and HARTMAN (1963) and MARTIN (1963). These results also suggest that protein synthesis must begin in the z gene-copy of this messenger before proceeding into the y gene-copy. There must then be a site in between the two gene-copies which signals the protein synthesizing machinery to start new protein synthesis at the beginning of the y gene-copy.

The O^o mutants do not appear to define a site involved in the initiation of either gene transcription or protein synthesis. Since revertant M 12 actually deletes the O^o mutation (JACOB, personal communication) and yet restores almost complete permease activity, this site could not be essential to either of these processes. If the other deletions are found not to extend out of the operon, then there is very little of the z gene that is required for initiation of a reading process.

If O^o mutants do not define any special site, it seems likely, as AMES and HATRMAN (1963) have proposed, that these mutants are merely extreme examples of the polar mutants which have been detected both in the lactose and histidine operons (FRANKLIN and LURIA, 1961; JACOB and MONOD, 1961; AMES and HARTMAN, 1963). Polar mutants which occur in the z region abolish β-galactosidase activity and result in lowered levels of galactoside permease and galactoside transacetylase. An explanation for the effects of these mutations follows from the conclusion that the operon messenger-RNA produced by O^o mutants is unusually unstable and that these mutations create „nonsense" triplets. The „nonsense" triplet in the operon slows up protein synthesis along the messenger or prevents it from proceeding further. The free segment of the messenger-RNA, not involved in protein synthesis, is then much more susceptible to the degradative action of RNAases. In O^o mutants this would mean that almost all of the messenger would be rapidly destroyed since very little of it is involved in protein synthesis. It is not immediately obvious why different polar mutants allow different amounts of permease to be made. It would be premature to enter into a more detailed discussion of these mutants until more extensive data on the genetic location and on the levels of activity of polar mutants are available.

The methods of detecting messenger-RNA developed by ATTARDI *et al.* (1962) and by HAYASHI *et al.* (1963) would not provide information on operon messenger-RNA synthesis in O^o mutants, if this messenger is unusually unstable, as has been proposed. Similarly, the absence of *lac* operon messenger-RNA in bacteria which have not been exposed to a β-galactosidase inducer (ATTARDI, *et al.*, 1962 HAYASHI *et al.*, 1963) may only reflect a decreased stability of the gene product in the presence of active repressor. Although the conclusions concerning messenger-RNA detection do not disprove the model of a repressor acting at the gene level, they would eliminate the main piece of evidence which was thought to distinguish between this model and one in which repression occurs at the messenger-RNA to protein level. If, in fact, repression is occurring at the RNA level rather than at the genetic level, there are two possibilities for the mode of action of the repressor. (1) The i^+ repressor is a highly specific RNAase which degrades only the *lac* operon messenger-RNA because of the particular base sequence in its operator. (2) The repressor acts by binding to the operator site of the operon messenger-RNA thus preventing protein synthesis from proceeding, and causing the messenger to be much more sensitive to RNAase degradation.

Literature Cited

AMES, B. N., and P. E. HARTMAN, 1963: The histidine operon. Cold Spring Harbor Symp. Quant. Biol. **28**, 349–356.

AMES, B. N., P. E. HARTMAN, and F. JACOB, 1963: Chromosomal alterations affecting the regulation of histidine biosynthetic enzymes in *Salmonella*. J. Mol. Biol. **7**, 23–42.

ATTARDI, G., S. NAONO, F. GROS, S. BRENNER, and F. JACOB, 1962: Effet de l'induction enzymatique sur le taux de synthése d'un RNA messager specifique chez *E. coli*. C. R. Acad. Sci. **255**, 2303–2305.

BECKWITH, J. R., 1963: Restoration of operon activity by suppressors. Biochim. Biophys. Acta **76**, 162–164.

BENZER, S., and S. P. CHAMPE, 1962: A change from nonsense to sense in the genetic code. Proc. Nat. Acad. Sci. **48**, 1114–1121.

FRANKLIN, N. C., and S. E. LURIA, 1961: Transduction by bacteriophage P1 and the properties of the lac genetic region in *E. coli* and *S. dysenteriae*. Virology **15**, 299–311.

HAYASHI, M., S. SPIEGELMAN, N. C. FRANKLIN, und S. E. LURIA, 1963: Separation of the RNA message transcribed in response to a specific inducer. Proc. Nat. Acad. Sci. **49**, 729–736.

JACOB, F., and J. MONOD, 1961: On the regulation of gene activity. Cold Spring Harbor Symp. Quant. Biol. **26**, 193–209.

MARTIN, R. G., 1963: The one operon-one messenger theory. Cold Spring Harbor Symp. Quant. Biol. **28**, 357–361.

PARDEE, A. B., 1957: An inducible mechanism for the accumulation of melibiose in *E. coli*. J. Bact. **73**, 376–385.

PARDEE, A. B., and J. R. BECKWITH, 1962a: Control of constitutive enzyme synthesis. In: Informational Macromolecules, ed. Henry Vogel, pp. 255–269. Academic Press: New Brunswick.

PARDEE, A. B., and J. R. BECKWITH, 1962b: Genetic determination of constitutive enzyme levels. Biochim. Biophys. Acta **60**, 452–454.

The Mechanism of Messenger RNA Replication in Bacteria

S. E. Bresler, R. A. Kreneva, V. V. Kushev, and M. I. Mosevitskii

Institute of High Molecular Weight Compounds of the Academy of Sciences of USSR. Leningrad. USSR

During protein synthesis genetic information coded in the DNA structure is transferred into ribosomes by means of m-RNA (Hayashi and Spiegelman, 1961; Brenner, Jacob and Meselson, 1961; Jacob and Monod, 1961). Lately biochemists have succeeded in purifying enzymes which synthesize RNA on a DNA primer (Stevens, 1960; Weiss and Nakamoto 1961; Furth, Hurwitz and Goldman, 1961). It was shown that RNA in this case is complementary to both strands of DNA and in favorable conditions it is able to form double helices of the Watson-Crick kind (Geidushek, Moohr and Weiss, 1962). It is obvious that the chemical composition of RNA in the case of double helix DNA primer is a copy (with the replacement of thymine by uracil) and in the case of a single stranded DNA primer (DNA of ΦX 174) is complementary to the template (Chamberlin and Berg, 1962; Furth, Hurwitz and Anders, 1962). So both chains of the DNA double helix are copied during the enzymatic *in vitro* synthesis. The RNA obtained *in vitro* is able to stimulate amino acids incorporation into proteins in cell-free ribosomal preparations (Wood and Berg, 1962; Ning and Stevins, 1962).

A new question arises, if we consider m-RNA synthesis in the cell: are both strands of DNA active as primer or only one of them? Existing data are discrepant. Analytical information shows that m-RNA from very different sources has mostly the same composition as DNA and conforms to Chargaff's rule (Volkin and Astrachan, 1956; Volkin, Astrachan and Countryman, 1958; Nomura, Hall and Spiegelman, 1960; Sibatani, de Kloet, Allfrey and Mirsky, 1962). This is an evidence for the replication of both DNA strands. On the other hand it is a current opinion that in the living cell where DNA is integrated into the chromosome structure and regulation mechanisms act on the genetic level, only one of the DNA chains is the template for m-RNA synthesis, the copying of the second chain being blocked (Bautz and Hall, 1962; Champe and Benzer, 1962).

This work was undertaken to study the role of both DNA strands during the m-RNA synthesis in the cell. The method was to use bacterial transformation by two linked genetic markers whose loci are placed in a single molecule of DNA. The transforming DNA consisted of molecular hybrids having one active genetic marker on one strand and the other marker in the second strand of the double helix. The method of obtaining such hybrids was developed by Marmur and Lane (1960) and Doty, Marmur, Eigner and Schildkraut (1960) and comprises thermal denaturation of a mixture of two DNA species having each one genetic marker and the renaturation of the mixture by slow cooling (annealing). During this procedure double strands are broken and reformed at random. Herriott (1961) used molecular hybrids of DNA taken from two strains of *Haemophilus influenzae* resistent to two different poisons – streptomycin and catomycin. These markers are genetically linked and their transmission is simultaneous. Using hybrid molecules for the transformation of wild type cells, Herriott obtained double transformants for both markers. This result shows that both strands of the DNA-molecule can be integrated into the genome of the recipient cell.

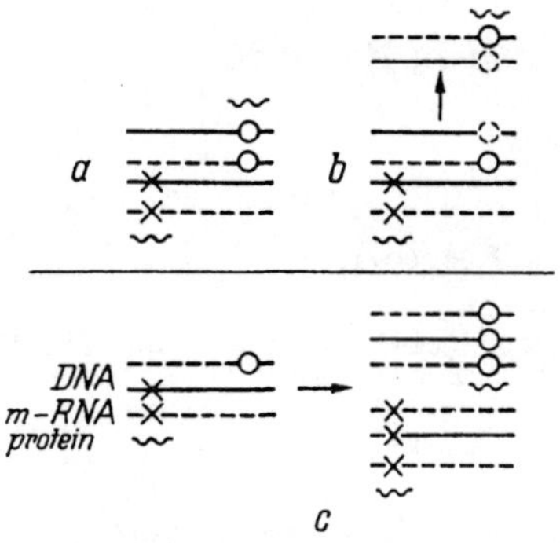

Fig. 1. Possible mechanisms of m-RNA copying in the cell.
a) Both strands of DNA are copied and both are active
b) Both strands of DNA are copied, but only one of two copies is used directly; to use the second m-RNA chain it must be re-copied once more
c) Only one strand of DNA is copied forming m-RNA. For the realisation of genetic information for both enzymes, the hybrid DNA molecule must previously reduplicate

In the course of the DNA replication they give recombinants resistant to both poisons. Nevertheless this experiment could not determine whether the m-RNA replication takes place from one DNA strand or from both (Fig. 1c).

We used the transformation of a recipient strain of *Bacillus subtilis* which was a double auxotroph for two linked markers: histidine and tryptophane dependence. The transforming DNA was a molecular hybrid obtained by simultaneous denaturation and renaturation of two DNA species. One of them was obtained from a *Bac. subtilis* strain auxotrophic for histidine only and the second one from a strain deficient in tryptophane. The conditions of the selection of the transformants excluded the presence of traces of both tryptophane and histidine in the growth medium. The transformed cell will proliferate on this medium only in the case when both kinds of m-RNA needed for the histidine and tryptophane enzymes synthesis are formed. The prerequisite of our experiment is the inability of the cell to reduplicate DNA if protein synthesis is blocked (Maaløe, 1961; Ryan, Nakada and Schneider, 1961). So in this case DNA reduplication cannot precede the formation of the enzymes which stimulate the tryptophane and histidine synthesis. If we find that immediately after the transformation procedure the recipient cell behaves like a double transformant, it means that both new types of m-RNA were synthesized previously to the DNA reduplication. Therefore the system we have chosen is suitable for answering the fundamental question about the copying of m-RNA from one or both strands of DNA.

Materials and methods

Bacterial strains

In this work we used following strains of *Bacillus subtilis*: *SHgw wild, H25 his*$^-$, *168 tr*$^-$, *SB25 his tr*$^-$ and a strain of *E. coli B wild*.

Isolation of DNA

DNA was prepared from all bacterial strains according to the following procedure. Cells harvested at the end of the exponential phase were lysed by lysozyme (50 μg/ml) at 37 °C for 30 min followed by the action of sodium dodecylsulphate at 20 °C for 10 min. After two phenol deproteinisations (phenol pH 8) and precipitation with 96% ethanol, the DNA was dissolved in 0,15 M NaCl, subjected to the action of RNA'ase (30 min at 37°) and a final phenol deproteinisation followed. By this treatment a DNA preparation is obtained with OD_{260}/OD_{230} ratio 1,8–2,2.

Hybridisation

The hybridisation of DNA molecules followed closely the method of MARMUR *et al.* (1960) and DOTY *et al.* (1960). DNA from *Bac. subtilis* strain *168* (DNA_{168}) and DNA_{H25} were mixed in the ratio 1 : 1 or 1 : 10 at a final concentration 20 μg/ml. Aliquots of this mixture were subjected to heating for 10 min at 100 °C and annealed at 68 °C for 90 min. For control experiments both DNA_{168} and DNA_{H25} were denatured and annealed separately and only after this treatment mixed together.

Conditions of transformation

Competent cultures of recipient cells were obtained after the prescription of SPIZIZEN (1959). The saltglucose medium of SPIZIZEN used for transformation is designated SGM.

Preparation of silicate gel plates

Equal volumes of solutions of sodium metasilicate (Na_2SiO_3 of density $\varrho = 1{,}1$) and HCl ($\varrho = 1{,}1$) were mixed. The mixture was deaerated by vacuum-pumping and poured into Petri-dishes. A transparent gel obtained was washed for several days with distilled water and impregnated with SGM medium. Autoclaving was made at 0,5 atm during 20 min.

Measurement of DNA concentration

The quantity of DNA in cells was measured by means of the diphenylamine reaction under standard conditions. For better release of DNA the cells were opened by lysozyme.

Ultrasonic experiments

Sonication of DNA preparations was performed in 0,15 M NaCl-0,03 M Na-citrate solution at the DNA concentration 20 μg/ml. The frequency was 480 kc, power output 20 w/cm².

Experimental results

I. Transformation of *Bacillus subtilis SB25* by two linked genetic markers (*his* and *tryp* dependence) under the action of hybrid molecules of DNA

Bac. subtilis SB25 cells in the state of competence were concentrated 10-fold (to $5 \cdot 10^9$ cells/ml) and subjected to the action of transforming DNA preparations. The latter were hybrids of DNA_{168} and DNA_{H25} in the ratio 1 : 1 and 1 : 10. In our experiments double transformants could be formed not only after absorption by a recipient cell of hybrid DNA molecule, but also when markers *his*⁺ and *tryp*⁺ were brought into the cell by two different molecules of DNA. It was shown earlier that the distribution of donor DNA between recipient cells is not even (BRESLER, MOSEVITSKII, and TIMKOVSKII, 1963). Some cells adsorb several hundreds molecules and therefore are transformed with the efficiency 20% or more times higher, comparing to random distribution of donor DNA between all recipient cells, this phenomenon increases many times the probability of penetration into the same highly competent cell of two different molecules with active *his*⁺ and *tryp*⁺ markers. For control we used the corresponding mixtures of both DNA which were previously subjected separately to the denaturation-renaturation procedure. After a 20 min time of contact with transforming DNA at a concentration 1 μg/ml, DNA'ase was used (20 μg/ml) for 5 min and the cells were plated on minimal plates (0,5 ml of cell suspension on each *Petri*-dish) for the determination of double transformants. The same culture was assayed after dilution for single transformants on minimal plates with the addition of histidine (50 μg/ml) or tryptophane (50 μg/ml).

The data in Table 1 show that the hybrids of DNA_{168} and DNA_{H25} give approximately 10 times more double transformants than the mixture of both DNA's. The appearance of double recombinants in control experiments is explained by random penetration of two different molecules with active *his*⁺ or *tryp*⁺ markers into the same recipient cell. The efficiency of transformation for a single marker was the same in both cases.

Table 1

Transformation of *Bacillus subtilis SB 25* by two linked genetic markers (of *tryp* and *his* dependence) under the action of hybrid molecules of DNA

DNA_{168}/DNA_{H25} ratio	DNA preparation	Number of transformed cells per ml *tryp*⁺ *his*⁺	*his*⁺	*tryp*⁺
1:10	hybrid	$2{,}3 \cdot 10^2$	$1{,}0 \cdot 10^4$	
	mixture	10	$1{,}0 \cdot 10^4$	
1:1	hybrid	$1{,}2 \cdot 10^2$	$1{,}4 \cdot 10^4$	$7{,}1 \cdot 10^3$
	mixture	6	$1{,}5 \cdot 10^4$	$7{,}1 \cdot 10^3$

Each value given in the Table is the mean of 10—12 identical experiments

The highest number of double transformants in these experiments with hybrid DNA constituted 2% of the number of single transformants. Similar results were obtained by HERRIOTT (1961) for *Haemophilus influenzae*. To explain these results we must remember that the inclusion of a hybrid DNA molecule into the cell is only one of the necessary conditions for the formation of double transformant. There must be a subsequent semiconservative reduplication of the hybrid DNA which results in two double helices having each only one active genetic marker. Finally genetic recombination must take place and after that both markers are reunited in one molecule of DNA, but now it is not a hybrid but a common double helix (RAVIN, 1961). As an alternative possibility is the segregation of both features, which can occure during the cell division. Both genetic loci of histidine and tryptophane are closely linked. Therefore recombination between them has a low probability. This fairly explains the poor yield of double transformants, compared to the single ones.

II. Exploration of the structure of hybrid DNA

The above results can be explained also if the simultaneous inclusion of both genetic markers into the recipient cell is caused by bimolecular complexes formed by the matching on short regions of complementary strands of two DNA double helices distorted and rearranged during the fusion-annealing process. It wold be difficult to distinguish these four stranded complexes from the double stranded hybrids both in genetic and physico-chemical tests (even in a density gradient centrifugation). It must be mentioned that in a recent paper by PEACOCK and WALKER (1962) the preservation of double strands in denatured DNA was claimed. It is obvious that such a structure would be incompatible with the formation of double stranded hybrids.

To elucidate this question we undertook two series of experiments. The first one aimed to verify the separation of both DNA strands in the course of thermal denaturation. For this purpose we added to the DNA of a prototrophic *Bac. subtilis SHgw* strain used as donor a 10 fold excess of DNA extracted from the recipient culture or an equal excess of heterologous DNA isolated from *E. coli B*. Transforming activities of both DNA preparations were measured as function of the time of annealing. As recipient *Bac. subtilis H25* strain was used. If there is no strands separation during denaturation, the transforming activity of the genetically

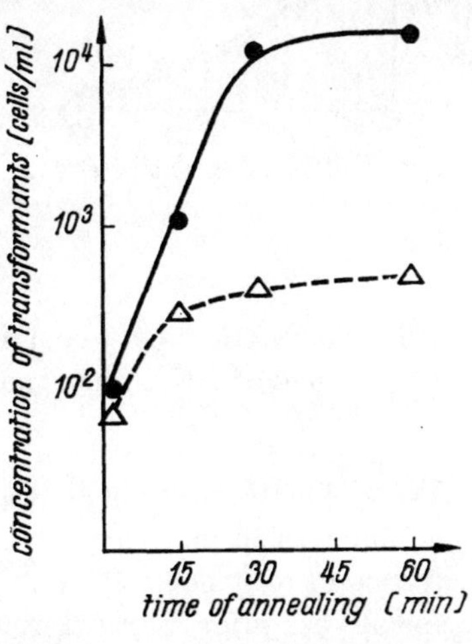

Fig. 2. Transformation of *Bacillus subtilis H25* under the action of prototrophic DNA (0,1 μg/ml) renatured in the presence of a 10-fold excess of DNA from *Bacillus subtilis H25* (——o——) or DNA from *E. coli B* (- - - △ - - -)
Each point is the mean of 3 identical experiments

marked DNA must not depend on the origin of the diluting DNA. But in reality, as is seen in Fig. 2, the transforming activity of DNA decreases scores of times in the presence of heterologous molecules. This fact is in agreement with a complete separation of both DNA strands, which must reunite during the time of annealing. The presence of heterologous DNA decreases the rate of collisions of complementary strands; hence the probability of renaturation is also decreased. The second experiment was aimed to study the possibility of formation of the four stranded complexes mentioned above. For this purpose we measured the rate of inactivation of the hybrid DNA by ultrasonic vibrations according to one or both genetic markers. Ultrasonic vibrations are well known to break simultaneously both strands of DNA (Litt, Marmur, Ephrussi-Taylor and Doty, 1958). The inactivation of a genetic marker is effected if the break hits the corresponding cistron. Closely linked markers as a rule are inactivated in one hit (Stuy, 1961; Bresler, Perumov and Kalinin, 1963). If both genetic markers are united in a four stranded complex, it is quite probable that under the action of ultrasonic vibration they would separate into two single active cistrons (Fig. 3). In this case we could expect a much higher rate of decrease of the double transformants number as compared with single transformants after the action of ultrasonic vibration. But our data (Fig. 4) show that both rates are practically identical. This result corroborates the formation of true double stranded hybrids – molecular heterozygotes – according to the mechanism proposed by Doty, Marmur *et al.*

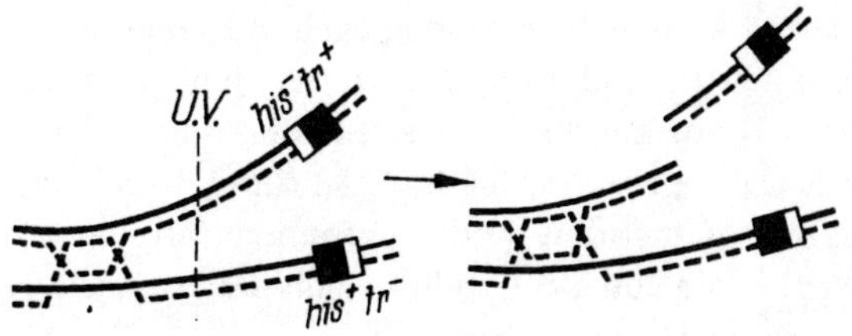

Fig. 3. The scheme of the separation of four stranded complexes by the action of ultrasonic vibration

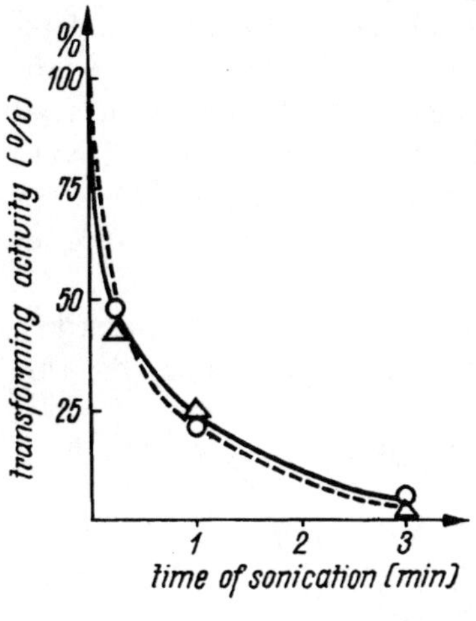

Fig. 4. Decrease of transforming activity of hybrid DNA for single *his*$^+$ (- - - ○ - - -) and double *his*$^+$, *tryp*$^+$ (—— △ ——) transformants after the action of ultrasonic vibrations Each point is the mean of 8 identical experiments

III. Transformation by two linked markers (*his*$^-$, *tryp*$^-$) under the action of hybrid molecules of DNA when the synthesis of DNA in recipient cells is excluded

As was pointed out above, the ultimate aim of this work is to investigate the possibility of double transformation by heterozygous molecules of DNA in such conditions when DNA synthesis in recipient cells is impossible. To fulfil this condition we washed thoroughly the recipient cells prior to transformation. The washing was done in SGM and was followed by 10 minutes starvation at 37° with aeration at a cell concentration 5×10^9 per ml. Then the transforming DNA was added. After 15 minutes of incubation with DNA the culture was washed still once to eliminate DNA and traces of proteins. To make sure that in such conditions the DNA synthesis is stopped, we used as a control the DNA from the recipient strain instead of transforming DNA. After incubation with genetically inactive DNA (1 μg/ml) and washing in SGM the suspension of recipient cells was divided into two parts. One of them was stored at −10°, the second one was aerated for 15 hours at 37°. Then the concentration of DNA was measured in both samples using the diphenylamine method. As can be seen from data listed in Table 2 there was no increase and therefore no replication of DNA in the culture after aeration at 37°.

For a precise realisation of transformation in the absence of DNA synthesis it was necessary also to guarantee a complete absence of amino acids in the solid medium during the titration of double transformants. For this reason we did not use agar plates where traces of nutrients can not be excluded, and developed special minimal medium plates based on a silicate gel. The preparation of these plates was described above in the section „Materials and methods".

Table 2
Comparison of the DNA contents in a suspension of washed cells before and after the 15 hours aeration in SGM

NN of runs	Quantity of DNA (per ml of suspension) suspension kept at −10°	suspension aerated at 37°
1	120	115
2	90	90
3	88	88
4	89	89

The general scheme of the experiment follows. A suspension of competent cells of strain SB25 after washing and starvation in SGM at a concentration 5×10^9 cells per ml, was distributed in tubes with 0,03; 0,1; 0,3 and 1,0 μg/ml of hybridized DNA_{168} and DNA_{H25} with a ratio of components 1 : 1 and in a series of control tubes which contained the same quantities of a mixture of both DNA's, denatured and annealed separately. After 15 minutes of contact with DNA at 37° the cells were washed and resuspended in SGM at the same concentration. 0,5 ml of every sample with hybridized DNA was plated on the plates with silicate gel impregnated with SGM and similar plates, supplemented with very low amounts of limiting amino acids (1 μg/ml of each). The control samples with mixture of DNA's were also plated on the medium, containing microquantities of amino acids. These microquantities of limiting amino acids were sufficient to start the synthesis of DNA in the cells, but they did not allow auxotrophic cells to give visible colonies. On the plates we can see in these conditions the formation of a film of recipient cells. This film does not prevent the counting of double transformant colonies.

If the realisation of information transferred into a cell by a hybrid DNA molecule requires reduplication of DNA, we must find on the plates lacking the limiting amino acids only a few double transformants equal in number to the background measured in the same run by

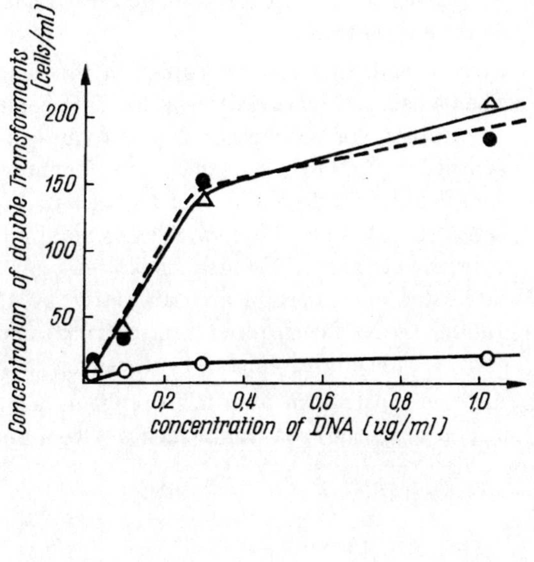

Fig. 5. Transformation of *Bacillus subtilis SB 25* by two linked markers *his* and *tryp* under the action of:

a) hybrid DNA; the synthesis of DNA in recipient cells is possible (---●---),
b) hybrid DNA; the synthesis of DNA is excluded (—— △ ——),
c) control mixture of DNA_{168} and DNA_{H25} (—— ○ ——)

Each point is the mean of 6 identical experiments

means of a mixture of DNA's. The results of these experiments are plotted in Fig. 5. We see that the number of double transformants after the interaction of cells with hybrid DNA is much higher then the background and does not depend on the presence of limiting amino acids. It follows that hybrid DNA molecules stimulate the ability of the cell to synthesize histidine and tryptophane and this phenomenon does not require a preceding reduplication of DNA.

Discussion

The above data seem to show that both strands of DNA are copied in the cell to make m-RNA molecules. The main point is that in our conditions of cell growth there could not be DNA replication prior to the synthesis of enzymes leading to histidine and tryptophane. The silicate gel plates contained a medium free of these amino acids. It was shown by aeration of auxotrophic bacteria in a similar but liquid medium that the amount of DNA remained constant after 20 hours. The analytical method has a precision of 1–3% and we can not exclude a DNA synthesis of this magnitude. Therefore, if the replication of hybrid DNA molecules is necessary prior to the formation of both enzymes, the amount of double transformants would be 30–100 times less then in conditions of allowed DNA replication. But that is not consistent with the data. There remains the possibility that the particular fragment of donor DNA integrated in the cell genome is replicated first. There are no plausible models to take into account this assumption. Can remain the objection that a DNA turnover may exist in starved cells without overall DNA synthesis. But this point was checked by RYAN, NAKADA and SCHNEIDER (1961), who showed that in 300 hours of amino acid starvation there was no noticeable isotope exchange of DNA in a bacterial culture with external medium. So DNA turnover may be excluded with the same precision as DNA synthesis. Therefore we think that our results give a proof of m-RNA synthesis, using both strands of DNA as templates. To explain how this is possible we may choose one of the alternatives:

1. Presumably both genes could be read in opposite directions which would make different strands of DNA active for these particular enzymes. This explanation seems not very plausible.

   The reduplication of DNA, prior to m-RNA synthesis is possible in the presence of both amino acids. This would give a doubling of the number of double transformants (curve 5a) comparing with the case without amino acid addition (curve 5b). Experiment does not confirm this idea.

2. Both strands of DNA are copied in the cell to make complementary m-RNA molecules. Then a new problem arises: whether both complementary m-RNA molecules are equivalent or in other words, whether any of them can serve as a template in ribosomes for protein synthesis (Fig. 1a). Available data for more than 40 codons are incompatible with the complementary degeneracy of the genetic code (JONES and NIRENBERG, 1962; WAHBA, GARDNER, BASILIO, MILLER, SPEYER and LENGYEL, 1963). Therefore we must suppose that only one of the m-RNA strands is used directly for protein synthesis; the second must be replicated once more to give an active m-RNA molecule (Fig. 1b). We can apply to the finding by NAKAMOTO and WEISS (1962) and FOX, ROBINSON and WEISS (1963) of an enzyme in bacteria, which is synthesizing complementary RNA chains on RNA templates.

3. Another mechanism of m-RNA replication is possible by which a third polyribonucleotide strand is synthesized complementary to a double helix of DNA. It means that a base of

newly synthesized m-RNA molecule is determined by both complementary bases of double stranded DNA template (Zubay, 1962). If a base pair in the DNA macromolecule is not complementary, as it is in molecular hybrids, it can nevertheless give the right base in the third m-RNA strand and an active enzyme will issue.

Summary

The role of both strands of the DNA double helix in the process of the information transfer for protein synthesis in living cell was investigated. For this purpose the transformation of *Bacillus subtilis SB25 his⁻ tryp⁻* by two linked genetic markers under the action of hybrid molecules of DNA was used. The molecular hybrids were obtained by thermal denaturation and annealing of a mixture of two DNA's, each one extracted from a single auxotrophic strain (*H25 his⁻* and *168 tryp⁻*). The formation of the heterozygous DNA double helices was proved by special experiments. The transformation procedure excluded DNA synthesis by recipient cells prior to the formation of enzymes for histidine and tryptophane synthesis. It was found that hybrid DNA molecules are able to transform in these conditions the double auxotrophic cells to prototrophic ones. Therefore we must assume that both strands of the DNA double helix can serve as templates for the m-RNA synthesis.

References

1. Bautz, E., and B. Hall, 1962: Proc. Nat. Acad. Sci., Wash. **48**, 400.
2. Brenner, S., F. Jacob and M. Meselson, 1961: Nature, **190**, 576.
3. Bresler, S. E., M. I. Mosevitskii and A. L. Timkovskii, 1963, Doklady Akademii Nauk SSSR, **149**, 721.
4. Bresler, S. E., D. A. Perumov and W. L. Kalinin, 1963: Biokhimya **28**, 907.
5. Chamberlin, M., and P. Berg, 1962: Proc. Nat. Acad. Sci., Wash. **48**, 81.
6. Champe, S., and S. Benzer, 1962: Proc. Nat. Acad. Sci., Wash. **48**, 532.
7. Doty, P., J. Marmur, J. Eigner and C. Schildkraut, 1960: Proc. Nat. Acad. Sci., Wash. **46**, 461.
8. Fox, C. F., W. S. Robinson and S. B. Weiss, 1963: Fed. Proc. **22**, 463.
9. Furth, J., J. Hurwitz and M. Goldman, 1961: Biochem. Biophys. Res. Comm., **4**, 362.
10. Furth, J., J. Hurwitz and M. Anders, 1962: Fed. Proc. **21**, 371.
11. Geiduschek, E., J. Moohr and S. Weiss, 1962: Proc. Nat. Acad. Sci., Wash. **48**, 1078.
12. Hayashi, M., and S. Spiegelman, 1961: Proc. Nat. Acad. Sci., Wash. **47**, 1564.
13. Herriott, R., 1961: Proc. Nat. Acad. Sci., Wash. **47**, 146.
14. Jacob, F., and J. Monod, 1961: J. Mol. Biol. **3**, 318.
15. Jones, O., and M. Nirenberg, 1962: Proc. Nat. Acad. Sci., Wash. **48**, 2115.
16. Litt, M., J. Marmur, H. Ephrussi-Taylor and P. Doty, 1958: Proc. Nat. Acad. Sci., Wash. **44**, 144.
17. Maaløe, O., 1961: Cold Spring Harbor Symposia Quant. Biol. **26**, 45.
18. Marmur, J. and D. Lane,. 1960: Proc. Nat. Acad. Sci., Wash. **46**, 453.
19. Nakamoto, T. and S. Weiss, 1962: Proc. Nat, Acad. Sci., Wash. **48**, 880.
20. Ning, C., and A. Stevens, 1962: J. Mol. Biol. **5**, 650.
21. Nomura, M., B. Hall and S. Spiegelman, 1960: J. Mol. Biol. **2**, 306.

22. PEACOCKE, A. and J. WALKER, 1962: J. Mol. Biol. **5**, 564.
23. RAVIN, A., 1961: J. Chim. Phys. **58**, 1107.
24. RYAN, F., D. NAKADA, and M. SCHNEIDER, 1961: Zeitschrift für Vererbungslehre **92**, 38.
25. SCHILDKRAUT, C., J. MARMUR, and P. DOTY, 1961: J. Mol. Biol. **3**, 595.
26. SIBATANI, A., S. de KLOET, V. ALLFREY and A. MIRSKY, 1962: Proc. Nat. Acad. Sci., Wash. **48**, 471.
27. SPIZIZEN, J., 1959: Feder. Proc. **18**, 957.
28. STEVENS, A., 1960: Biochem. Biophys. Res. Comm. **3**, 92.
29. STUY, J., 1961: Doctoral thesis. Utrecht. Netherlands.
30. VOLKIN, E., and L. ASTRACHAN, 1956: Virology **2**, 149.
31. VOLKIN, E., L. ASTRACHAN and J. COUNTRYMAN, 1958: Virology **6**, 545.
32. WAHBA, A., R. GARDNER, C. BASILIO, R. MILLER, J. SPEYER and P. LENGYEL, 1963. Proc. Nat. Acad. Sci., Wash. **49**, 116.
33. WEISS, S. and T. NAKAMOTO, 1961: Proc. Nat. Acad. Sci., Wash. **47**, 694.
34. WOOD, W. and P. BERG, 1962: Proc. Nat. Acad. Sci., Wash. **48**, 94.
35. ZUBAY, G., 1962: Proc. Nat. Acad. Sci., Wash. **48**, 456.

Zum Mechanismus der Proteinsynthese

Alfred Gierer

Max-Planck-Institut für Virusforschung, Tübingen

I. Einleitung

Orte der Proteinsynthese in der Zelle sind bekanntlich die Ribosomen, die zu je etwa der Hälfte aus Protein und Ribonukleinsäure bestehen. Es handelt sich um annähernd kugelförmige Partikel, die frei oder an Reticulum gebunden vorkommen können. Das Molekulargewicht beträgt 3–4 Millionen. Der Proteinanteil setzt sich aus vielen verschiedenartigen Molekülen zusammen; die Ribonukleinsäure liegt in Form eines oder zweier großer Moleküle vor.

Die Aktivierung der Aminosäure für die Peptidsynthese erfolgt außerhalb der Ribosomen im Zellplasma. Die Aminosäuren werden enzymatisch über eine Zwischenreaktion, bei der Adenosintriphosphat gespalten wird, an für die jeweiligen Aminosäuren spezifische kleine RNS, die Transfer-RNS, gebunden. Transfer-RNS besteht aus einer Kette von 80 Nukleotiden. Der RNS-Strang ist vermutlich rückgefaltet, so daß ein großer Teil des Moleküls ähnlich wie DNS zweisträngig ist. Die Länge des Moleküls wäre bei einer derartigen Struktur 140 Å, der Durchmesser etwa 20 Å. Das mit einer Aminosäure beladene Transfer-RNS-Molekül wird vom Ribosom gebunden und gibt die aktivierte Aminosäure an die wachsende Peptidkette ab.

Die Bestimmung der Reihenfolge der Aminosäuren im Protein erfolgt primär durch die Struktur des genetischen Materials, d. h. durch die Nukleotidsequenz von Zell- bzw. Virusnukleinsäure. Dies geschieht jedoch nicht direkt; vielmehr wird das genetische Material abschnittsweise durch neusynthetisierte RNS, die Messenger-RNS, kopiert. Sie vereinigt sich mit den Ribosomen und bestimmt dort die Sequenz des an den betreffenden Ribosomen synthetisierten Proteins. Ribosomen sind also selbst unspezifisch in bezug auf das zu synthetisierende Protein und nur in Verbindung mit Messenger-RNS aktiv. Messenger-RNS ist kein konstitutiver Bestandteil des Ribosoms, zeigt einen wesentlich höheren Umsatz in der Zelle als die Struktur-RNS der Ribosomen und kann leicht (durch Mg^{++}-Entzug oder Ribonuklease) von den Ribosomen abgelöst werden.

Die Rolle der Ribosomen bei der Proteinsynthese, das Zusammenspiel von Ribosom, Transfer-RNS, Messenger-RNS und wachsender Peptidkette, ist noch weitgehend ungeklärt. Die folgenden Abschnitte befassen sich mit zwei Aspekten der Ribosomenfunktion, der Bindung der wachsenden Peptidkette an das Ribosom und der Bindung von Ribosomen an Messenger-RNS. Anschließend werden mögliche Modelle der Ribosomenfunktion diskutiert.

II. Bindung der wachsenden Peptidketten an Ribosomen

Zum Studium der Proteinsynthese haben sich neben Bakterienzellen die Reticulocyten von Kaninchen als besonders geeignet erwiesen. Diese Zellen enthalten keinen Kern und keine DNS. Dagegen enthalten sie Ribosomen und synthetisieren Protein, wovon 85% Haemoglobin sind. Ribosomen werden jedoch nicht neu synthetisiert, so daß bei Einbauversuchen mit radioaktiven Aminosäuren in der Ribosomenfraktion nur die wachsenden Peptidketten, nicht aber die Strukturproteine der Ribosomen radioaktiv markiert werden. Die Proteinsynthese wurde in Versuchen mit ganzen Zellen (Kruh und Borsook, 1956) und mit isolierten Zellkomponenten (Schweet *et al.*, 1958) nachgewiesen.

Aus den Untersuchungen von Dintzis (1961) über die Proteinsynthese in Reticulocyten ergab sich, daß die Peptidketten vom Amino- zum Carboxylende linear wachsen. Die polymerisierenden Aminosäuren werden also jeweils mit ihrer (unaktivierten) Aminogruppe, nicht mit ihrer aktivierten Carboxylgruppe an die wachsende Kette angelagert. Um die Peptidbindung zu schließen, muß daher das Carboxylende der wachsenden Kette selbst aktiviert sein. Diese Aktivierung stammt ursprünglich von der Bindung der jeweils endständigen Aminosäure an ihre Transfer-RNS. Ist die Bindung zur nächsten aktivierten Aminosäure auf Kosten der Aktivierung der endständigen Carboxylgruppe der wachsenden Kette geschlossen, so ist das neue Carboxylende durch die Bindung der neuen Aminosäure an ihre Transfer-RNS wiederum aktiviert, und der Wachstumsprozeß kann in gleicher Weise weitergehen. Verschiedene Möglichkeiten des Wachstumsmechanismus sind zu diskutieren:

1. Im einfachsten Fall hängt die wachsende Peptidkette immer an Transfer-RNS. Am Elementarschritt des Wachstums um eine Aminosäure sind zwei Transfer-RNS Moleküle direkt beteiligt, die beide an das Ribosom gebunden sein müssen: die Transfer-RNS, an der die Peptidkette und die Transfer-RNS, an der die nächste Aminosäure hängt. Das Wachstum besteht in einer direkten Übertragung der Kette von der einen Transfer-RNS auf die Aminosäure der nächsten (Nathans und Lipmann, 1961):

$$\begin{aligned} &\mathrm{AS_1\,AS_2 \cdots AS_n\ T\text{-}RNS_n + AS_{n+1}\ T\text{-}RNS_{n+1}} \\ \longrightarrow\ &\mathrm{AS_1\,AS_2 \cdots AS_{n+1}\ T\text{-}RNS_{n+1} + T\text{-}RNS_n} \end{aligned} \tag{1}$$

   (AS_n n-te Aminosäure der Peptidkette, T-RNS_n zugehörige Transfer-RNS).

2. Neben diesem einfachsten Schema sind Zwischenreaktionen denkbar. Insbesondere könnte die wachsende Kette von der Transfer-RNS auf eine Komponente X des Ribosoms übertragen werden:

$$\begin{aligned} &\mathrm{AS_1\,AS_2 \cdots AS_n\text{-}X + AS_{n+1}\ T\text{-}RNS_{n+1}} \\ \longrightarrow\ &\mathrm{AS_1\,AS_2 \cdots AS_{n+1}\ T\text{-}RNS_{n+1} + X} \\ \longrightarrow\ &\mathrm{AS_1\,AS_2 \cdots AS_{n+1} - X + T\text{-}RNS_{n+1}} \end{aligned} \tag{2}$$

   Daraus folgt, daß zu jedem Zeitpunkt ein Teil der wachsenden Peptidketten an Transfer-RNS gebunden ist.

Wir haben zusammen mit Dr. F. Herzfeld (1963) eine Bindung der Peptidketten an kleine RNS von der Größe der Transfer-RNS nachgewiesen. Dies steht in Einklang mit ähnlichen Ergebnissen von Gilbert (1963b) bei Bakterien.

Um diese Bindung nachzuweisen, wurden Reticulocyten mit radioaktiven Aminosäuren inkubiert und die Ribosomen daraus isoliert. Die Ribosomen wurden bei 70° 1 min. mit einer Lösung von 40% Phenol und 4 M Harnstoff behandelt, sodann wurde 8 M Harnstoff zugegeben und abgekühlt. Ein Teil des Ribosomenproteins fiel dabei aus und wurde abzentrifugiert. Aus dem Überstand wurde durch Alkoholfällung und Lösung des Präzipitats in 0.02 Phosphatpuffer eine Fraktion gewonnen, die neben ribosomaler RNS und Protein etwa die Hälfte der ursprünglich in den Ribosomen enthaltenen Radioaktivität aufwies. Der größte Teil der wachsenden Kette lag demnach in löslicher Form vor und konnte weiter untersucht werden. Die ribosomale RNS war nur bis herab zu einem Molekulargewicht von 300000 degradiert. Transfer-RNS konnte infolge ihres kleineren Molekulargewichtes nicht degradiert sein.

Untersuchungen des Sedimentationsverhalts der radioaktiven Komponente in der analytischen Ultrazentrifuge und im Saccharosegradienten zeigen, daß die Peptidketten in einer Fraktion enthalten sind, deren Sedimentationskonstante 5–6 S beträgt. Diese Fraktion enthält auch RNS: Behandlung mit RNase macht einen Teil der radioaktiven Komponenten unlöslich, während der lösliche Teil so langsam (1–2 S) sedimentiert, wie man es von isolierten Peptiden erwartet. Entsprechende Ergebnisse wurden nach Behandlung mit Hydroxylamin erhalten.

Es wird geschlossen, daß die wachsenden Peptide an RNS gebunden sind. Die Spaltbarkeit der Bindung durch Hydroxylamin deutet auf eine Bindung des Carboxylendes der Peptidkette an RNS hin (ähnlich der Bindung von Aminosäuren an Transfer-RNS). Das Molekulargewicht der gebundenen RNS ist von mindestens der gleichen Größenordnung wie das der Peptide: in CsCl-Lösung sedimentieren radioaktive Komponenten noch bei Dichten bis zu 1,8. Reines Protein besitzt in CsCl eine Dichte von etwa 1,3, RNS von etwa 2,1. Verbindungen von Peptiden und RNS mit einer Dichte, die größer als 1,8 ist, bestehen vermutlich überwiegend aus RNS. Da die Sedimentationskonstante der Verbindung 5–6 S, die der Peptide 1–2 S beträgt, erwartet man etwa 4–5 S für die Nukleinsäurekomponenten allein. Dies entspricht der Größe von Transfer-RNS. Somit ist die Bindung der wachsenden Peptidketten an RNS von der Größe der Transfer-RNS gezeigt. Daß es sich chemisch um Transfer-RNS handelt, ist nicht bewiesen. Das Resultat ist konsistent mit den oben beschriebenen einfachen Vorstellungen vom Mechanismus des Peptidkettenwachstums (Gleichungen 1 und 2).

III. Aggregation von Ribosomen durch Messenger-RNS

Messenger-RNS verbindet mehrere Ribosomen zu aktiven Aggregaten (GIERER, 1963). Das gleiche Resultat erhielten unabhängig SPYRIDES und LIPMAN (1962) sowie GILBERT (1963a) für Bakterien und WARNER, KNOPF und RICH (1963) für Reticulocyten.

In Lysaten von Reticulocyten bzw. in deren frisch präparierten Ribosomenfraktion finden sich im Sedimentationsdiagramm neben monomeren Ribosomen mit einer Sedimentationskonstante von 80 S und kleineren Bruchstücken (40 S und 60 S) eine Reihe von mindestens fünf schneller sedimentierenden Komponenten (120–220 S). Entsprechende Resultate erhält man bei der Trennung der Ribosomen durch Zentrifugation im Saccharosegradienten. Etwa ein Drittel bis die Hälfte der Ribosomen ist in den schneller sedimentierenden Komponenten enthalten. Ribonuklease bringt die schnell sedimentierenden Komponenten zum Verschwinden. Der größte Teil des Materials erscheint dann in der 80 S Fraktion; weniger als 4% der Gesamtnukleinsäure bzw. weniger als 10% der Nukleinsäure der schnellen Komponenten, erscheinen in einer sehr langsam sedimentierenden Fraktion als kleine Nukleotide und Polynukleotide. Es kann geschlossen werden, daß es sich bei den schnell sedimentierbaren Fraktionen um Aggregate von 2 bis zu mindestens 6 Ribosomen handelt, deren Aggregation durch Nukleinsäure bewirkt wird. Die durch Ribonuklease ablösbare Nukleinsäure entspricht höchstens einem Molekulargewicht von 200000 je aggregiertes Ribosom.

Die Funktion der Aggregate läßt sich sowohl durch Einbauexperimente mit ganzen Zellen und anschließender Trennung der Ribosomenfraktionen im Saccharosegradienten, als auch durch zellfreie Einbauversuche mit Ribosomen, die zuvor im Saccharosegradienten fraktioniert worden sind, untersuchen. In beiden Arten von Experimenten zeigen die Aggregate hohe, die einzelnen Ribosomen hingegen geringe Aktivität. Proteinsynthese erfolgt also überwiegend an Aggregaten.

Polyuridilsäure (Poly-U) ist bekanntlich Messenger-RNS für Polyphenylalanin. Die Stimulierung des Einbaus von radioaktivem Phenylalanin, die zuerst mit Bakterienribosomen nachgewiesen wurde, ergibt sich auch im Reticulocytensystem. Trennt man die Ribosomen vor der Inkubation mit Poly-U und Phenylalanin in die einzelnen Fraktionen, so weisen die Aggregate eine sehr geringe, die monomeren Ribosomen hingegen relativ und absolut eine sehr starke Stimulation des Phenylalanin-Einbaus durch Poly-U auf. Wenn man die monomeren Ribosomen mit Poly-U und radioaktivem Phenylalanin inkubiert, sodann isoliert und erneut fraktioniert, so findet sich ein großer Teil der Aktivität in Aggregaten.

Die Versuche führen zu folgenden Schlüssen:

1. Ein großer Teil der Ribosomen liegt in Aggregaten vor.
2. RNase wirkt desaggregierend, also sind die Ribosomen im Aggregat wahrscheinlich durch RNS verknüpft.
3. Nur die Aggregate synthetisieren Protein, also enthalten vermutlich nur die Aggregate Messenger-RNS.
4. Nur die einzelnen Ribosomen, die noch nicht mit Messenger-RNS beladen sind, nehmen neue Messenger-RNS auf.
5. Poly-U als Messenger-RNS verbindet einzelne inaktive Ribosomen zu aktiven Aggregaten.

Diese Experimente ebenso wie die parallelen Resultate der genannten anderen Arbeitsgruppen weisen somit daraufhin, daß bei der Proteinsynthese mehrere Ribosomen an ein und demselben Messenger-RNS-Molekül operieren.

IV. Zum Mechanismus der Proteinsynthese

Hinsichtlich der Rolle der Ribosomen bei der Proteinsynthese ist zwischen den Möglichkeiten einer statischen und einer dynamischen Beziehung des Ribosoms zur Messenger-RNS zu unterscheiden:

1. Die Messenger-RNS ist in ihrer ganzen Länge an Ribosomen gebunden, die Lage der Messenger-RNS zu den Ribosomen verändert sich im Laufe der Peptidsynthese nicht. Das Ribosom hat viele Zentren, an denen Transfer-RNS mit Messenger-RNS in Verbindung treten kann. Im Laufe der Peptidsynthese wird der Punkt des Wachstums von einem Zentrum zum nächsten verschoben. Ist die Zahl der Aminosäuren im Peptid größer als die Zahl der aktiven Zentren im Ribosom, so müssen mehrere Ribosomen hintereinander geschaltet sein, um ein Peptid zu synthetisieren. Auf diese Weise ließen sich die durch Messenger-RNS verbundenen Aggregate von Ribosomen erklären.

2. Messenger-RNS ist nur mit einer kleineren Gruppe von Nukleotiden an das Ribosom gebunden. Die Ribosomen bewegen sich mit ihren Transfer-RNS bindenden Zentren an der Messenger-RNS entlang, um Transfer-RNS in der durch die Messenger-RNS bestimmten Reihenfolge zu binden. Besitzt das Ribosom mehrere solche Zentren, so könnte es an der Messenger-RNS entlangrollen und ein Zentrum nach dem anderen mit ihr in Verbindung bringen.

Von besonderem Interesse erscheint die einfachste Lösung, daß die Synthese nur an einer spezialisierten Stelle stattfindet. Sie bindet Transfer-RNS, zieht den Nukleotidstrang der Messenger-RNS hindurch bzw. wandert an ihm entlang und verlängert mit jedem Elementarschritt – Versetzung gegenüber der Messenger-RNS um eine codierende Nukleotidgruppe, Bindung der entsprechenden nächsten Transfer-RNS – die Peptidkette um eine Aminosäure. Das Ribosom operiert gleichzeitig mit den beiden Strängen der Messenger-RNS und des Peptids in entfernter Analogie zum Mechanismus einer Nähmaschine. Es ist nicht notwendig, daß die Stellen der Peptidverknüpfung und der Messenger-RNS-Bindung nahe benachbart sind. Da ein Transfer-RNS-Molekül die gleiche Lineardimension (ca. 140 Å) besitzt wie das Ribosom selbst, könnten sich die beiden Vorgänge auch an entgegengesetzten Seiten des Ribosomenpartikels abspielen.

Obwohl andere Modelle nicht ausgeschlossen sind, bietet das zuletzt beschriebene Modell die einfachste Erklärung für die Rolle der Aggregate bei der Proteinsynthese: da die Bindung jeweils mit nur wenigen Nukleotiden erfolgt, können viele Ribosomen an einer Messenger-RNS zugleich operieren, um sie von einem Ende zum anderen her „abzulesen".

Für dieses Modell lassen sich die beiden im Abschnitt II diskutierten Mechanismen des Elementarschritts der Proteinsynthese, die mit der Bindung von Peptidketten an Transfer-RNS verträglich sind, wie folgt spezifizieren:

a) Bei der direkten Übertragung der Peptidkette von einem Transfer-RNS-Molekül zur Aminosäure des nächsten Transfer-RNS-Moleküls (Gleichung 1) besitzt das Ribosom zwei funktional gleiche Anlagerungsstellen für Transfer-RNS. Im Laufe seiner Synthese alterniert der Wachstumspunkt des Peptids zwischen diesen beiden Stellen am Ribosom.

b) Gibt es einen Zwischenschritt der Aminosäure-Anlagerung, bei der die Peptidkette von Transfer-RNS jeweils auf eine Komponente X des Ribosoms übertragen wird (Gleichung 2), so ist nur eine Anlagerungsstelle für Transfer-RNS auf dem Ribosom nötig. Nach der Übertragung der wachsenden Peptidkette von Transfer-RNS auf die Anlagerungsstelle X wird die Transfer-RNS freigesetzt, so daß dort die nächste, mit einer Aminosäure beladene Transfer-RNS gebunden werden kann.

Literaturzitate

DINTZIS, H., 1961: Proc. nat. Acad. Sci. U. S. A. **47**, 247.
GIERER, A., 1963: J. Mol. Biol. **6**, 148.
GILBERT, W., 1963a: J. Mol. Biol. **6**, 374.
GILBERT, W., 1963b: J. Mol. Biol. **6**, 389.
HERZFELD, F., 1963: Dissertation, Tübingen.
KRUH, J., and H. BORSOOK, 1956: J. Biol. Chem. **220**, 905.
NATHANS, D. and F. LIPMANN, 1961: Proc. nat. Acad. Sci. U. S. A. **47**, 497.
SCHWEET, R., H. LAMFROM, and E. ALLEN, 1958: Proc. nat. Acad. Sci. U. S. A. **44**, 1029.
SPYRIDES, G. J., and F. LIPMANN,, 1962: Proc. nat. Acad. Sci. U. S. A. **48**, 1977.
WARNER, J. R., P. M. KNOPF, and A. RICH, 1963: Proc. nat. Acad. Sci. U. S. A. **49**.

Untersuchungen über Mutanten und Stämme des Tabakmosaikvirus

H. G. Wittmann und B. Wittmann-Liebold

Max-Planck-Institut für Biologie, Abt. Melchers, Tübingen

Mit der Erkenntnis, daß die Nukleinsäuren das einzige – bisher bekannte – genetische Material darstellen, tauchte sehr bald die Frage auf, auf welche Weise die Primärstruktur der Proteine von den Nukleinsäuren determiniert wird. Es fehlte jedoch jahrelang ein erfolgreicher Zugang zur experimentellen Lösung dieses Problems. Er ist erst seit einigen Jahren möglich geworden, und zwar vor allem durch biochemische und genetische Forschungen auf sehr verschiedenen Gebieten, die hier in zeitlicher Reihenfolge aufgeführt sind: a) Proteinchemische Untersuchungen an Mutanten des Haemoglobins (Ingram, 1958) und des Tabakmosaikvirus (Wittmann, 1959, 1961, 1962; Tsugita und Fraenkel-Conrat, 1960, 1962); b) Polynukleotid-induzierte Peptidsynthese in einem zellfreien System von *Escherichia coli*, das zuerst von Matthaei und Nirenberg (1961) entwickelt und später von den Arbeitsgruppen um Ochoa und um Nirenberg sehr intensiv für Fragen des genetischen Codes benutzt wurde (Jones und Nirenberg, 1962; Wahba *et al.*, 1963); c) genetische Untersuchungen an der rII-Region des Bakteriophagen T4 (Crick *et al.*, 1961; Benzer und Champe, 1962); d) Untersuchungen über die Heterogenität der Transfer-RNS (Weisblum *et al.*, 1962; Sueoka und Yamane, 1962).

Die Untersuchungen an Mutanten des Tabakmosaikvirus (TMV), über die hier berichtet werden soll, wurden folgendermaßen ausgeführt: Man verändert die Nukleotidsequenz in der TMV-RNS durch Umwandlung einzelner Basen, isoliert nach Infektion geeigneter Wirtspflanzen die durch die Basenumwandlung entstandenen Mutanten und sucht im Hüllenprotein dieser Mutanten nach Aminosäureaustauschen. Durch Vergleiche der Art der Basenänderung in der RNS mit der Art der dadurch induzierten Aminosäureaustausche im Protein von zahlreichen Mutanten lassen sich eine Reihe von Schlüssen über den genetischen Code ziehen.

Vorraussetzung dafür sind u. a. mutagene Agentien, deren Wirkung auf die TMV-RNS möglichst genau bekannt ist. In den von uns durchgeführten Untersuchungen wurden TMV-Mutanten analysiert, die mit einer der drei folgenden mutagenen Substanzen erzeugt worden sind: 1. Salpetrige Säure: Die chemische Wirkung von salpetriger Säure auf die TMV-RNS und deren Inaktivierung wurde von Schuster und Schramm (1958) untersucht. Mundry und Gierer (1958) wiesen die Entstehung von Mutationen beim TMV durch salpetrige Säure nach und bewiesen den Eintreffer-Mechanismus. Die mutagene Wirkung beruht sehr wahrscheinlich: a. auf der Umwandlung von Cytosin in Uracil (C→U) und b. auf der von Adenin in Hypoxanthin und dessen Ablesung als Guanin (A→(H)→G). 2. Hydroxylamin: Die Behandlung von TMV-RNS mit Hydroxylamin ist je nach dem pH-Wert verschieden:

bei pH 6 wird vor allem Cytosin umgewandelt und zwar in Reaktionsprodukte, die als Uracil abgelesen werden können; bei pH 9 tritt eine Spaltung des Uracil-Ringes ein (SCHUSTER, 1961). Die Veränderungen bei pH 6 (C→U) sind mutagen, während nach Behandlung bei pH 9 keine Erhöhung der Mutationsrate nachgewiesen werden konnte (SCHUSTER und WITTMANN, 1963). 3. 5-Fluoruracil: Der Einbau von 5-Fluoruracil statt Uracil in die TMV-RNS, wobei über 50% des Uracils ersetzt werden können, führt zu Mutationen (KRAMER, WITTMANN und SCHUSTER, 1963) und zwar wahrscheinlich dadurch, daß das 5-Fluoruracil in seltenen Fällen als Cytosin statt als Uracil abgelesen wird.

Alle drei genannten mutagenen Substanzen wirken auch bei der DNS mutagen, wie bei Bakterien und Phagen nachgewiesen wurde (vgl. Übersichtsartikel von FREESE, 1963; ferner CHAMPE and BENZER, 1962).

Material und Methoden

Die methodischen Einzelheiten zur Erzeugung, Isolierung und Proteinanalyse der untersuchten Mutanten sind ausführlich beschrieben worden (WITTMANN, 1962; SCHUSTER und WITTMANN, 1963; KRAMER, WITTMANN und SCHUSTER, 1963). Daher soll hier nur auf das Prinzip der Methodik eingegangen werden.

Die Erzeugung der Mutanten geschieht bei den durch Nitrit bzw. Hydroxylamin induzierten Mutanten durch Behandlung in vitro und bei den durch 5-Fluoruracil induzierten Mutanten durch Vermehrung des Virus in Gegenwart von 5-Fluoruracil und Einbau des Basenanalogen in die TMV-RNS. Die Isolierung der Mutanten erfolgt über Läsionen (auf *Nicotiana tabacum* var. „Xanthi n. c.") und Einzelherdübertragungen auf einen systemischen Wirt (*Nicotiana tabacum* var. „Samsun").

Zur Gewinnung einer für die Analysen ausreichenden Virusproteinmenge werden die Mutanten im Gewächshaus auf *Nicotiana tabacum* var. Samsun vermehrt, das Virus wird isoliert, gereinigt und die RNS von dem Protein abgetrennt. Danach wird das Protein mit Trypsin gespalten, und die tryptischen Peptide werden säulen- und papierchromatographisch isoliert und gereinigt. Nach der Hydrolyse wird die quantitative Aminosäurezusammensetzung eines jeden Peptids in Aminosäureanalysatoren bestimmt und mit der des entsprechenden Peptids des Ausgangsstammes verglichen. Ergeben sich Unterschiede, so wird die genaue Position des Aminosäureaustauschs mit den Methoden der Sequenzanalyse lokalisiert.

Ergebnisse und Diskussion

Mit diesen Methoden wurden bisher etwa 150 Mutanten untersucht, wovon die weitaus meisten Nitritmutanten sind (Tab. 1). Dazu kommen noch die durch 5-Fluoruracil induzierten Mutanten, die in Tab. 1 nicht aufgeführt sind, da die Analyse dieser Mutanten noch nicht abgeschlossen ist.

Es ist auffallend, daß ein großer Teil der Mutanten keine Aminosäureaustausche aufweist, obgleich die Symptome oft sehr stark von denen des Ausgangsstamms verschieden sind (WITTMANN, 1959). Dieser Befund führte zu der Erkenntnis, daß nicht die gesamte TMV-RNS mit 6500 Nukleotiden für die Determinierung des TMV-Hüllenproteins notwendig ist, sondern nur ein Anteil. Die TMV-RNS besteht also aus mehreren Cistra, von denen nur eines das Hüllenprotein determiniert. Nur dann, wenn ein oder mehrere Nukleotide in diesem Cistron geändert werden, kann sich dies in einem Austausch von Aminosäuren im Hüllenprotein bemerkbar machen.

Tabelle 1
Zusammenstellung der bisher analysierten TMV-Mutanten

Austausche	Zahl der Mutanten		
	Nitrit-	Hydroxylamin-	Spontan-
0	96	5	8
1	33	1	5
2	7	0	2
3	0	0	1
>3	0	0	0
Summe:	136	6	16

Aus der durchschnittlichen Zahl von Nukleotidveränderungen pro RNS-Strang, die experimentell bestimmbar ist, und der durchschnittlichen Zahl von Aminosäureaustauschen pro Mutante läßt sich unter Berücksichtigung von Selektionsfaktoren die Größe des Cistrons für das Hüllenprotein und damit auch das Kodierungsverhältnis abschätzen. Diese Abschätzung (Wittmann, 1962) ergibt eine unabhängige Bestätigung für die aus genetischen Untersuchungen an der rII-Region des Bakteriophagen T4 erhaltene Folgerung, daß ein Triplett-Code wahrscheinlicher ist als ein Code mit einer Zahl von Nukleotiden pro Kodierungseinheit, die ein Mehrfaches von drei ist.

Die Verteilung der Aminosäureaustausche auf die Zahl der Nitritmutanten entspricht der Poisson-Verteilung. Es ist bemerkenswert, daß wir bislang nie eine chemisch induzierte Mutante mit mehr als zwei Austauschen gefunden haben. Bei den von Tsugita und Fraenkel-Conrat (1962) untersuchten angeblichen Mutanten mit zahlreichen Austauschen dürfte es sich aus verschiedenen Gründen (Wittmann, 1962) höchstwahrscheinlich um in der Natur vorkommende Stämme handeln, die in geringer Menge in dem Ausgangsmaterial vorhanden waren, und die durch die angewendete Isolierungsmethode herausselektioniert wurden.

Bei denjenigen Nitritmutanten, die zwei Austausche pro Proteinkette aufweisen, liegen diese Austausche in keinem Fall in benachbarten, sondern stets in weit voneinander entfernten Positionen (Abb. 1). Dieser Befund spricht sehr stark für einen nicht überlappenden Code.

Wie aus Tab. 2 hervorgeht, ist bei Nitritmutanten eine Häufung von bestimmten Aminosäureaustauschen zu beobachten. So ist Threonin insgesamt zwölfmal ausgetauscht, doch nur gegen zwei Aminosäuren und zwar gegen Isoleucin (neunmal in vier verschiedenen tryptischen Peptiden) und gegen Methionin. Ähnliches gilt auch für andere Austausche der Tab. 2. Bei Spontanmutanten und bei Fluoruracil-Mutanten wurden auch andere Austausche als bei den Nitritmutanten gefunden.

Aus der Kombination der in Tab. 2 aufgeführten Aminosäureaustausche mit den durch Nitritbehandlung möglichen Triplettveränderungen folgt, daß der genetische Code, mindestens für einen Teil der Aminosäuren, degeneriert ist (Wittmann, 1961). Über den Grad der Degeneration lassen sich aus dem Vergleich der Zahl der durch Nitritbehandlung theoretisch möglichen mit der Zahl der tatsächlich beobachteten Aminosäureaustausche folgende Schlüsse ziehen: Entweder ist das Ausmaß der Degeneration nicht sehr hoch, oder aber im Falle eines hoch degenerierten Codes sind diejenigen Tripletts, die dieselbe Aminosäure

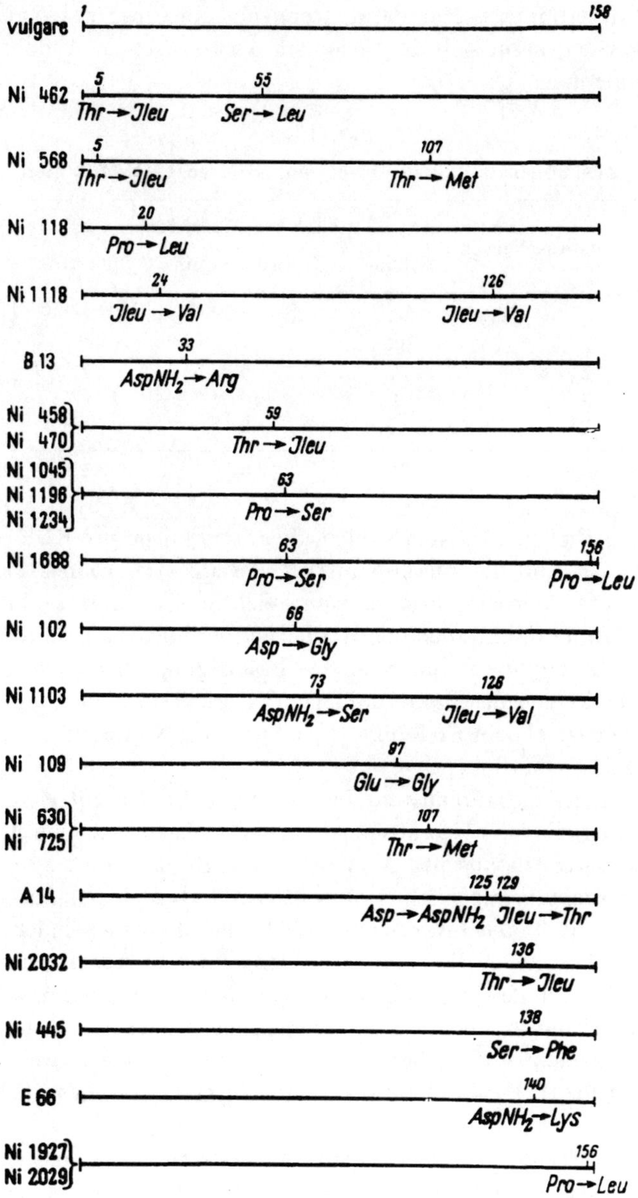

Abb. 1. Lokalisierung der Aminosäureaustausche bei TMV-Mutanten

Die mit Ni . . . bezeichneten Mutanten sind durch Behandlung mit salpetriger Säure isoliert, die übrigen sind Spontanmutanten

determinieren, nicht eine zufallsgemäße Auswahl von den 64 möglichen Tripletts (Wittmann, 1962). Die neuen, aus Versuchen im zellfreien *E. coli*-System gewonnenen Ergebnisse (Jones und Nirenberg, 1962; Wahba *et al.*, 1963) sprechen stark für die zweite Alternative. Dasselbe gilt für die von Crick *et al.* (1961) durchgeführten genetischen Untersuchungen am Bakteriophagen T4.

Die zahlreichen beobachteten Aminosäureunterschiede im Hüllenprotein von TMV-Mutanten und Stämmen lassen sich in Kombination mit der aus dem zellfreien *E. coli*-System erschlossenen Nukleotidzusammensetzung der Tripletts dazu benutzen, eine Nukleotidreihenfolge innerhalb der Tripletts in erster Annäherung festzulegen (WITTMANN-LIEBOLD und WITTMANN, 1963b).

Aus dem Vergleich der Ergebnisse, die an Nitritmutanten des TMV und bei der polynukleotid-induzierten Peptidsynthese im zellfreien System gewonnen wurden, folgt, daß der infizierende TMV-RNS-Strang (oder ein Strang mit identischer Nukleotidsequenz) und nicht ein komplementärer Strang als Matrize für die Synthese des TMV-Hüllenproteins dient (WITTMANN, 1962).

Die Aminosäuresequenz des TMV-Stamms *dahlemense*, der von einer Freiland-Tomatenkultur durch MELCHERS (1940) isoliert wurde, unterscheidet sich bei gleicher Zahl der Aminosäuren pro Proteinkette von dem TMV-Stamm *vulgare* in insgesamt 30 der 158 Aminosäurepositionen (WITTMANN-LIEBOLD und WITTMANN, 1963a). Es handelt sich hierbei um den ersten Fall, in dem die vollständige Aminosäuresequenz zweier Virusstämme verglichen werden kann.

Tabelle 2
Aminosäureaustausche bei Nitritmutanten

Austausch	im Peptid	Zahl der Mutanten
Thr → Ileu	I	2
,, → ,,	III	2
,, → ,,	X	4
,, → ,,	XI	1
,, → Met	VIII	3
Ser → Phe	I	1
,, → ,,	XI	3
,, → Leu	I	1
,, → ,,	III	1
Asp* → Ser	I	2
AspN → ,,	VI	1
,, → ,,	XI	1
Asp* → Gly	I	2
Asp → ,,	IV	2
,, → Ala	I	4
Ileu → Val	I	1
,, → ,,	X	2
,, → Met	I	1
Pro → Ser	IV	4
,, → Leu	I	1
,, → ,,	XII	3
Leu → Phe	I	1
Glu* → Val	I	2
Glu → Gly	VIII	1
		46

*) Amid oder freie Carboxylgruppe

Literatur

BENZER, S., and S. W. CHAMPE, 1962: Proc. Nat. Acad. Sci. **48**, 1114.
CHAMPE, S. W., and S. BENZER, 1962: Proc. Nat. Acad. Sci. **48**, 532.
CRICK, F. H. C., L. BARNETT, S. BRENNER, and R. J. WATTS-TOBIN, 1961: Nature **192**, 1227.
FREESE, E., 1963: in: Molecular Genetics, ed. by J. H. Taylor, Acad. Press, New York, p. 207–270.
INGRAM, V. M., Proc. IV. Internat. Congr. Biochem. Vienna 1958, Symposium VIII, p. 95–106.
JONES, O. W., and M. W. NIRENBERG, 1962: Proc. Nat. Acad. Sci. **48**, 2115.
KRAMER, G., H. G. WITTMANN und M. W. SCHUSTER, Z. Naturforschg. **19b**, 46.
MATTHAEI, J. H., and M. W. NIRENBERG, 1961: Proc. Nat. Acad. Sci. **47**, 1580.
MELCHERS, G., 1940: Biol. Zbl. **60**, 527.
MUNDRY, K. W. und A. GIERER, 1958: Z. f. Vererbungslehre **89**, 614.
SCHUSTER, H., 1961: J. mol. Biol. **3**, 447.
SCHUSTER, H., und G. SCHRAMM, 1958: Zeitschr. f. Naturforschg. **13** b, 697.
SCHUSTER, H., and H. G. WITTMANN, 1963: Virology **19**, 421.
SUEOKA, N., and T. YAMANE, 1962: Proc. Nat. Acad. Sci. **48**, 1454.
TSUGITA, A., and H. FRAENKEL-CONRAT, 1960: Proc. Nat. Acad. Sci. **46**, 636; 1962: J. mol. Biol. **4**, 73.

WAHBA, A. J., R. S. MILLER, C. BASILIO, R. S. GARDNER, P. LENGYEL, and J. F. SPEYER, 1963: Proc. Nat. Acad. Sci. **49**.

WEISBLUM, B., S. BENZER, and R. W. HOLLEY, 1962: Proc. Nat. Acad. Sci. **48**, 1449.

WITTMANN-LIEBOLD, B., und H. G. WITTMANN, Zeitschr. f. Naturforschg. (im Druck) 1963: Zeitschr. f. Vererbungsl. **94**, 427.

WITTMANN, H. G., 1959: Z. f. Vererbungslehre **90**, 463; 1961: Naturwissenschaften **48**, 729; 1962: Zeitschr. f. Vererbungsl. **93**, 491.

Studies on Rapidly Labelled RNA in HeLa Cells

M. Hill*, D. Winkelmans**, A. Miller-Faurés and M. Errera

Laboratoire de Biophysique et Radiobiologie, Faculté des Sciences, Université libre de Bruxelles

The problem of the biosynthesis of ribonucleic acids is far from being solved in spite of the great progress made in recent years. After the clear demonstration by Brachet (1957) of the role of the cell nucleus in cytoplasmic RNA synthesis, many authors have approached the problem from a variety of angles which have led to the concept of three major classes of RNA's, which it is no more necessary to define (Grunberg-Manago, 1962): messenger RNA's (m RNA), ribosomal RNA's (r RNA) and aminoacid transfer RNA's (s RNA).

The requirement of a DNA primer for m RNA synthesis seems obvious, as does its dependency on nuclear function. These relationships do not seem quite as clear for r RNA and s RNA. In the case of r RNA synthesis it was shown by Perry (1960) and Perry *et al.* (1961a, b) that the nucleolus plays an important role in cytoplasmic RNA synthesis which is mostly ribosomal, but this does not exclude the participation of nucleolar associated DNA, as pointed out by the authors and as shown on plant cells by Rho and Bonner (1961). The fact that r RNA is capable of hybridizing with DNA reinforces the idea that its synthesis is DNA dependent (Yanofsky and Spiegelman, 1962). In the case of s RNA the situation is still less clear, but as the incorporation of pseudouridine triphosphate into an s RNA-like molecule is DNA dependent, and since s RNA also hybridizes with small sequences of DNA, there are some reasons to believe that a least part of s RNA synthesis is also DNA dependent (Goldberg and Rabinowitz, 1961; Spiegelman, 1963).

We therefore thought that it might be worth-while to approach the problem of RNA synthesis by studying the distribution of cellular RNA in various cell fractions after a brief exposure to the tracer, and to investigate its ultimate fate. The present study concerns only the rapidly formed RNA components (5–30 minutes) analyzed by sedimenting a whole cell homogenate in a sucrose gradient; therefore, in these experiments all the rapidly labelled RNA can be accounted for. Furthermore, some of the cell fractions analyzed were studied by electron microscopy and demonstrated the existence of polysomes.

---

* Research fellow of the International Atomic Energy Agency (Vienna), present address: Institute of Biophysics, Czechoslovak Academy of Sciences, Brno, Czechoslovakia.

** Present address: Laboratorio Internazionale di Genetica e Biofisica, Napoli, Italy.

Material and Methods

Cell Cultures

HeLa cells are used in all the present studies and we are grateful to the Institut Pasteur du Brabant for giving us the cell line and for helping us in making the culture media. The cells are cultured in the media described previously (Perry *et al.*, 1961a, b; Srinivasan *et al.*, 1963) in Roux flasks. The complete medium ($\varnothing_{10}$) used for breeding the cells is changed to Eagles medium 2 hours before the start of an experiment. Cells are usually taken when they are nearing the end of the logarithmic phase of growth, but are still in monocellular layers.

RNA labelling

The cells are labelled in Roux flasks for the appropriate time with adenine ^{14}C, dissolved in Eagles medium (1 μc/ml). They are incubated with the precursor in a water bath at 37 °C and are chilled to 0–2 °C immediately after, and washed twice with cold Eagles solution containing 200 μg/ml of non labelled adenine.

Reagents used routinely

Tris Mg buffer: 0.05 M Tris (hydroxymethyl) aminomethane 0.025 M KCl, $5 \cdot 10^{-3}$ M $MgCl_2$, pH 7.45.
Phosphate Mg buffer: 0.0011 M Na phosphate, $5 \cdot 10^{-4}$ M $MgCl_2$, pH 7.45.
Deoxyribonuclease: Nutritional Biochemicals (2 × crystallized).
Ribonuclease: Sigma (5 × crystallized).
Adenine 8 ^{14}C sulphate (Amersham), 28.3 mC/mM.
L. Lysine ^{14}C monohydrochloride (Amersham), 307 mC/mM.
Actinomycin D was a generous gift from Dr. K. Folkers of Merck, Sharp and Dohme Research Laboratories

Homogenization

After washing the labelled monolayers of cells in Eagles medium, they are harvested with glass beads, collected by a 5 minutes centrifugation at 1.500 rpm, then washed again with cold Eagles solution containing non labelled adenine. Usually, for good optical density measurements of the centrifugation fractions, about $5 \cdot 10^7$ cells are needed. They are dispersed in 1.2 to 1.5 ml tris Mg buffer or phosphate Mg buffer to which is added sodium desoxycholate

(5 p. c. in H_2O) and Bentonite (5 mgr per ml), prepared according to FRAENKEL-CONRAT *et. al.* (1961) in a final concentration of 1 p. c. and 0.5 mgr/ml respectively. The buffers are adjusted to pH 7.45. The cells are dispersed by pipetting and a few crystals of deoxyribonuclease are added in order to decrease the viscosity; after 30 to 60 minutes, the homogenate is ready for gradient centrifugation.

Sucrose gradient centrifugation

Linear sucrose gradients are prepared, according to BRITTEN and ROBERTS (1960), from 14.2 ml of 5 p. c. (or 15 p. c.) sucrose and 13.4 ml of 20 p. c. (or 30 p. c.) sucrose made up in the same buffer used for homogenization. The cell homogenates are layered on top of the sucrose gradients and are centrifuged in 34 ml lucite tubes in the swinging bucket rotor 25 of a Spinco model L preparative ultracentrifuge at 24.000 rpm. When 5–20 p. c. sucrose gradients were used, the duration of centrifugation was of 4.5 hours; with the 15–30 p. c. sucrose gradients, the centrifugation lasted for only 2 hours. After centrifugation, 45 to 50 fractions are collected in 10 ml test tubes and assayed for optical density (0.15 ml + 0.75 ml H_2O) and the remaining ($\pm$ 0.35 ml) are prepared for radioactivity counting. To enable the comparison of the graphs, the abscissae representing the gradient were always taken of a constant length independently of the number of fractions. Afterwards, for simplicity's sake, the abscissae were divided into 50 arbitrary fractions.

Radioactivity counting

To an aliquot of each fraction ($\pm$ 0.35 ml), 0.3 ml of a bovine serum albumin solution (0.4 mgr/ml in tris or phosphate buffer) and 2.0 ml of 5 p. c. trichloracetic acid are added. The total suspensions are filtered on 25 mm Millipore filters (HA 0.45 μ), washed twice with 2 ml of 5 p. c. trichloracetic acid, then dried at 37 °C in the oven (2 hours). The Millipore filters carrying the radioactive precipitates are then put into standard counting vials containing 5 ml of scintillation solution (0.5 p. c. P. O. P. and 0.05 P. O. P. O. P.). The counting is made in a model 725 Nuclear Chicago scintillation counter.

Fixation for electron microscopy

After having established the O. D. profile in the gradient by analyzing the fractions in the usual manner, small aliquots of the selected fractions (0.2–0.4 ml) are dispersed in an equal volume of the following fixing solution: phosphate Mg buffer containing 12 p. c. sucrose and 1 p. c. osmium tetroxide. Fixation lasts for 10–20 hours at 4 °C after which a droplet of the suspension is carefully transferred to a grid coated with collodion and carbon, and air dried. In order to get rid of the dried sucrose the grids are transferred successively for 30 seconds in sucrose solutions of decreasing concentration (12 p. c., 10 p. c., 5 p. c.,

3 p. c.) followed by a wash in buffer and lastly in distilled water. The grids are finally platinum shadowed by the standard procedure. All the observations were made on a Hitachi model HS-G microscope at a magnification of $\times$ 16.000.

Results

A. Pulse labelling

Typical profiles of the centrifugation gradients are presented in Fig. 1. These result from 5 and 10 minutes adenine ^{14}C incorporation and the total cell homogenate is fractionated on a 5 to 20 p. c. sucrose gradient. The peak of optical density lies in the 74 S region (ribosomes) (Penman *et al.*, 1963), the optical density in the light part of the gradient is obscured by the digestion products of DNA. A preliminary run with the analytical ultracentrifuge kindly performed by Dr. Hamers indicated that the major peak of cytoplasmic ribosomes has a sedimentation constant of 73.5 S and it is assumed that in these runs the major peak consists essentially of this type of ribosomes. The smaller peaks in the lighter region have sedimentation constants of $\sim$ 50 S and $\sim$ 30 S (ribosomal constituents). Another peak at 16 S was also detected (free RNA?).

It can be seen that 2 distinct radioactivity regions are observed. A light fraction remains near the surface of the gradient in the 4–20 S region and contains almost certainly some s RNA either in its final form or as a precursor of s RNA. The lighter part of the gradient has not been further studied and it is not possible for us to identify the heterogeneous 6–20 S fractions with a base distribution reminiscent of HeLa DNA demonstrated by Penman *et al.* (1963), because these RNA's would probably be confluent with the lighter peaks. A heavy fraction contains radioactivity which sediments as far as the bottom of the tube and consists of a heterogeneous component with a wide and irregular peak in the region sedimenting between the 50 S and the 30 S particles (Fig. 1a, b, c). This RNA is very sensitive to ribonuclease (Fig. 1c) and the heavy fractions disappear when the cells are homogenized in the absence of an inhibitor of this enzyme. This was observed repeatedly in attempts to characterize nuclear and cytoplasmic rapidly labelled RNA by density gradient centrifugation. In the nuclear fraction the main peak is in the 4 S region with irregular tailing towards 25–30 S. In the cytoplasmic fraction only a small 4 S peak is observed in 10 minutes incubated cells.

This newly formed RNA (fraction 1–35) can reasonably be assumed to be the heavy RNA of Perry (1962) and the 45 S and 35 sRNA's of Scherrer *et al.* (1963). There could still be some free RNA sedimenting as far as the 74 S zone because both these authors found that „nex" RNA still sediments down to the bottom of their gradients. The heavier part of this heterogeneous fraction (> 74 S) has further been analyzed in a 15–30 p. c. sucrose gradient in order to obtain more details. Fig. 2 shows that an important part of the rapidly labelled RNA ($\sim$ 40 to 50 p. c.) still migrates faster than the 74 S components. This is unlikely to be free RNA, because the single stranded regions would probably be mechanically broken for such heavy molecules during the preparation of the samples. This RNA could be bound to cellular structures or other macro-molecules. Perry (1962, 1963) showed that in the presence of very small amounts of actinomycin D ($5 \cdot 10^{-8}$ M) there was a decrease of all the radioactivity of 30 minutes labelled RNA's sedimenting faster than 10 S, as well as an

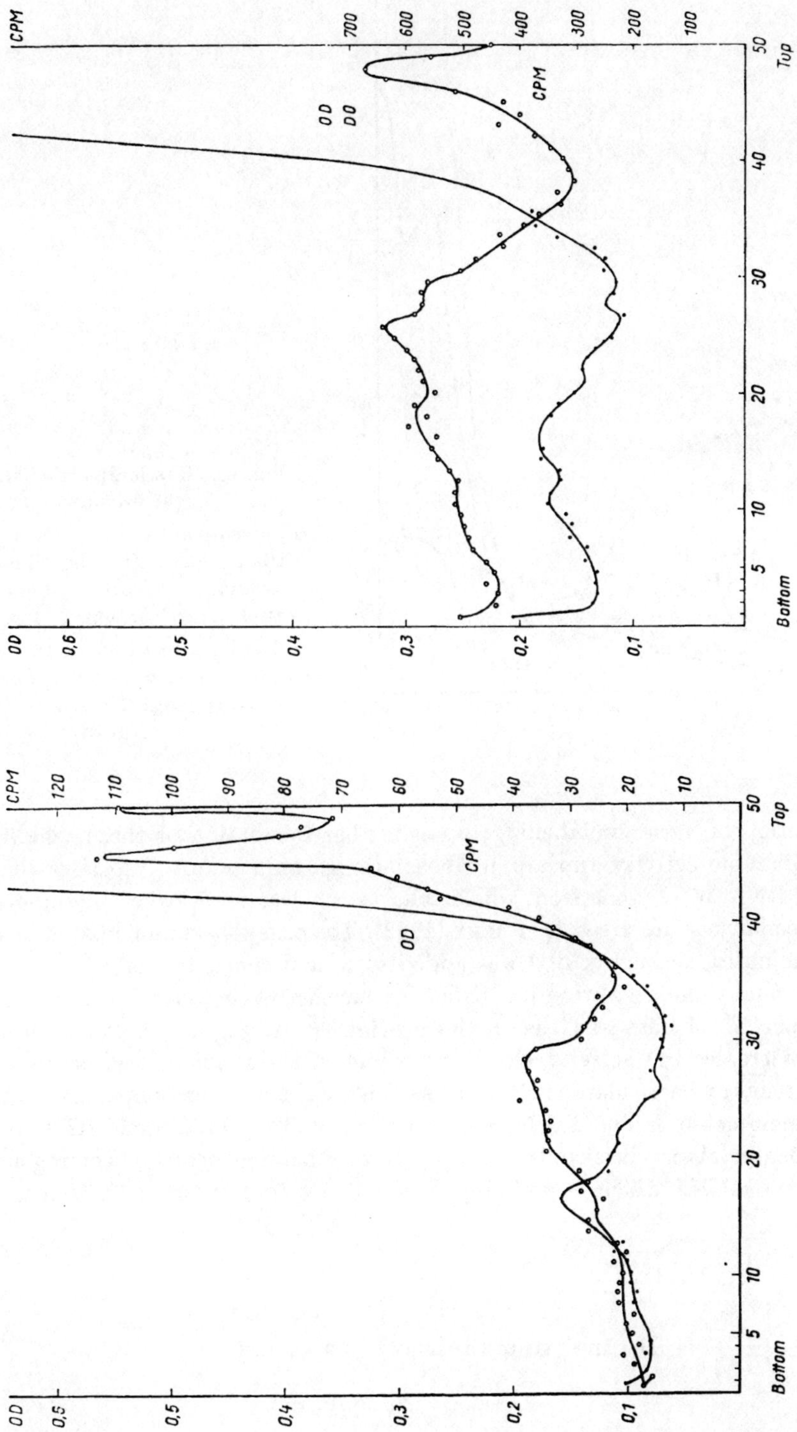

Fig. 1 a and b. Adenine-8-^{14}C labelled HeLa cells homogenized and centrifuged for 4.5 hours in a 5—20 p. c. sucrose gradient at 24,000 rpm. (1a: five minutes pulse, 1b: ten minutes pulse)

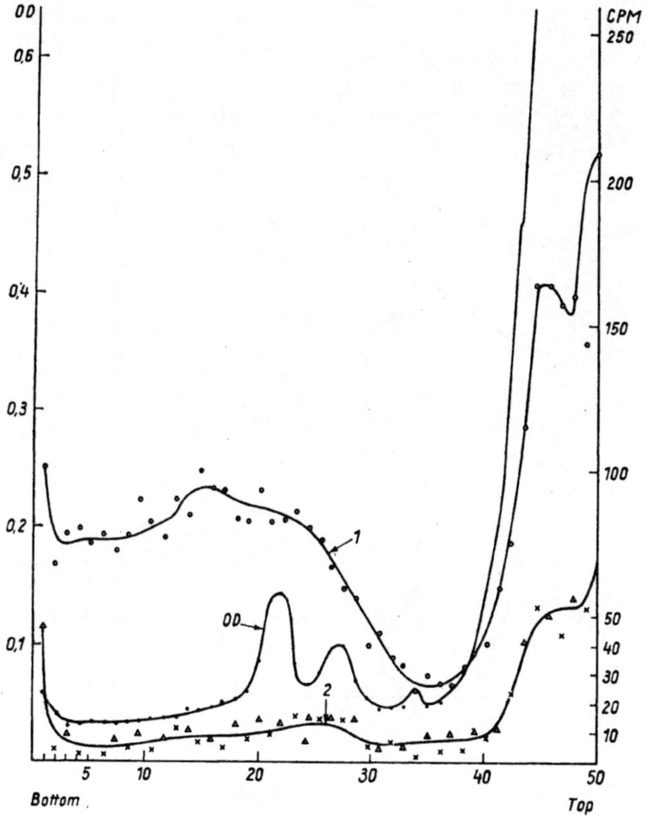

Fig. 1c. ^{14}C-adenine labelled cells (30 minutes)
o untreated,
× ribonuclease after centrifugation,
△ deoxyribonuclease + ribonuclease after centrifugation;
abscissae: normalized fraction number (see text), ordinates: left, optical density (O. D.). right, counts per minute (cpm)

important inhibition of *nucleolar* labelling; upon further incubation of these cells in non-radioactive medium no activity appears in ribosomes. In an attempt to localize this ribosomal precursor RNA in fractions from whole cells, a run was made where actinomycin D was used in the conditions described by Perry (1962): The cells were preincubated in Eagles solution for 90 minutes, actinomycin D was added to a final concentration of $5 \cdot 10^{-8}$ M for 30 minutes, and finally the cells were incubated for another 30 minutes in the presence of actinomycin D and of adenine-8-^{14}C as in the previous runs (Fig. 2). It can be seen that actinomycin D decreases the activity along the whole of the gradient sedimenting faster than 4—10 S without any particular localisation. As this treatment is presumed, as in Perry's experiments, to completely inhibit the formation of 28 S and 16 S ribosomal RNA, one can conclude that adenine after a brief pulse goes partly to a heterogeneous or heterogeneously bound precursor of r RNA which is probably remodelled before entering the ribosomes in its final form.

B. Analysis of the heavy components

Further experiments were done in order to obtain information on these heavy fractions and find out what cell constituents they might contain and which might bind some of the new RNA.

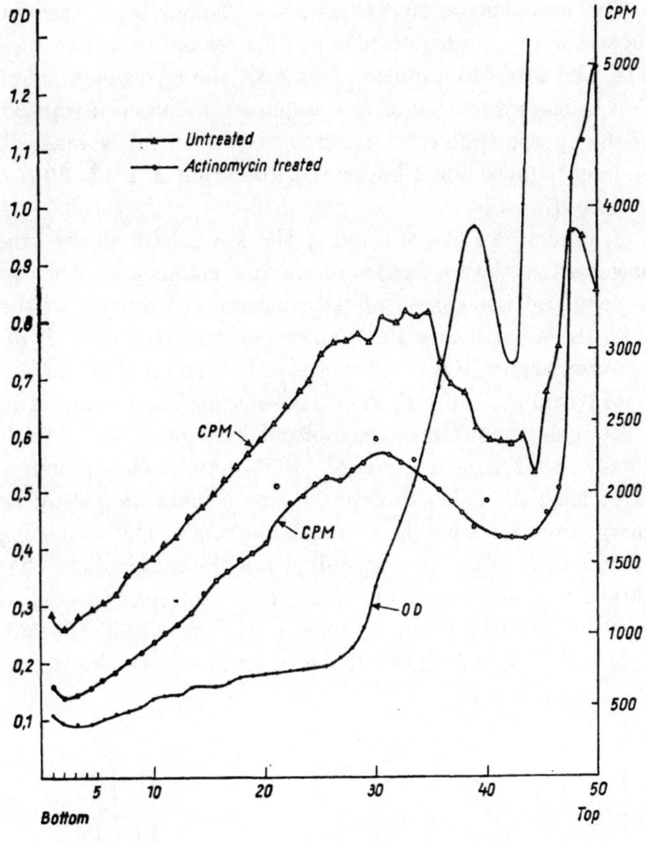

Fig. 2. Adenine-8-^{14}C labelled HeLa cells (30 minutes pulse) with and without actinomycin D homogenized and centrifuged in a 15–30 p. c. sucrose gradient for 2 hours at 24,000 rpm. Coordinates: as in Fig. 1

Evidence for polysomes by electron micrososcopy

a) Total cell homogenates

Whole cell preparations are made in the presence of bentonite (prepared according to Fraenkel-Conrat *et al.*, 1961) to avoid the action of intracellular ribonuclease. The cells from 10 Roux flasks ($\pm 4 \cdot 10^8$ cells) are dispersed in 1.5 ml tris Mg buffer containing 0.5 mg/ml bentonite + 1 p. c. Na deoxycholate and a few crystals of deoxyribonuclease. When the drop in viscosity of the suspension is complete (approximately 30 minutes) the homogenate (1.5 ml) is then layered on a 28 ml 15–30 p. c. sucrose gradient made in tris Mg buffer and centrifuged for 2 hours in the SW 25 rotor of the Spinco L preparative ultracentrifuge at 24.000 rpm. The sedimentation profile is the same as in Fig. 2 and fraction 4 is presented in plate 1: One can see many ribosomal aggregates of various sizes including chain like formations in addition to a few isolated ribosomes.

b) Cytoplasmic polysomes

$4 \cdot 10^8$ cells are homogenized by the method of Harris *et al.* in a 0.1% solution of Tween 80 at 4 °C for 25 to 45 minutes. The nuclei are separated by centrifugation for 5 minutes at 200 g.

The cytoplasmic ribosomes are collected from the supernatant which is further centrifuged for 15 minutes at 3000 g. This second supernatant is treated with 0.2% Na deoxycholate, and after 30 minutes at 0–2 °C, the ribosomes are concentrated by 2 hours centrifugation in the rotor n°40 of the preparative Spinco ultracentrifuge at 105.000 g. Up to 85 p. c. of the cytoplasmic RNA is recovered in the ribosomal pellet. It is taken up in tris Mg buffer and centrifuged for 2 hours at 24.000 rpm in a 15–30 p. c. sucrose gradient prepared in the same buffer.

Fractions can be collected in the lower half of the gradient and the electron microscopic observations show a variety of clumps, chains and other types of ribosomal association (polysomes), and also some isolated ribosomes of the size of the 74 S category (Fig. 4).

In these polysomes the diameter of the 74 S units is of the order of 400 Å like in nuclear or cytoplasmic 74 S ribosomes (Winkelmans *et al.*, 1963); these units are very closely associated, and not more than 4–5 Å separate each member of a chain.

Rough estimations of the molecular weight of the RNA formed rapidly (Penman *et al.*, 1963, Perry, 1962, Scherrer *et al.*, 1963) and probably bound to several ribosomes, give a value of at least $2 \cdot 10^6$ M; this would give a chain length of the order of 20.000 Å, which could carry some forty or more ribosomal units. The larger aggregates of Fig. 3 could very well consist of at least as many units, but the ones in Fig. 4 have probably been partly desaggregated. If the cytoplasmic ribosomal fraction is treated with 0.5 μg/ml of ribonuclease *after* gradient centrifugation, no more chains are observed, and with the exception of a few minor aggregates of 2–3 units, all the ribosomes have the size of 74 S ribosomes (Fig. 5).

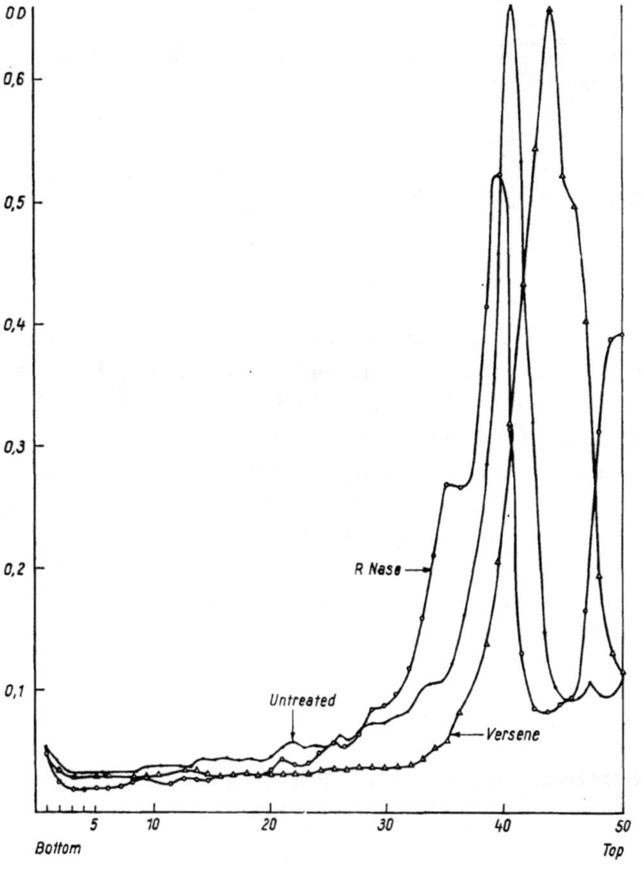

Fig. 6. Sedimentation profile O. D. of cytoplasmic ribosomes, prepared

a) in Tris Mg buffer (untreated),

b) in the same buffer to which ribonuclease is added before centrifugation, or

c) in Tris buffer containing versene instead of $MgCl_2$.

Coordinates: as in Fig. 1

When the O. D. profile of the sedimentation pattern of a RNase treated homogenate is studied, it can be seen (Fig. 6) that after ribonuclease treatment the O. D. is lower in the peak (74 S region). This effect of RNase has been observed several times and the relative proportion of U. V. absorbing constituents in 3 zones of the gradient has been tabulated (Table 1). These experiments support the view that the various ribosomal units of the polysomes are held together by RNA and the preceding experiments show that this RNA becomes labelled very rapidly by radioactive precursors (m RNA ?).

Table 1
Percent of U. V. absorbing material in different regions of the centrifugation gradients

	Polysomes	74 S region	Surface
1 Control	27,9	61,3	10,8
RNase	17,3	49,6	33,1
2 Control	30,9	53,6	15,5
RNase	20,8	49,4	29,8
3 Control	29,6	58,2	12,2
RNase	17,7	41,3	41,0

The 74 S region consisted of 5 fractions on each side of the 74 S peak; the other 2 regions being the heavier fractions (polysomes) and the lighter ones (surface).
The ribonuclease was added before gradient centrifugation and the incubation was done for 1 hour at 4° C.
In experiments 1 and 2, 0,5 μg/ml of enzyme was used, and in experiment 3, 5 μg/ml.
In another experiment, the last ribosomal pellet before gradient centrifugation was taken up in 0.01 M versene and centrifuged in a sucrose gradient made up in tris buffer containing no $MgCl_2$ (Fig. 3).

It can be seen that the O. D. of the heavy part of the gradient has dropped and, in addition, all the 74 S region has dissociated into lighter components (50 S and 30 S).

This experiment suggests that the link between the RNA strand, which unites the 74 S ribosomes, takes place at or near the contact surface between their 30 S and 50 S constituents and that cations (Mg^{++}?) participate in this union.

Evidence for amino acid uptake in the heavy parts of the gradient

It has been shown in reticulocytes that hemoglobin synthesis takes place in polysomes (Warner *et al.*, 1963): These are associations of ribosomes, presumably along a messenger RNA strand (Penman *et al.*, 1963, Noll *et al.*, 1963, Wettstein *et al.*, 1963, Zimmerman 1963). It was therefore important to study the pattern of protein synthesis or at least of amino acid uptake in the various parts of the gradient. To this effect, the cells after having been incubated in Eagles medium for 2 hours, were further incubated for 2.5, 5, 10 and 30 minutes in Eagles medium (prepared without lysine) to which was added 10 μc/ml of 3H-lysine. After 2.5 minutes, the uptake was hardly above background, but for the other incubation times there was a measurable uptake of lysine in the region where ribosomal complexes were found in the electron microscope studies.

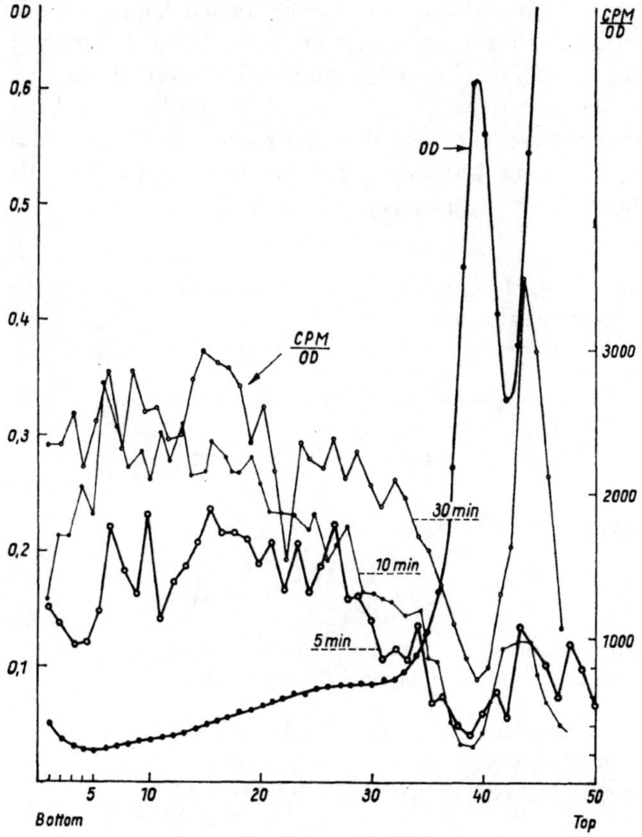

Fig. 7. Kinetics of lysine uptake by HeLa cells

The cells are homogenized and centrifuged for 2 hours on a 15—30 p. c. sucrose gradient. The results are plotted as relative specific activity $\left(\frac{\text{cpm}}{\text{O.D.}}\right)$ for each run. Other coordinates as in Fig. 1

The results are shown in Fig. 7 and lysine uptake is calculated for unit optical density in the same fraction („relative specific activity"). It can be seen that maximum relative activity is found in the heavier fractions and reaches almost 60 p. c. of the 30 minutes value after 5 minutes incubation. These results are very similar to those mentioned above and confirm the fact that polysomes are the site of protein synthesis. The minimum of specific activity in the 74 S ribosome region is striking.

In the lighter parts of the gradient (difficult to analyze on account of DNase digestion products) the relative specific activity increases with time, the highest increase taking place in the part of the gradient where the O. D. is minimum ($\sim$ 30—50 S). It is not yet possible to discuss the nature of this radioactivity peak – but this new protein remaining bound to physical structures obviously needs further investigation. Lysine being one of the prominent ribosomal amino acids (10—12 p. c. of the total amino acid composition of the ribosomes according to WANG, 1962) it would not be astonishing that part of this radioactivity consists of new ribosomal proteins. At the surface of the gradient are appreciable amounts of labelled acid insoluble material, probably representing newly released proteins.

Kinetics of polysome formation in cell homogenates

To study the kinetics of adenine uptake into polysomes, cells were given ^{14}C-adenine for various periods of time and thereafter analyzed by density gradient centrifugation in a 15–30 p. c. sucrose gradient. The results are shown in Figures 8 and 9. It can be seen that

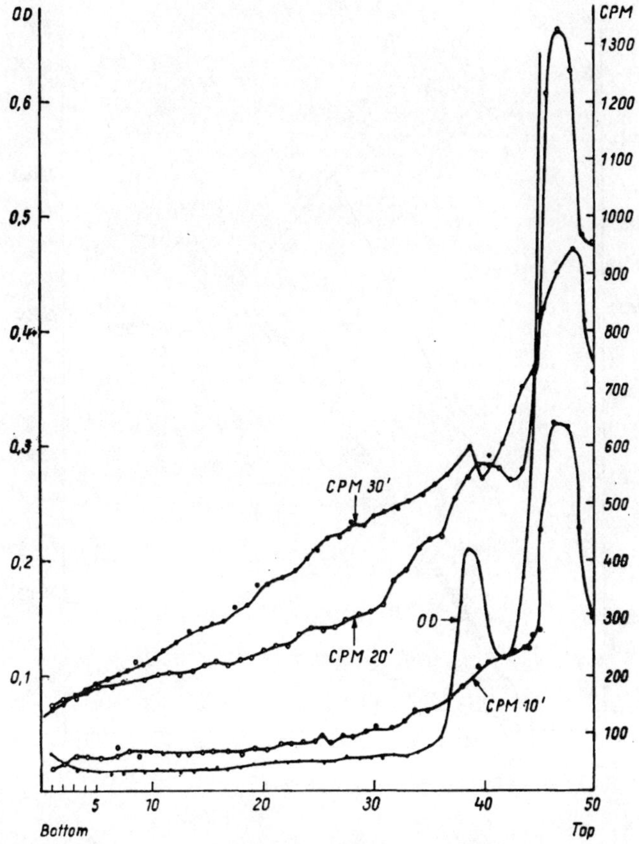

Fig. 8. Kinetics of polysome formation in HeLa cells

Cells are incubated for 10, 20, 30 minutes with adenine-8-^{14}C, homogenized and put on a 15–30 p. c. sucrose gradient and centrifuged for 2 hours at 24,000 rpm. Coordinates: as in Fig. 1

after 10 minutes incubation, the radioactivity is still relatively low, but a rough graphic calculation shows that 40 p. c. sediments in the region of the gradient heavier than the 74 S ribosomes. After 20 min., approximately 47 p. c. is in this region, and after 30 minutes, approximately 65 to 70 p. c. The kinetics of uptake in fractions 15, 25, 35, 38 and 47 is plotted in Fig. 9. These fractions are chosen arbitrarily, except for fraction 35 which is in the region where ribosome dimers are expected to sediment, and for fraction 38 (74 S monomers). If one extrapolates these various curves for zero uptake into the heavy fractions, they all extrapolate down to 4–5 minutes, after which the activity begins to rise. This indicates that it takes approximately 5 minutes for the formation of polysomes from existing ribosomes and new RNA.

The present experiments do not prove that inside the living cell, the polysomes are formed in such little time. The newly labelled RNA could very well become attached in polysomal form to ribosomes, which become accessible only after the homogenization. Experiments to determine if the labelling of the polysomes occur before or after homogenization are under way. The rise in relative specific radioactivity of fraction 38 (74 S) is slower than in the polysomal fractions on account of the bulk of pre-existing 74 S ribosomes. In fraction 42 (20–50 S ?) the rise in radioactivity apparently starts from time zero – it might well be free RNA before it becomes bound to the polysomes, however we believe that more refined kinetic studies than the present ones are needed in order to discover the relationship, which may exist between lighter and heavier fractions.

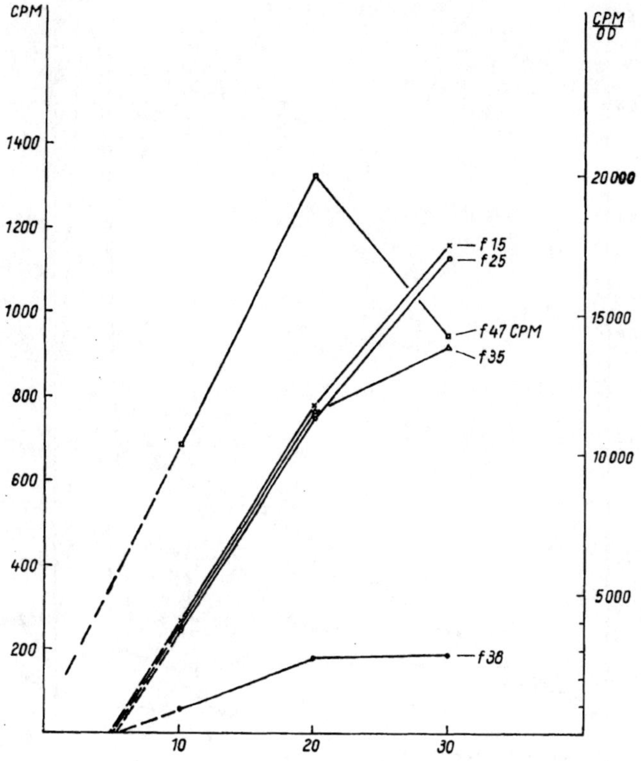

Fig. 9. Kinetics of polysome formation in HeLa cells
Fractions 15, 25, 35, 38 and 47 plotted as relative specific radioactivity $\left(\frac{\text{cpm}}{\text{O. D.}}\right)$
The uptake of adenine into polysomes seems to follow identical kinetics for dimers or polymers and indicates that these have presumably all been formed during the experiment. The lower relative specific activity of the monomers is taken to indicate that many monomers present at the beginning of the labelling period have not become attached to newly formed RNA
Fractions 42 (sedimenting in the 10—16 S region) cannot be expressed in relative specific activity on account of the high absorption due to DNA digestion products. Abscissae: time in minutes, ordinates: left, cpm (fraction 42); right, $\frac{\text{cpm}}{\text{O. D.}}$ (other fractions)

Could polysomes be formed in the cell nucleus?

Earlier radioautographic experiments (SRINIVASAN *et al.*, 1963) have demonstrated that, after 10 minutes incubation, more than 95 p. c. of the radioactivity of labelled adenine or other nucleosides resides in the nucleus. Table 2 gives a comparison of the cytological and gradient distribution of rapidly labelled RNA.

Table 2
Per cent radioactivity in cell nucleus, compared to activity of polysomes

	Radioautography [1] p. c. in nucleus	Ultracentrifugation [2] p. c. in heavy fraction
10	< 97 p. c.	40 p. c.
20	~ 97 p. c.	47 p. c.
30	~ 95 p. c.	63—73 p. c.

[1]) Values taken from SRINIVASAN *et al.* (1963) in runs where the cells were incubated for 10 minutes in ^{14}C-adenine and transferred for 10 and 20 minutes in non labelled medium.

[2]) Values computed graphically from the radioactivity sedimenting in the heavy (H) and lighter (L) parts of the gradient.
H: integral radioactivity in fractions 1—35
L: ,, ,, ,, ,, 36—50
(Fraction 35 is in the region where ribosome dimers are presumed to sediment).

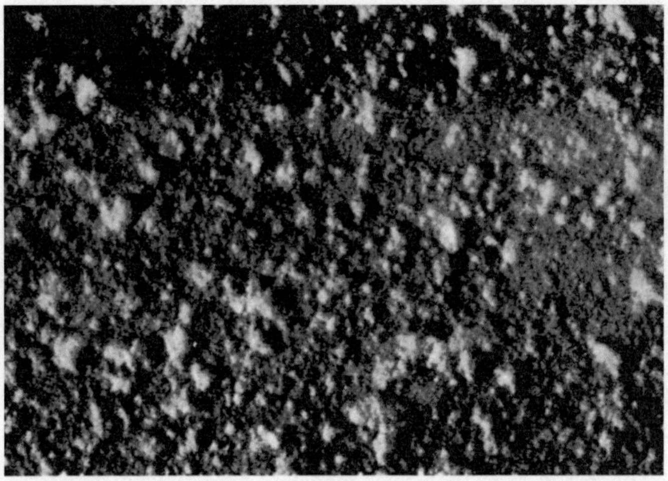

Fig. 3. Whole cells, fraction 4 (Fig. 1) (46,000 x)

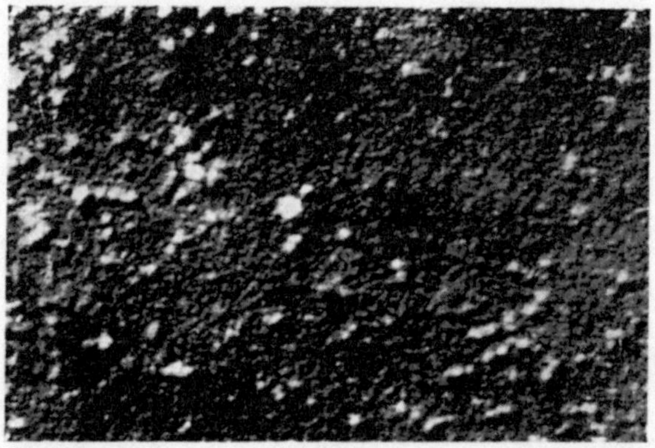

Fig. 4

Fig. 5

Fig. 4 and 5. Cytoplasmic polysomes (fraction 7) without (Fig. 4) and with ribonuclease treatment (Fig. 5) after density gradient centrifugation (46,000 x)

If the labelling of polysomes, as studied in the experiments described in figures 8 and 9, really represent their rate of formation inside the cell, this comparison would indicate that most of the newly formed polysomes are in the cell nucleus. This would, however, not be a proof that cytoplasmic ribosomes or polysomes are formed inside the nucleus.

Conclusions

The RNA formed during a short pulse of adenine-^{14}C in a dividing cellular population, where a great variety of proteins and other constituents are duplicated at each generation, can be expected to be complex. In the present density gradient analysis, RNA species sedimenting slowly in both types of gradients probably consists of a variety of transfer RNA's, and a heavier species of RNA sedimenting up to ~ 20 S, which could contain „polysomal" RNA's with DNA-like base ratios, as found recently by Penman *et al.* (1963). But, as stated earlier, a more refined analysis of the lighter part of the gradient as well as base analysis are still required to check these points. In the heavier fraction (fraction 1–40) of a 5–20 p. c. sucrose gradient a heterogeneous sedimentation pattern is found and treatment of the homogenate with ribonuclease results in an important loss of this radioactivity. From the phenol purified RNA analysis of Perry (1962) and of Scherrer *et al.* (1963), the labelling of HeLa cells by RNA precursors appears rapidly in high molecular RNA's sedimenting around 45 S, presumably of molecular weights above $2 \cdot 10^6$. Afterward sbegins to appear a 35 S species followed by the 16 and 28 S ribosomal RNA's. The 45 S and 35 S species might well be in the free state in our analysis, on account of the maximal radioactivity found in these regions of the gradients. Electron microscopical analysis of fractions taken in this area shows the existence of rather pure $\sim$ 50 S and 30 S ribosomes (Winkelmans *et al.*, 1963), which are not labelled (preliminary data). The absence of other morphologically identifiable components and the non parallelism between ribosomal O. D. and radioactivity supports the view that free RNA might well be what sediments in these regions.

In the denser regions (1–20 of the light gradient or 1–35 of the heavier one), electron microscopy as well as the demonstration of amino acid uptake indicate the presence of polysomes: This is a confirmation of what has been found for reticulocytes by Warner *et al.* (1963), by Noll *et al.* (1963), and Wettstein *et al.* (1963), and more recently by Penman *et al.* (1963) for HeLa cells. The fact that these associated ribosomes break up in ribonuclease also confirms the fact that the mode of union of these units involves RNA (messenger RNA as postulated by the various authors just cited). Unfortunately the resolution of the electron microscope used has not enabled us to observe with any certainty any RNA strand between the various units of the polysomes. The fact that these polysomes break up into 50 S and 30 S ribosomes when cations are removed suggests a close association of the linking RNA strand with the contact surfaces of the ribosomal subunits. A rough calculation presented in the text leads to the idea that association of as many as 40 ribosomal units per polysome might exist.

The uptake of RNA precursors in these fractions as well as the absence of uptake in the ribosome monomers after such short times (preliminary experiments of this laboratory) or in ribosomal RNA (Perry, 1962, Scherrer *et al.*, 1963), indicate that the rapid sedimentation of these newly formed RNA's is chiefly due to polysomal formation from new RNA combining with older unlabelled ribosomes. Ribosomal dimers and heavier polysomes becoming labelled only after 5 minutes incubation, it cannot be excluded that after these short times of incubation some RNA is bound to other cell structures. A search for DNA-RNA hybrids was inconclusive – but our preliminary evidence indicates that a further investigation is needed.

Finally, there is a dip in the 4–30 S region which could nevertheless contain small amounts of r RNA's, and polysomal RNA's of the type described by PENMAN *et al.* (1963).

It is difficult at present to see how these various RNA species are related to each other; the only certain common denominator is that they are all synthesized in the cell nucleus and probably all DNA primed. The heterogeneity of the newly labelled RNA gives the impression either that DNA primed synthesis leads to the detachment of long RNA chains which break up afterwards, or that a variety of RNA's of heterogeneous chain lengths are produced. In the case of m RNA it is not at all certain if the 6–22 S polysomal RNA's discovered by PENMAN *et al.* (1963) are the original RNA's, or if these arise from natural or artificial breakdown of original components of higher molecular weight. Low concentrations of actinomycin D have been shown by PERRY (1962, 1963) to inhibit both nucleolar and ribosomal RNA formation; the sedimentation data indicate that ribosomal RNA seems to come also from heavy heterogeneous RNA. When total cell homogenates are similarly studied with low concentrations of actinomycin D, no particular inhibition pattern is found and it is not possible to localize the possible r RNA precursors in any particular region of the sedimentation gradient. Transfer RNA probably also has its origin in the nucleus and could also be DNA primed (GOLDBERG and RABINOWITZ, 1961), although the methylation of its rare bases occurs presumably as an independent step (MANDEL and BOREK, 1963). One of the many questions remaining open is the possibility of some of the RNA's being synthesized away from the chromosomes with RNA primers. This would not be astonishing on account of the RNA primed replication of viral RNA (HOLLAND, 1962), and of the evidence for natural RNA primed RNA polymerases (BURDON and SMELLIE, 1962). The primers necessary for these RNA dependent RNA polymerases might themselves be formed on DNA: These polymerases could perhaps remodel some of the RNA's formed initially on the chromatin, as suggested by PERRY for ribosomal RNA's which could undergo such a transformation in the nucleoli. Such remodelling of RNA's might also occur in other cell sites, as in the cytoplasm, where some incorporation of RNA precursors might take place (SRINIVASAN *et al.*, 1963). It is not impossible therefore that „early RNA", a part of which would be m RNA, would correspond to one operon: this would be in line with present concepts on the regulation of protein synthesis. The exact nature of the polysome complexes as well as their mode of functioning will probably throw some light on these problems.

Acknowledgments

We would like to thank most heartily Professor J. BRACHET for having given us permission to use his electron microscope and Professor R. JEENER and Dr. HAMERS for the analytical centrifuge.

We are very grateful for Drs. F. VANDERHAEGHE and P. VAN GANSEN for their advice for preparing the samples for electron microscopy.

This work was supported by the National Institutes of Health, U.S. Public Health Service, Grant R. G. 6214 and by Euratom, Contract 016.61.10 ABIB.

Summary

A study of the sedimentation pattern in sucrose gradients of rapidly labelled RNA (5–30 minutes labelling with adenine-^{14}C) was done on whole extracts of HeLa cells. Two regions of radioactivity have been found: a lighter region sedimenting in the range of 4–20 S particles and a heavier, very heterogeneous region sedimenting from 30 S to the bottom of the gradients, even when 30 p. c. sucrose was used. The nature of the various types of RNA's likely to sediment in these regions has been discussed. The heavier heterogeneous region contains very small amounts of DNA, but no definite evidence for the existence of DNA-RNA hybrids could be obtained. On the other hand, the heavy heterogeneous region is active in amino acid incorporation and consists of a variety of polysomes; their characterization by electron microscopy is described. These polysomes after a short labelling period consist of unlabelled 74 S ribosomes to which is attached rapidly labelled RNA; it was shown that it takes roughly five minutes for adenine-^{14}C to become integrated into RNA sedimenting with the polysomes. Comparison of autoradiographic and sedimentation analysis shows that a large proportion of the polysomes could be formed in the cell nucleus.

References

BRACHET, J., 1957: Biochemical Cytology. Academic Press, New York.
BRITTEN, R. J., and R. B. ROBERTS, 1960: Science 131, 32.
BURDON, R. H., and R. M. S. SMELLIE, 1962: Biochim. biophys. Acta 61, 633.
FRAENKEL-CONRAT, H., B. SINGER and A. TSUGITA, 1961: Virology 14, 54.
GOLDBERG, I. H., and E. RABINOWITZ, 1961: Biochim. biophys. Acta 54, 202.
GRUNBERG-MANAGO, M., 1962: Ann. Rev. Biochem. 31, 301.
HOLLAND, J. S., 1962: Biochem. biophys. Res. Comm. 9, 556.
MANDEL, L. H., and E. BOREK, 1963: Biochemistry 2, 555.
NOLL, H., T. STAEHELIN and F. C. WETTSTEIN, 1963: Nature 198, 632.
PENMAN, S., K. SCHERRER, Y. BECKER and J. E. DARNELL, 1963: Proc. nat. Acad. Sci. U.S.A. 49, 654.
PERRY, R. P., 1960: Exper. Cell Res. 20, 216.
PERRY, R. P., 1962: Proc. nat. Acad. Sci. U.S.A. 48, 2179.
PERRY, R. P., 1963: Exper. Cell Res. 29, 400.
PERRY, R. P., M. ERRERA and A. HELL, 1961a: Biochim. biophys. Acta 49, 47.
PERRY, R. P., M. ERRERA, A. HELL and S. DÜRWALD, 1961b: J. biophys. biochem. Cytol. 11, 1.
RHO, J. H., and J. BONNER, 1961: Proc. nat. Acad. Sci. U.S.A. 47, 1611.
SCHERRER, K., H. LATHAM and J. E. DARNELL, 1963: Proc. nat. Acad. Sci. U.S.A. 49, 240.
SPIEGELMAN, S., 1963: Feder. Proc. 22, 36.
SRINIVASAN, P. R., A. MILLER-FAURÈS, M. BRUNFAUT and M. ERRERA, 1963: Biochem. biophys. Acta 72, 209.
WANG, T. Y., 1962: Arch. Biochem. Biophys. 97, 387.
WARNER, J. H., S. KNOLL and A. RICH, 1963: Proc. nat. Acad. Sci. U.S.A. 49, 122.
WETTSTEIN, F. C., T. STAEHELIN and H. NOLL, 1963: Nature 197, 430.
WINKELMANS, D., M. HILL and M. ERRERA, 1963: Biochim. biophys. Acta, submitted for publication.
YANOFSKY, J. A., and S. SPIEGELMAN, 1962: Proc. nat. Acad. Sci. U.S.A. 48, 1069.
ZIMMERMAN, E. F., 1963: Biochem. biophys. Res. Comm. 11, 301.

On the Structure of Ribosomes

A. S. Spirin

A. N. Bach Institute of Biochemistry, Academy of Sciences of the USSR, Moscow

It is established now that every cell contains a whole set of functionally different species of RNA and that the protein synthesis is achieved through complex processes of molecular interactions between various types of cellular polyribonucleotides and first of all between ribosomal, template and adaptor RNA's. Ribosomal particles are the centers of all these interactions. It is in the ribosomes that the information encoded in template RNA is being transcribed into amino acid sequence of polypeptide chain. All we know about the mechanism of these processes however is only some schematical ideas that a template (messenger RNA) and an adaptor („soluble" RNA) might somehow complementary interact; and the real role of a ribosome as a central point of the protein-synthesizing apparatus is completely obscure.

At the same time, since a ribosome is the center where all the three known species of cellular RNA meet with each other and perform their functions in the synthesis of specific polypeptide chain of protein the problem of structure and functioning of ribosomes is the general problem for all different RNA's in cells. The real role of the ribosomal, template and adaptor RNA's and the intimate relation between their structure and function may be expected to be understood through studies of structure and functions of ribosomes.

On the other hand the problem of ribosomes is of uttermost importance from the biological viewpoint. Ribosomes are universally occuring structures present in all types of cells and in all species of organisms. The central biochemical process of all living matter takes places in these particles. Every living form known up-to-date is characterized by the existence of ribosomes with their specific biochemical apparatus. The universal occurrence of ribosomes and of biochemical reactions associated with them is especially noteworthy. It seems to mean that the structural organisation of ribosomes and their mode of functioning rest on some most essential principles of general biological organization. It should be added that ribosomes are the smallest of all the cellular granules known and that their dimensions lie practically on the border between those of cellular organoids and macromolecules; at any rate all physical methods used for study of macromolecules are also applicable for ribosomes. Therefore this case seems to be of especial interest for attempts to reveal some general principles of biological organization immediately in the molecular organization of particles themselves.

Ribosomes are ribonucleoprotein particles (RNP-particles) consisting of high polymer ribosomal RNA and structural protein. Ribosomes of different origin contain 40 to 65% RNA and 60 to 35% protein. Molecular weight of individual ribosomes from different sources varies from 2.8 to 4.5 millions; the sedimentation coefficients are 70 to 85 S, respectively. Such ribosomal particles always consist of two unequal subunits; they dissociate into the subunits upon lowering the Mg^{++} concentration to a certain level. Thus, *E. coli* ribosomes with sedimentation coefficient 70 S (so called 70 S particles) dissociate into 50 S and 30 S subunits (50 S and 30 S particles). The increase in the Mg^{++} concentration makes two 70 S particles to aggregate and form one 100 S particle. These dissociation and association are all reversible. Each subunit (50 S and 30 S) includes only one molecule of ribosomal RNA (M. W. $1{,}2 \times 10^6$ for 50 S subunit and 0.5×10^6 for 30 S) and up to several dozens of molecules of structural ribosomal protein.

Detailed electron microscope investigations of normal ribosomal particles from *E. coli* were performed by Hall and Slayter (1959) using the shadow-casting method and by Huxley and Zubay (1960) who used the negative and positive staining technique. Recently the electron microscope analysis of *E. coli* ribosomes was made also by Dr. N. A. Kisselev (Institute of Crystallography, Academy of Sciences of the USSR, Moscow) in our work on the structure of ribosomes (Spirin, Kisselev, Shakulov and Bogdanov, 1963). Our observations are consistent with the results reported earlier and permit to make some further suggestions concerning the shape and size of ribosomal particles.

Fig. 1a shows the 70 S ribosomes of *E. coli* and their dimers, the 100 S particles. Each 70 S ribosome no matter whether it forms a dimer or is seen individually is distinctly divided into two unequal subunits: the larger one, approximately spherical (50 S subunit), and the smaller one (30 S), flattened and slightly concave on the side which faces the larger subunit. In general the micrographs show that dimensions of the 70 S ribosome are 190 Å in length and 150 Å in width. It can be easily seen that the dimerization of the 70 S ribosomes resulting in formation of the 100 S particles occurs through interaction of the smaller subunits. Such ribosome dimers, the 100 S particles, are about 400 Å in length and up to 150 Å in width.

The ribosomes dissociated into 50 S and 30 S subunits are shown on micrograph, Fig. 1b. It can be seen that part of the structures visible on the micrograph are roughly spherical particles with a diameter of about 140–160 Å. Occasionally they have polygonal, mainly pentangular, outlines. These structures may correspond to the 50 S subunits. Another type of particles corresponding probably to the 30 S subunits may be also observed. On the plates of shadowed preparations (which are not presented here) the 30 S subunits look like flattened particles with a height of about 70–90 Å. In Fig. 1b where negative staining with PTA was used the 30 S subunits are probably the particles which have rectangular shape in visible projection, with dimensions 120 × 140 Å. Thus if the 50 S particle may be thought as polygonal in its contour, similar to spherical structure the 30 S particle looks rectangular, at least when it is not associated with the 50 S particle. Probably the interaction between the 30 S and 50 S particles leading to the formation of the 70 S particle is accompanied by some alteration in the configuration of the 30 S subunit: it acquires the form of overlapping cap fitting onto one side of the larger subunit.

Morphology and dimensions of the *E. coli* ribosomal particles and their subunits are schematically presented in Fig. 2.

The data concerning the inner structural organization of ribosomal particles are quite scanty. The important results in this direction were obtained in electron microscope observations by Huxley and Zubay (1960) who used positive staining with uranyl acetate which binds mainly to RNA. No preferential concentration of ribosomal protein or ribosomal RNA on the periphery or in the center of the particle was observed. One gets an impression that ribosomal protein and RNA are mutually and more or less evenly impregnated with each other. Ribosomes seem to have no protein shell, in contrast with virus particles where RNA forms a nucleic core and is concentrated inside the particle while protein is located on the periphery and forms a shell. Therefore one may think that in ribosomes the protein molecules accompany the somehow folded RNA along all its length. Our experiments on the effect of exogeneous RNase on RNA within ribosomes (Shakulov, Ajtkhozhin and Spirin, 1962) also evidence in favour of the existence of some contact of the ribosomal RNA with environment and the absence of a dense protein shell. It has been shown that RNase present in the external solution can attack RNA within ribosomes acting on certain regions of the polynucleotide chain not sheltered by protein; the formal integrity of the particle in this case is not affected („the latent degradation of ribosomes").

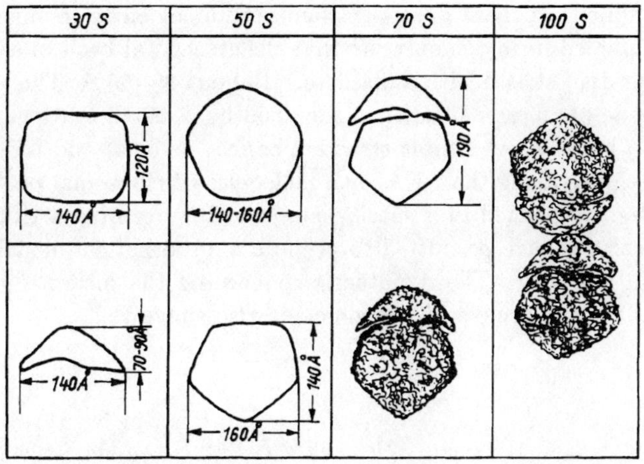

Fig. 2. Morphology and dimensions of *E. coli* ribosomal particles (scheme)

Some data on the state of RNA within ribosomes were obtained in X-ray diffraction studies (Zubay and Wilkins, 1960; Klug *et al.*, 1961) and in the investigations of ultraviolet hypochromicity of ribosomes (Zubay and Wilkins, 1960; Schlessinger, 1960; Bonhoeffer and Schaçhman, 1960). It was shown that the diffraction pattern of ribosomes is similar to that obtained by superimposing of X-ray pattern of isolated ribosomal RNA on diffraction pattern of free ribosomal protein. The analysis of diffraction patterns has indicated that RNA in ribosomal particles has helical regions of the same structure as isolated RNA in solution. Moreover as it follows from the study of hypochromicity the number of helical regions and the percentage of nucleotides in these regions in RNA of ribosomes are approximately similar to those of RNA in solution at moderate ionic strength. From these data one may suggest that RNA chains within ribosomes have numerous double-stranded regions due to interaction of the parts of the same chain with each other forming the secondary structure similar to that in isolated RNA.

On the whole it can be noticed that the available data on organization and structure of ribosomes are mainly descriptive. They concern chemical composition, size, morphology of ribosome subunits, chemical and physical-chemical properties of ribosomal protein and nucleic acid, etc., and cannot permit to make any conclusions on principles of molecular organization of ribosomes.

Two years ago we started to study the structure of ribosomes in our laboratory. At present this work is being performed in collaboration with Dr. N. A. Kisselev (Laboratory of Protein structure, Institute of Crystallography, Academy of Sciences of the USSR, Moscow). Dr. R. S. Shakulov and Dr. A. A. Bogdanov participated in this investigation from my laboratory. Three different approaches are used in the study of structure and formation of ribosomes: 1. controlled partial degradation of ribosomes and some other influences on ribosomal particles in solution with the aim to cause the structural changes allowing to elucidate some principles of structural organization of ribosomes; 2. study of possible natural intracellular precursors of ribosomes the structure of which might represent the simplified prototype of ribosomal subunits; 3. attempts to reconstruct the ribosomal particles in vitro.

Following these lines the combination of electron microscopy and physical analysis have enabled us to demonstrate that the structural basis of each ribosomal subunit is a ribonucleoprotein strand with a diameter of about 30–40 Å. The strand probably consists of the molecule of ribosomal RNA in the „rod-like" configuration, with developped secondary structure (a set of short double-stranded helical regions) and is stabilized by interaction of numerous regions along the RNA with molecules of ribosomal protein. The ribonucleoprotein strand is tightly packed in a specific manner thus forming a ribosomal subunit. A number of observations have permitted to propose a hypothetical model of the mode of RNP-strand folding in ribosome. The hypothesis concerning the intermediate stages of ribosome formation in a cell (biogenesis of ribosomes) is also suggested.

Controlled Influences on the Structure of Ribosome

It is known that the main difficulty in any attempt to make a controllable change in the structure of ribosomal particles in solution was always the presence of the latent ribonuclease within ribosomes: any disturbance in native structure of the particles immediately results in activation of the enzyme and this in turn leads to rapid non-controlled degradation of ribosomal RNA and the particle as a whole.

In order to surpass this difficulty we turned our attention first to formaldehyde as an agent which completely inhibits the activity of enzymes and at the same time provides a stable fixation of protein structures. Fixation of ribosome with formaldehyde for the purposes of electron microscopy was earlier described by Huxley and Zubay (1960). It was found that the fixation does not cause any visible change in the structure of ribosomal particles. The procedure we used for fixation of *E. coli* ribosomes involved the incubation of isolated ribosomes in 4–8% solution of formaldehyde for several hours in the cold and subsequent removal of excess of formaldehyde by dialysis. The ribosomes fixed in this manner were stable in Mg^{++}-free solution, displayed no ribonuclease activity and appeared to have normal sedimentation coefficients and normal morphology under electron microscope.

The first promising results were obtained in the experiments where the effect of urea on such ribosomes was studied. It was shown that when formaldehyde-fixed ribosomes were placed into 6 M urea some variable but essential decrease in sedimentation coefficients (extrapolated to standard conditions, water, 20 °C) was observed for both of the ribosomal subunits (the fixed particles dissociate into the subunits in the presence of urea). This decrease was accompanied by the increase in specific viscosity of the particles. No loss of protein was observed after treatment with urea. From this one may think that urea causes some loosening of originally compact particles but does not result in dissociation of them into RNA and protein. The electron microscope study has indicated some loss of the former clear contours of the particles, and what is the most important, one could observe short rod-like structures, or fibrils, like „wicks" sticking out of the main „bodies" of the particles. The diameter of the „wicks" was about 30–40 Å. The formation of similar „fibrils" or „strands" could also be observed after treatment of formaldehyde-fixed ribosomes with low concentrations of detergent (e. g. sodium dodecylsulphate) and with some other agents. Sometimes similar short „strands" sticking out of the particles were seen on electron micrographs of usual (non-fixed) ribosomes; for example, they appeared as a result of some spontaneous degradation of the ribosomes in the course of preparing the samples for electron microscopy, or degradation after chromatography of the ribosomes on DEAE-cellulose, etc. Typical micrograph of

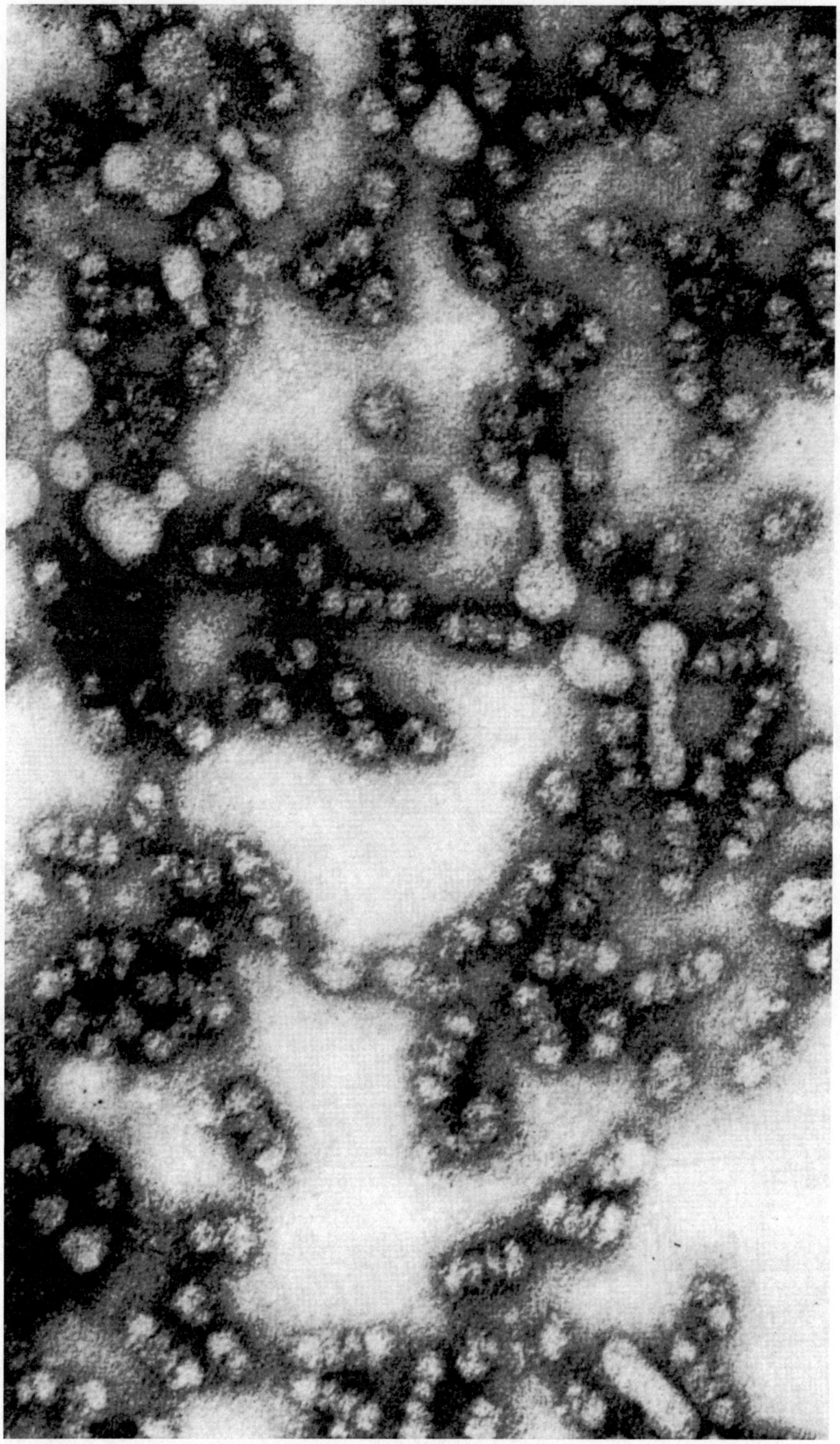

Fig. 1. Micrographs of *E. coli* ribosomes negatively stained with PTA. Magnification 330000 ×

a) 70 S and 100 S particles

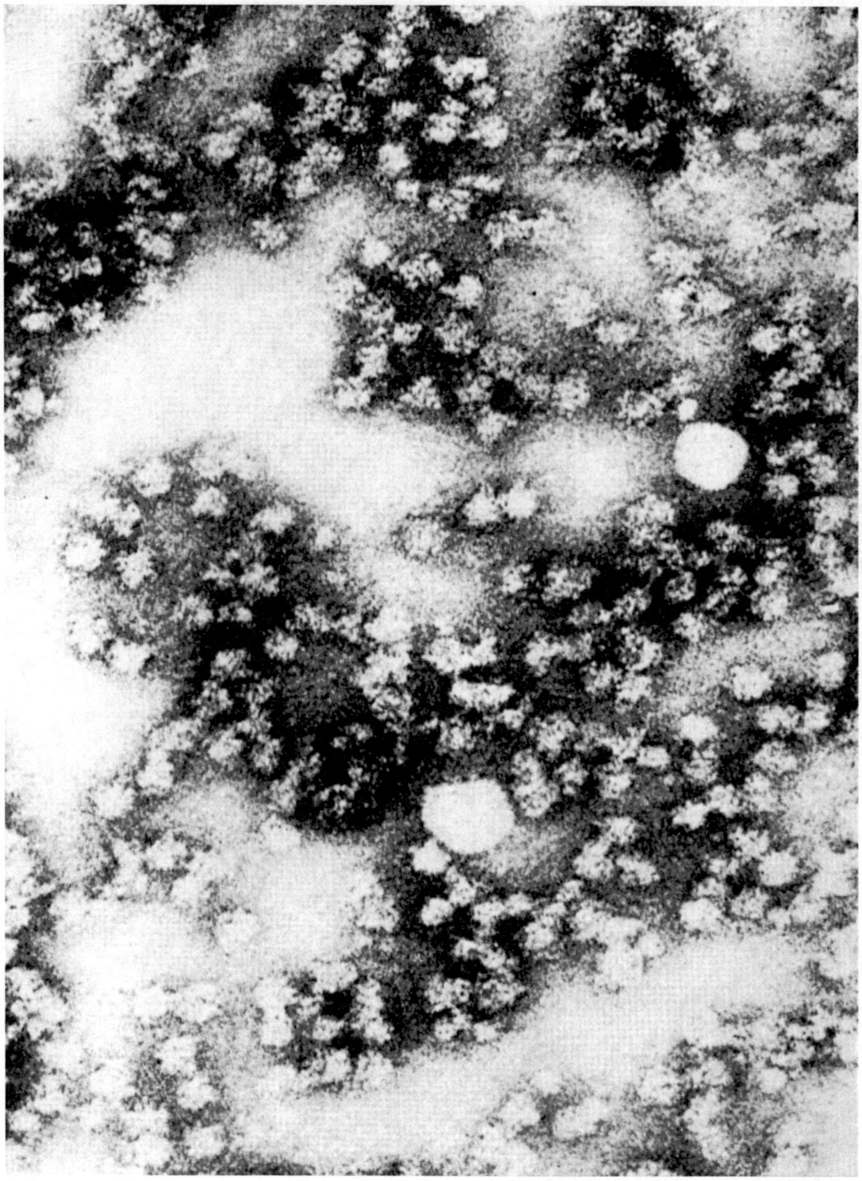

Fig. 1. Micrographs of *E. coli* ribosomes negatively stained with PTA. Magnification 330 000 ×

b) 50 S and 30 S particles; particles with rectangular and polygonal contours are seen

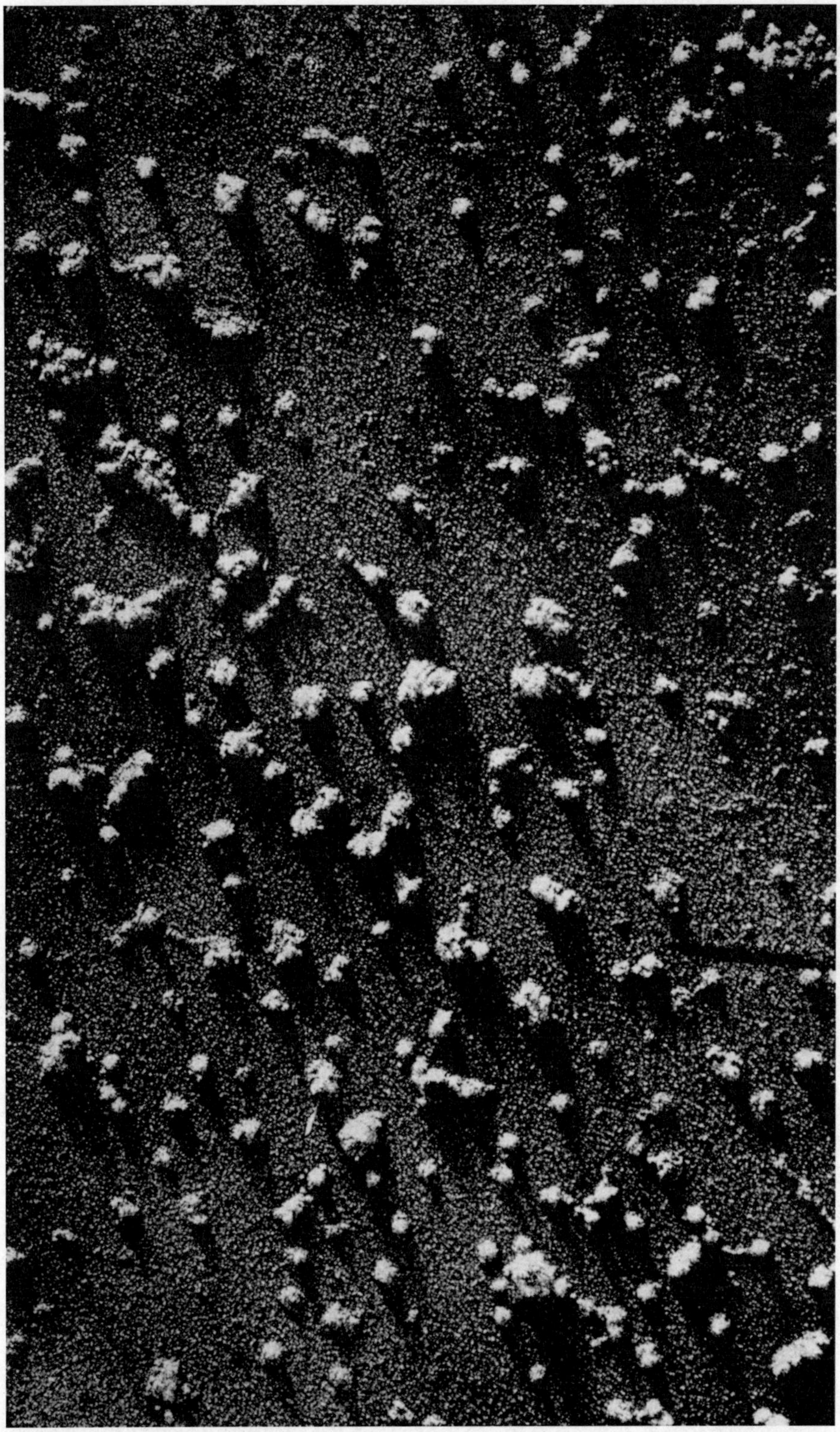

Fig. 3. A micrograph of shadowed ribosomes partially degraded; strands sticking out of the particles are seen occasionally. Magnification 100000 ×

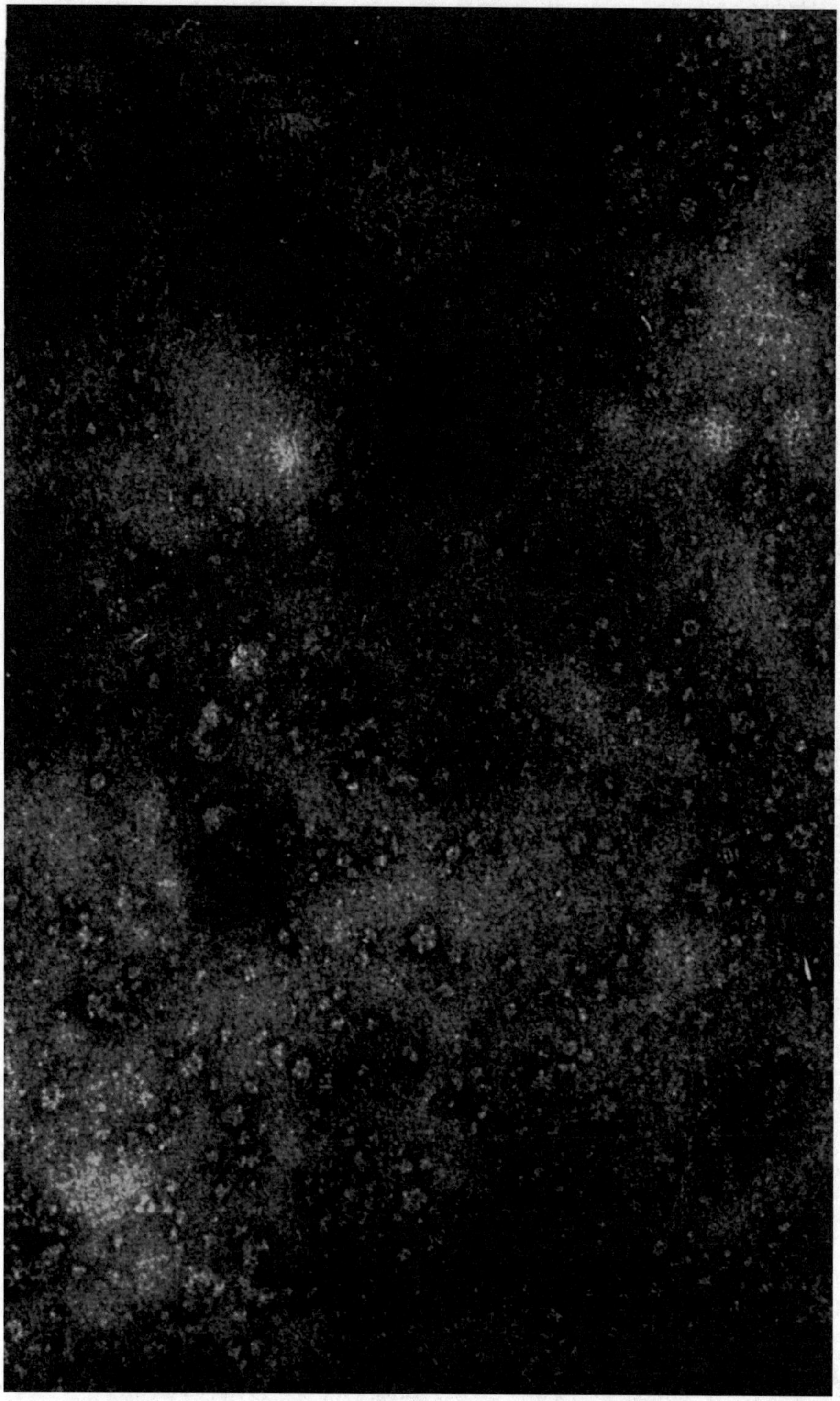

Fig. 6. A micrograph of CM ribonucleoprotein particles negatively stained with PTA. Magnification 220000 ×

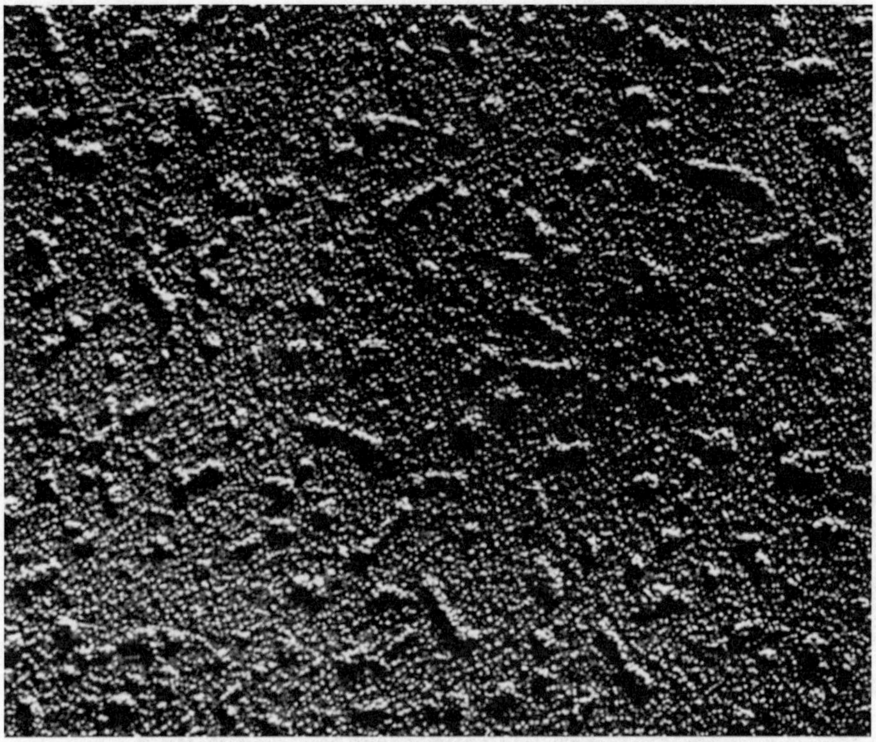

Fig. 5. A micrograph of shadowed ribonucleoprotein strands derived from ribosomal particles. Shadow-to-height ratio 9 : 1, Magnification 99000 ×

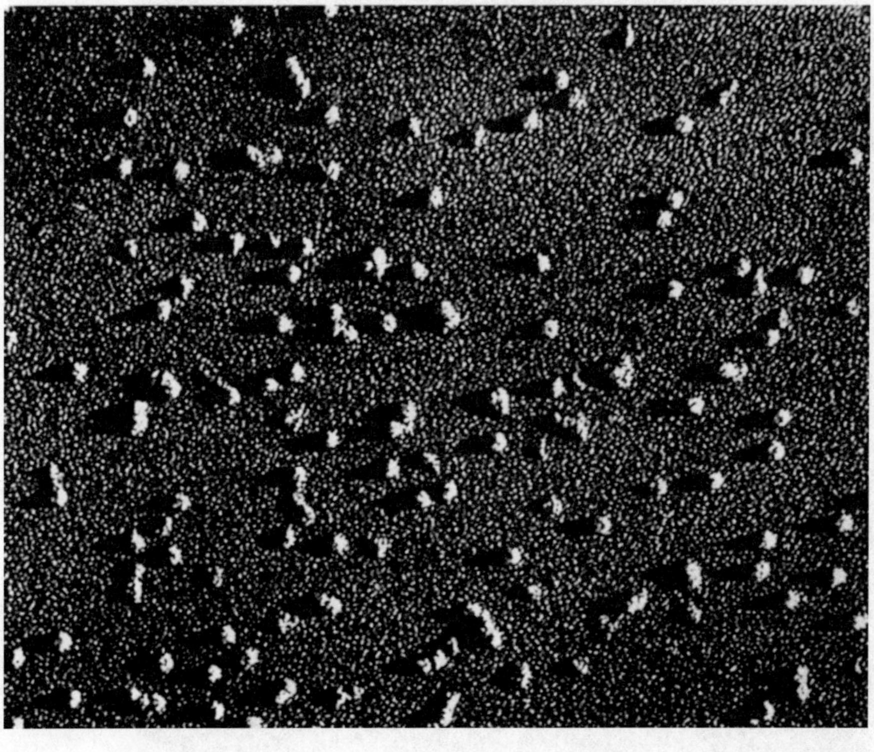

Fig. 8. A micrograph of „conversed“ CM-particles (30 S and 50 S) shadowed at shadow-to-height ratio 6 :1, Magnification 100000 ×. Two kinds of particles with dimensions and appearance of the normal 30 S and 50 S ribosomal particles are seen

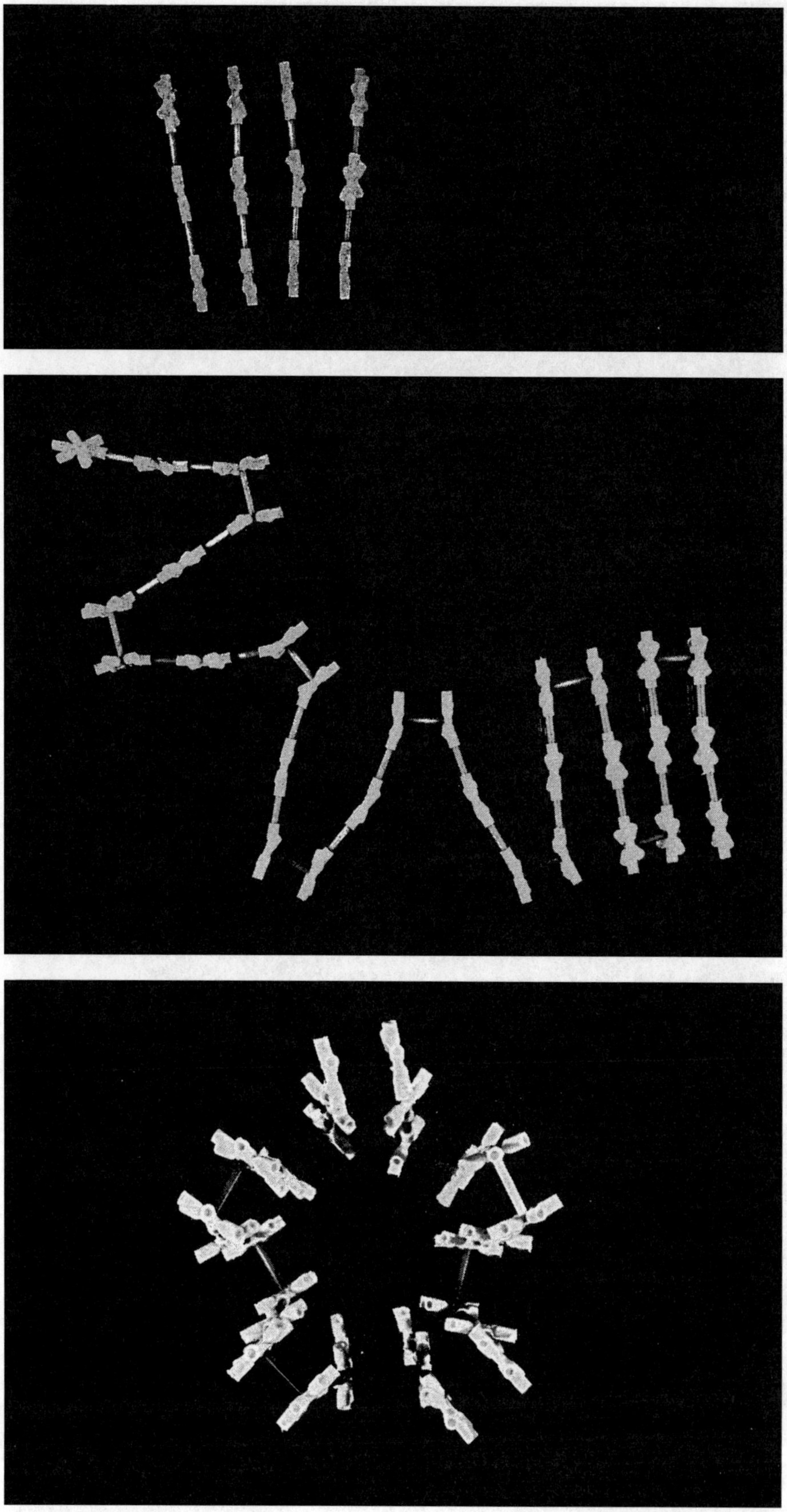

a)

b)

c)

Fig. 10. Photographs of the schematical models of ribonucleoprotein strand (a, b) and one of the variants of folding of this strand into 50 S particle or its precursor (c)

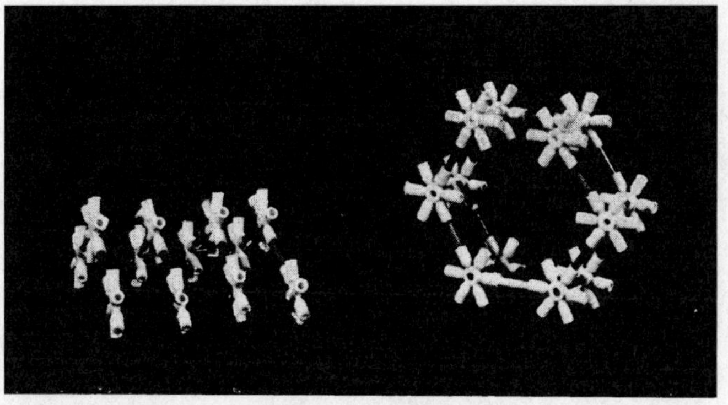

a)

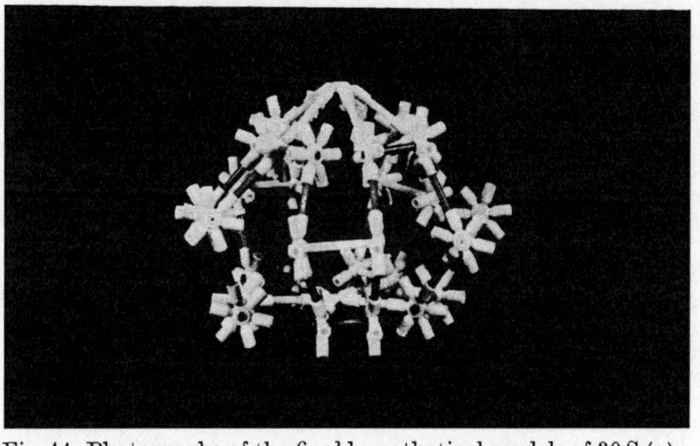

b)

Fig. 11. Photographs of the final hypothetical models of 30 S (a) and 50 S (b) particles

ribosomal particles with the short fibrils („wicks") sticking out of the particles is presented in Fig. 3. Since the formation of these short strands (for example after treatment with urea) was not accompanied by releasing of free ribosomal protein these strands were suggested to be not just RNA sticking out of the ribosomes but rather RNA with protein. In other words they might be of ribonucleoprotein nature. Therefore it was tempting to find out whether the ribosomal particles could be completely unfolded into ribonucleoprotein strands by treatment with some agents.

All attempts to use formaldehyde-fixed ribosomes for this purpose were not successful since the fixation with formaldehyde could probably cross-link the particles thus not permitting its complete unfolding. Fortunately Stanley and Bock (personal communication) developed a technique for removal of the latent ribonuclease from the native ribosomes by the treatment of the ribosomes with 0.5 M NH_4Cl. This procedure does not cause any visible chemical or structural changes of the ribosomal particles. We have used this method for preparation of „ribonuclease-free" 50 S and 30 S ribosomal subunits.

The usually purified 70 S ribosomes were suspended in 0.5 M NH_4Cl with 0.001 M Tris-buffer pH 7.8 and kept for 15 hours in refrigerator. Under these conditions the 70 S ribosomes dissociated completely into their 50 S and 30 S subunits which in this solution had sedimentation coefficients of about 45 and 30 S. The solution of the 45 S and 30 S ribosomal particles was centrifuged during 15 minutes at 20000 g to remove insoluble contaminations and aggregates. Then the ribosomal particles were spun down by 4 hour centrifugation at 105000 g. The particles pelleted from NH_4Cl solution contained 60% RNA and 40% protein, like the original preparation of 70 S ribosomes; thus no significant loss of ribosomal protein occurred during this treatment.

If the pellet of the „ribonuclease-free" ribosomes isolated by this procedure was suspended in deionized water or even in 0.01 M Tris-buffer without Mg^{++} (see scheme of the experiment, Fig. 4) the phenomenon of unfolding or loosening of the originally compact particles could be easily observed. This followed first of all from the changes in hydrodynamic properties: decrease of sedimentation coefficients from 45 and 30 S down to 24–26 and 12–15 S respectively (these values are experimental and not extrapolated to the infinite dilution), and at the same time significant increase in viscosity.

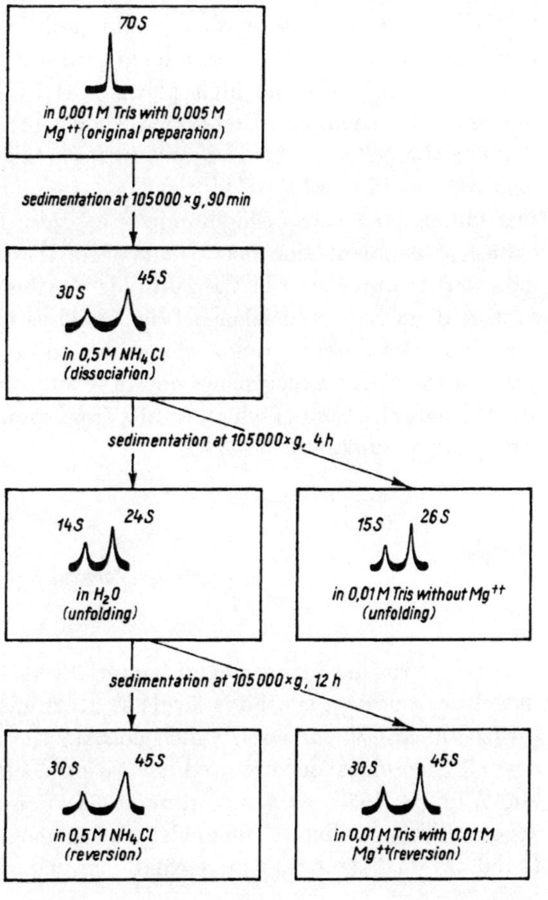

Fig. 4. Scheme of the experiment on the reversible unfolding of ribosomal particles into ribonucleoprotein strands (with corresponding sedimentation patterns)

For more detailed analysis of what happens with the ,,ribonuclease-free" ribosomes after their transfer into Mg^{++}-free solution of low ionic strength the solution of the 24 S and 14 S particles in deionized water was centrifuged during 12 hours at 105000 g. The chemical analysis of the pellet has showed the former RNA and protein content that was characteristic for the original 70 S ribosomes or the 45 S and 30 S particles: 60% RNA and 40 % protein. Hence the decrease in sedimentation coefficients and the increase in specific viscosity of the ribisomal particles after their transfer into water was really due to unfolding or loosening of the whole ribonucleoprotein particles without any loss or solubilization of ribosomal-protein. In other words this phenomenon was shown to be connected neither with partial or complete releasing of ribosomal RNA or protein nor with any other processes of ribonucleoprotein dissociation into RNA and protein. On the other hand, isolation of RNA from the pellet and its sedimentation analysis showed the presence of the two usual high molecular weight components (23 S and 17 S) characteristic for ribosomal RNA from native *E. coli* ribosomes. The isolated RNA preparations displayed the increase of specific viscosity upon heating solution indicating the presence of continuous polynucleotide chains. All this seems to prove directly that the drop in sedimentation coefficients of the ,,ribonuclease-free" ribosomal particles in water is not associated with any kind of unfolding or loosening of each particle as a whole the integrity and continuity of its RNA chain being preserved.

Unfolding of the 50 S and 30 S ribosomal subunits into ribonucleoprotein strands as a result of transferring ribosomes into Mg^{++}-free water solutions was finally evidenced by electron microscopy. A typical micrograph of shadowed preparation of the 24 S and 14 S particles after their pelleting from deionized water is presented in Fig. 5. One can see numerous strand-like particles with a height (a diameter of strand), calculated from the shadow length, of about 30 Å and with a length up to 1200–1300 Å. These ribonucleoprotein strands look very much like the high polymer RNA molecules in their ,,rod-like" configuration though, as it was already mentioned, they contain 40% protein (as in the normal ribosomes).

When the pellet of the 24 S and 14 S particles (that is of the ,,unfolded" ribosomes) was suspended not in water or diluted Mg^{++}-free buffer but either in 0.5 M NH_4Cl (with 0.01 M Tris-buffer) as solution of high ionic strength or in Tris-buffer (0.01 M) with 0.01 M Mg^{++} the values of sedimentation coefficients were found to be again 45 and 30 S. This evidently indicated the reversion of the ,,unfolded" ribonucleoprotein particles to the original compact configuration (see scheme, Fig. 4). Thus the unfolding of the ribosomal subunits into the ribonucleoprotein strands was shown to be a reversible process.

From the above experiments one may suggest that the 50 S and 30 S ribosomal subunits are the particles each of which results from some compact folding of a long ribonucleoprotein strand with a diameter 30–40 Å.

A Study of Natural Precursors of Ribosomes

It is known that incubation of bacterial cells in the presence of chloramphenicol, a specific inhibitor of protein synthesis, leads to accumulation in cells of the ribonucleoprotein particles (so called CM particles) which contain the normal ribosomal RNA but differ from the normal ribosomes in lower sedimentation coefficients and lower protein content (Nomura and Watson, 1959; Kurland *et al.*, 1962). Some other inhibitors of protein synthesis causes accumulation of similar ribonucleoprotein particles. ,,Light" ribosomal particles were also found in small amounts in normally growing bacteria (Roberts, 1960). All this suggests that these particles may be considered as normal precursors of ribosomes („neosomes") accumulating under the conditions of inhibited protein synthesis because of impossibility to be completed with protein into the normal ribosomes. This idea is supported by the results of our recent experiments indicating that in the presence of magnesium ions the CM-particles can bind additional protein in vitro resulting in formation of the particles indistinguishable from the normal 30 S and 50 S ribosomal particles in their sedimentation coefficients, protein content and appearance under electron microscope (SHAKULOV, BOGDANOV and SPIRIN, 1963).

One may logically suggest that being metabolic precursors of ribosomes the CM-particles are also their structural precursors i. e. they may bear all the principal features of structural organization of the normal ribosomes, may be in a „simplified" form. Hence a special electron microscope study of the CM-particles was undertaken in our laboratory in collaboration with Dr. N. A. KISSELEV (SPIRIN, KISSELEV *et al.*, 1963).

In accordance with the earlier observations by WATSON, NOMURA and KURLAND, our preparations of CM-particles contained 73–75% RNA and 27–25% protein. In the ultracentrifuge the preparations showed two components with sedimentation coefficients 25 and 19 S (25 S and 19 S-particles). RNA isolated from such preparations consisted of two components, 23 S and 17 S, i. e. it was analogous to the normal ribosomal RNA. Electron microscope study of shadowed preparations of the CM-particles showed the presence of two types of structures corresponding apparently to the 25 S and 19 S particles; in their size these particles were very similar to the 50 S and 30 S subunits of the normal ribosomes. There were roughly spherical particles with a height (calculated from a shadow length) about 120–150 Å and, on the other hand, flattened particles with a height from 50 Å to 80 Å.

The negative staining technique permits to reveal further details in the structure of the CM-particles. A corresponding electron micrograph is given in Fig. 6. First of all, two types of regular particles can be seen. The particles of the first type look as peculiar pentangular structures with a diameter up to 160 Å and with a hole in the center. They seem to consist as if of five large subunits arranged in a pentagon and joined by strands. The second type of the regular structures are rectangular particles; they consist of four rows of small subunits packed side-by-side. Each the row has a width about 35 Å and occasionally three small subunits may be distinguished in it. The dimensions of the rectangular particles are 120 × 140 Å. It should be also mentioned that strands of different length with a width of about 30 Å can be occasionally seen on the micrographs. In addition there are numerous small particles which represent probably the degradation products.

Comparing the results of the electron microscope investigation of the CM-particles (Fig. 6) with the data on the normal ribosomal subunits (Fig. 1b) one can first of all notice that the dimensions of the pentangular CM particles and of the rectangular particles are consistent with the corresponding values for the 50 S subunits and the 30 S subunits, respectively. It may be concluded therefore that the „pentangular" CM particles (probably, 25 S-particles) represent precursors of the 50 S ribosomal subunits whereas the „rectangular" CM particles (probably 19 S) are precursors of the 30 S subunits. This conclusion is also confirmed by comparison of the shape of the CM-particles with the appearance of the 50 S and 30 S ribosomal subunits: the 50 S subunits as it was already mentioned have more or less spherical or rather polyhedral contours and occasionally look like pentangular structures whereas the 30 S particles very often look more or less rectangular (Fig. 1b).

The structural regularity visible on the electron micrographs for the both types of CM particles permits to make certain conclusions concerning the mode of packing of protein molecules in the particles. First of all this holds for the „rectangular" particles identified as the 19 S component. It is known that the molecular weight of a single RNA molecule present in this particle is 0.5—0.6 million and that RNA is about 73—75% of the particle weight. Hence the share of ribosomal protein is 27—25%. According to the data available the molecular weight of ribosomal protein is about 17000—20000. This means that a 19 S particle should contain 10—13 protein molecules. On the electron micrograph the 19 S particles have 4 rows of small subunits, 3 subunits in a row, that is in total 12 subunits negatively stained with PTA. This leads to the conclusion that each visible small subunit is an individual protein molecule and that all the protein molecules (12) present in the 19 S subunit are located more or less in one plane so that they all are seen on the micrograph. Indeed, the 19 S particles (as well as the corresponding ribosomal 30 S subunits) look on the micrographs of shadowed preparations like flattened particles. On the other hand, theoretically calculated diameter of a spherical protein molecule with a molecular weight 20000 is about 36 Å this well corresponding to the dimensions of small subunits visible in Fig. 6. Thus the 19 S particles may be considered as more or less regular structures in which 12 protein molecules arranged approximately in the same plane so that they form four parallel side-by-side oriented rows each row consisting of 3 protein molecules. Evidently, all these molecules are associated with the single RNA molecule and so the arrangement of protein molecules discussed above should properly correspond to the mode of folding of the single continuous RNA molecule (RNA strand) in the 19 S and respectively, in the 30 S particles.

The analysis of the „pentangular“ structures which seem to be the 25 S component of the CM particles is much more complicated. Apparently, five large subunits visible on the micrographs can not be individual protein molecules, for they are too large. Besides the particles of this type are by no means flat and therefore the visible picture is actually a projection of structural elements located on different levels. Consequently the micrographs presented do not permit to make direct conclusions about the arrangement of protein in these particles; it would be more promising to use a complex approach and to try to construct a model of packing of RNA and protein which could explain the pictures observed (see below).

In vitro Reconstruction of Ribosomal Particles

It was noticed that after the first preparative sedimentation of the CM particles from starting *E. coli* cell free extract the preparations often contained, in addition to the typical 19 S and 25 S components, a slower moving protein component (Fig. 7a). If these preparations of the CM particles with protein were suspended in Mg^{++}-free Tris-buffer the repeated

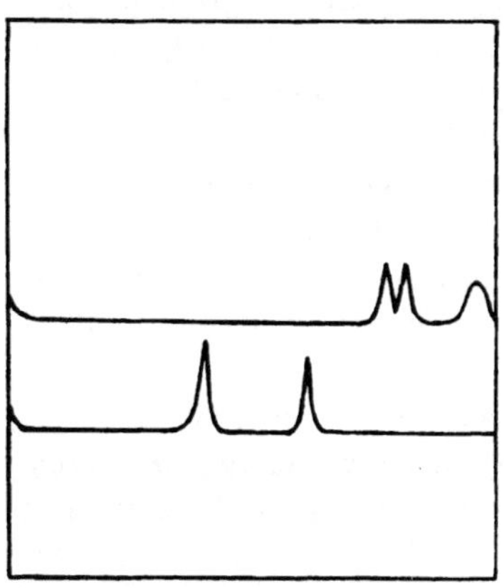

Fig. 7. Sedimentation patterns of preparation of CM particles with concomitant protein in 0.001 M Tris-buffer plus 10^{-4} M magnesium acetate. (Scheme)

a) upper part: before pelleting in preparative rotor; 25 S and 19 S components of CM particles and slowly moving protein component are seen

b) lower part: after pelleting in preparative rotor and subsequent resuspending in the same buffer; only 50 S and 30 S components („conversed“ CM particles) are seen

preparative sedimentation from this solution was essentially enough to get a significant purification of the CM particles from the concomitant protein. As it was mentioned above the purified preparations of the CM particles contained 25–27% protein and 75–73% RNA. If, however, the repeated preparative sedimentation of the CM particles was carried out in Tris-buffer containing Mg^{++}-ions (10^{-4} M magnesium acetate) neither the typical 19 S and 15 S particles nor the slowly moving protein component were found after resuspension of the pellet; instead two new heavier components with sedimentation coefficients 30 S and 50 S have appeared (Fig. 7b). The sedimentation coefficients found exactly corresponded to those of the normal ribosomal 30 S and 50 S subunits. The chemical analysis of these newly formed particles indicated that they contained 40% protein and 60% RNA, like normal ribosomes. Electron microscope study of these preparations performed by Dr. N. A. KISSELEV has revealed the presence of two types of particles indistinguishable morphologically from the 30 S and 50 S subunits of the normal *E. coli* ribosomes (Fig. 8).

Thus when the 19 S and 25 S CM particles and the concomitant protein component are pelleted together in the presence of Mg^{++}-ions at 100000 g binding of the protein to the CM particles occurs resulting in formation of new particles similar to the normal 30 S and 50 S ribosomal subunits in their physical chemical properties.

It should be noted that this conversion of the CM particles into ribosome-like particles in vitro was found to occur only when the concomitant slowly moving protein was present in the original preparation. Sedimentation of the purified 19 S and 25 S CM particles in the presence of Mg^{++}-ions at 100000 g had no effect on the particles. No reconstruction of ribosome-like particles was observed if the CM particles and the concomitant protein were incubated together without ultracentrifugation. And finally, reconstruction did not occur when the CM particles and the protein were spun down in the absence of Mg^{++}-ions.

Certain conclusions may be drawn from data presented. First, the possibility of in vitro formation of ribosome-like particles from the CM particles is consistent with the idea that the CM particles are precursors of ribosomes (i. e. they are „neosomes") which accumulate in the cell when protein synthesis is inhibited. Further, these results may indicate that the formation of ribosomes in the cell may be a stepwise process and that one of the last steps, conversion of „neosomes" into final ribosomes, may occur as spontaneous interaction of soluble ribosomal protein with the „neosome". Finally, these observations permit to distinguish at least two classes of protein in ribosomes: the first may be called *basal* structural ribosomal protein; it is the protein component of the „neosomes" and the CM particles; no Mg^{++}-ions are needed to bind this protein to RNA molecule; the second is *additional* ribosomal protein which can be bound only to completed „neosome", probably by means of Mg^{++}-ions. It is tempting to suggest that it is this additional protein that is responsible for the enzymatic activities found in ribosomes (and particularly for the latent ribonuclease activity) whereas the basal structural protein is purely structural nonenzymatic protein of ribosomal particles.

A Possible Model of Ribosome Structure

The most important observation made so far in our experiments is that the compact ribosomal particles can be reversibly unfolded into long ribonucleoprotein strands with a diameter 30–40 Å without any degradation of the nucleic acid or protein components. Basing on a number of other observations one may try to discuss the possible structure of such ribonucleoprotein strand and the mode of its packing in a ribosomal particle.

Two independent groups of observations, the study of hypochromicity of the ribosomal RNA within ribosomes and the X-ray diffraction analysis of ribosomes (ZUBAY and WILKINS, 1960; SCHLESSINGER, 1960; BONHOEFFER and SCHACHMAN, 1960; KLUG *et al.*, 1961) indicate that ribosomal RNA in ribosomes possesses the secondary structure i. e. a set of helical regions probably of the same structure as exist in isolated RNA in solution.

It is known that isolated high-polymer RNA in solution has the compact conformation that includes numerous relatively short helical regions alternating with flexible single-stranded regions. According to our data, under certain conditions the axes of these helical regions can become oriented in parallel planes and therefore helical regions would stack over each other forming a strand or ,,rod-like" structure with the helical regions oriented approximately perpendicularly to the long axis of this strand or ,,rod" (SPIRIN, 1960, 1963). Fragment of such strand or rod is shown on the upper part of Fig. 9. It is understood that the diameter

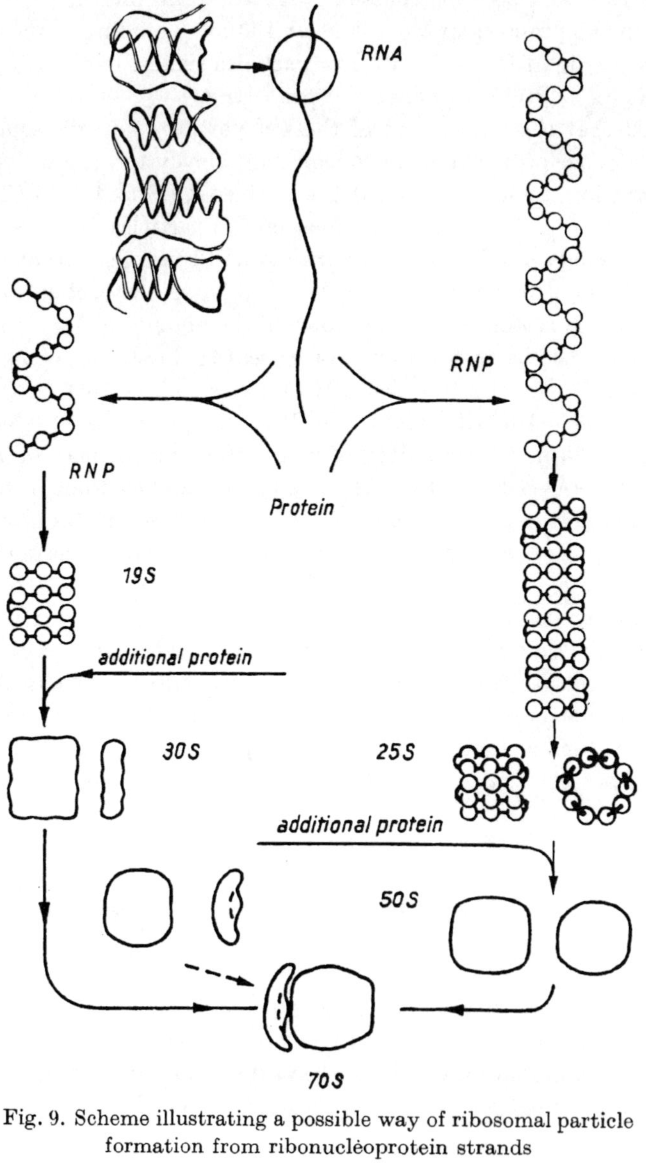

Fig. 9. Scheme illustrating a possible way of ribosomal particle formation from ribonucleoprotein strands

of the RNA strand (that is of RNA in the ,,rod-like" configuration) should correspond to the average length of helical regions forming the structure. The diameter of the RNA rod measured by electron microscope determination of the height of shadowed particles was found to be around 30 Å thus corresponding to the average length of a helical region of about one complete turn of a double-helix (KISSELEV, GAVRILOVA and SPIRIN, 1961). According to the electron microscope data presented here the diameter of ribonucleoprotein strands resulting from the unfolding of ribosomal particles is also about 30 Å.

On the other hand, HUXLEY and ZUBAY (1960) using the positive staining of RNA in ribosomes with uranyl acetate have demonstrated that RNA and protein are mutually impregnated in the ribosomes i. e. that the protein molecules are more or less equally distributed along the somehow folded RNA molecule and do not form any kind of shell for the ,,coil" of ribosomal RNA. If to assume that the protein molecules are bound to the mentioned long flexible ,,rod" of ribosomal RNA along all its length (being located between helical regions, for instance) and in turn this ribonucleoprotein strand is folded into a compact, almost spherical particle, called ribosome, the apparent mutual impregnation of RNA and protein within ribosomes may be understandable.

Thus as it follows from our experiments each ribosomal particle or to say it more precisely each 30 S and 50 S subunit consists of a single specifically folded ribonucleoprotein strand. It is suggested that the basis of the strand is a molecule of ribosomal RNA in the ,,rod-like" (strand-like) configuration with the helical regions oriented probably perpendicular to the long axis of the strand. The molecules of ribosomal protein are bound to the RNA molecule in such a way that the conformation of RNA is not significantly disturbed as they are located between the helical regions ,,impregnating" the RNA strand more or less evenly along all its length.

Constructing the models of folding of the ribonucleoprotein strands into ribosomes we used mainly the electron microscope observations on the CM particles because the regularity in the arrangement of individual elements in this case is especially evident. The morphological similarity between the CM particles and the normal ribosomal particles seems to permit to extrapolate some visible regularities found for the CM particles to modelling of the 50 S and 30 S ribosomal subunits.

Formation of the 30 S particle (or its precursor, the 19 S particle) from the RNP strand may be thought to be as if a result of three-fold bending of the strand and subsequent parallel arrangement of the resultant sections side-by-side, in the same plane. The compact packing of the four parallel sections (bends) may be provided by the protein-to-protein interaction between them. All this results in formation of a flat rectangular particle, this morphology being characteristic for the 30 S ribosomal subunit (Fig. 1b) and for its precursor, the 19 S particle (Fig. 6). The formation of the 30 S particle from the RNP strand is schematically shown on the left part of Fig. 9. Fig. 10 gives a photograph of the model of the 30 S subunit.

For construction of models of the 50 S particle we have attempted to proceed from the same packing principle that was found in the case of the 19 S and 30 S subunits. What I mean is the regular bending of the strand on itself each 120 Å and the parallel adhesion of the resultant 120 Å sections (possibly due to tendency of the molecules of ribosomal protein to interact with each other). Applying this principle for the case of a strand with a length of about 1200 Å (the possible length of the ribonucleoprotein strand in the 50 S subunit) one would not have four sections as it holds for the 30 S or 19 S particle but ten sections i. e. ten parallel rows which all are parts of the same strand. This structure consisting of 10 rows formed by bending of a continuous strand and arranged in a parallel fashion is shown in Fig. 9 right. The principle of formation of such structure from a single many times bent strand is given on the photograph, Fig. 10b. If to assume now that this flat particle will tend to roll up forming a cylinder due to interaction of its marginal rows (the length of the 10 bends particle seems to permit that) the model prototype of the 25 S and respectively 50 S particle (Fig. 9 right) is constructed. On looking at this cylinder from the base (from above) each two stand-up sections (or bends) connected above will look like one large subunit; there will be seen as if five large subunits altogether arranged in a pentagon with a hole in the center (see the photo of the model, Fig. 10c). That is exactly how the ,,pentangular" 25 S CM particles look under electron microscope (Fig. 6).

In conclusion it should be pointed out that the models proposed, a ,,flat rectangle" for 30 S particle and a ,,cylinder" or, more exactly, ,,pentahedron" for 50 S particle, are only rough approximations to describe some principles of strand folding and not necessarily reflect the actual detailed structure of the particles in question. Most likely the formation of the particles involves some additional bendings within each bend making the shape of the particles more complicated. In particular the 30 S particle is probably not completely flat but, due to additional bending in the middle of each bend of the strand it rather may resemble something like a span roof (see the general view of the model, Fig. 11a). Due to similar bending inside of each bend of the strand the 50 S particle might easily acquire a form resembling a polyhedron or a sphere (see the general view of the model, Fig. 11b).

A Possible Way of Ribosome Formation in a Cell

One can hardly doubt that the formation of normal ribosomal particle in a cell goes through a number of successive intermediate steps. The first step should include two independent and spatially separated sequences of biochemical reactions: synthesis of ribosomal RNA (on DNA) and synthesis of ribosomal proteins (probably in nuclear ribosomes). This is purely a biosynthetic step resulting in the synthesis of ribosomal components. Next steps of ribosome formation should include some processes of assembling of the synthesized RNA and protein and their certain packing into specific structures. I would like to discuss now these ,,non-biosynthetic" steps, i. e. steps of assembling of the ribosome structure from RNA and protein.

For elucidation of events which take place in the course of ribosome formation two groups of observations are of especial interest. The first is the possibility to find in bacterial cells a special type of ribonucleoprotein particles representing probably ,,half-finished" ribosomes, or ribosome precursors. I mean first of all so called ,,neosomes" of Roberts' group and CM particles accumulating in cells under conditions of inhibited protein synthesis. These particles contain only about half of the protein content of the normal ribosomes. At the same time these RNP particles seem to have constant and well-defined characteristics of their chemical composition and physical chemical properties thus representing the discrete group of particles. No gradual transitions or intermediates between them and free ribosomal RNA or Roberts' ,,eosomes", on one hand, and between them and the normal ribosomal particles, on the other, was ever observed. All this gives an impression that the formation of the ribosomal particles (50 S and 30 S subunits) from RNA and protein molecules is a two-stage process that may be written as follows:

eosome (RNA?) + protein molecules → neosome (CM particle);
neosome (CM particle) + protein molecules → ribosomal subunit.

Chloramphenicol blocks the second stage of this process and the accumulation of the CM particles takes place. It is characteristic that preparations of the isolated CM particles are equally stable in the presence and in the absence of magnesium ions, in contrast with normal ribosomes requiring magnesium for their stability. This fact may indicate that the binding of protein during the first stage and the formation of the „neosome" does not involve magnesium ions. It is likely that magnesium ions are necessary only for the second stage of the assembling of the ribosomal particles.

The second series of observations favouring these ideas is our experiments on in vitro reconstruction of ribosome-like particles from CM particles and protein. Practically in these experiments we managed to perform the second stage of the ribosome assembling process artificially, outside the cell. Magnesium ions were indeed necessary for this process. These experiments have evidenced further that CM particles are most likely to be normal ribosome precursors, i. e. normal intermediates in the formation of ribosomes in vivo. In the in vitro experiments the binding of protein to CM particles and formation of ribosome-like particles was observed as an „all-or-none" process; no intermediate states between the CM-like and ribosome-like particles were detected. Thus if the amount of protein was not enough to complete all CM particles present in a preparation only four discrete types of particles appeared in ultracentrifuge as a result of the reconstruction experiments: 50 S, 30 S, 25 S and 19 S, and no intermediates between them. On the whole the experiments on the in vitro reconstruction of ribosome-like particles from CM particles and protein most strongly support the idea that the formation of ribosomes from RNA and protein is not a one-step interaction but involves several, at least two, successive stages.

The idea of multi-stage formation of ribosomes in the cell permits to reconsider the possibilities of total reconstruction of ribosomes from isolated RNA and protein in vitro. Many unsuccessful attempts along this line were undertaken in different laboratories and, as we understand now, they were to be failed, for the necessity of reconstruction in several steps was not taken into consideration. Apparently the reconstruction should be attempted to be made at least in two steps. Moreover in each step a proper fraction but not the total ribosomal protein is probably to be used. The difficulty now is to carry out the first steps, i. e. the combination of free ribosomal RNA and the basal structural protein into „neosome" (CM-like particle).

In agreement with what was said above the process of formation of ribosomal subunits in a normal cell may be thought like follows. Ribosomal RNA is synthesized on certain DNA cistrons and then appears in a free state. Hereabouts, probably also in nuclear structures, the synthesis of the basal structural protein constantly occurs and a certain concentration of this protein exists in this part of the cell. As the synthesis of the RNA goes on, its molecules immediately combine, with the basal structural protein forming the ribonucleoprotein precursors of ribosomes, the neosomes. At the same time the synthesis of the additional ribosomal protein also takes place somewhere in the cell and hence a certain level of its exists in cellular sap. When newly formed neosomes leave the nuclear structures they can combine with the additional ribosomal protein in the presence of magnesium ions and form the normal ribosomal subunits. Two unequal ribosomal subunits unite in the presence of Mg^{++} and form the ribosome.

What happens, from this point of view, during the inhibition of protein synthesis with chloramphenicol? The ribosomal RNA synthesis goes on. The synthesis of ribosomal protein is blocked or at least strongly inhibited. All this does not mean however that the process of ribosome formation ceases. It can proceed for some time owing to the presence of some cellular pool of the already synthesized ribosomal protein. In some time, however, constantly synthesized ribosomal RNA will decrease the concentration of ribosomal protein in the cell to the level that will be too low to provide its binding to precursors so that the formation of new ribosomal particles will stop. Since there are two different classes of ribosomal proteins their threshold levels of concentrations should be probably different. The apparent effect of chloramphenicol is the accumulation of „neosomes", i. e. the products of association of RNA with the basal structural protein; the second stage, binding of the additional protein, does not occur. Consequently the minimum threshold level of concentration of the additional ribosomal protein in the cell may be thought to be attained earlier than in the case of the basal structural protein. So when the second stage of the ribosome assembling begins to stop the first stage still proceeds for some time and this leads to accumulation of the CM particles. As the synthesis of ribosomal RNA continues the minimum threshold concentration of the basal structural protein is soon achieved too and the accumulation of the CM particles ceases. However, since RNA within the particles, in contrast with the normal ribosomes, is not properly protected and therefore can be attacked by external nucleases the CM particles may constantly degrade. The released basal structural protein may be reutilized combining with newly synthesized RNA molecules and forming new CM particles. Under these conditions the apparent level of concentration of the CM particles in the cell would be constant.

The assumption that a living cell has a certain level of concentration of free ribosomal proteins and that below some minimum threshold concentration the protein is not effective in the ribosome formation is favoured by our experiments on the in vitro reconstruction of ribosome-like particles. Indeed as it should be expected the ordinary incubation of the CM particles in original cell extract in the presence of magnesium ions have not resulted in any conversion of the CM particles. When, however, the CM particles were spun down together with free protein into the pellet where concentration of the protein should be much higher than in the original extract the conversion of the CM particles into the ribosome-like particles occurred. This experiment proves that the protein needed for conversion of the CM particles into ribosomes was present in extract in a free state but its concentration was not high enough for the second stage of ribosome formation to occur.

References

Bonhoeffer, F., and H. K. Schachman, 1960: Biochem. Biophys. Research Communs. **2**, 366.

Hall, C. E., and H. S. Slayter, 1959: J. Mol. Biol. **1**, 329.

Huxley, H. E., and G. Zubay, 1960: J. Mol. Biol. **2**, 10.

Kisselev, N. A., L. P. Gavrilova, and A. S. Spirin, 1961: J. Mol. Biol. **3**, 778.

Klug, A., K. C. Holmes, and J. T. Finch, 1961: J. Mol. Biol. **3**, 87.

Kurland, C. G., M. Nomura, and J. D. Watson, 1962: J. Mol. Biol. **4**, 388.

Nomura, M., and J. D. Watson, 1959: J. Mol. Biol. **1**, 204.

Roberts, R. B., 1960: Ann. N. Y. Acad. Sci. **88**, 752.

Schlessinger, D., 1960: J. Mol. Biol. **2**, 92.

Shakulov, R. S., M. A. Ajtkhozhin, and A. S. Spirin, 1962: Biokhimiya **27**, 744.

Shakulov, R. S., A. A. Bogdanov, and A. S. Spirin 1963: Doklady Akad. Nauk S. S. S. R. **153**, 224.

Spirin, A. S., 1960: J. Mol. Biol. **2**, 436.

Spirin, A. S., 1963: In „Progress in Nucleic Acid Research" (eds. J. N. Davidson, and W. E. Cohn), v. **1**, p. 301. Acad. Press. N. Y., 1963.

Spirin, A. S., N. A. Kisselev, R. S. Shakulov, and A. A. Bogdanov, 1963: Biokhimiya **28**, 920.

Zubay, G., and M. H. F. Wilkins, 1960: J. Mol. Biol. **2**, 105.

Über die Rolle der Aminosäuren bei der Synthese der Ribosomen-RNS

R. LINDIGKEIT

Institut für Zellphysiologie, Abt. Zellregulation, der Deutschen Akademie der Wissenschaften zu Berlin

Der Aufbau der löslichen Eiweiße in der Zelle der heute dank der zahlreichen Untersuchungen der letzten Jahre weitgehend überschaubar geworden ist, geschieht bekanntlich mit Hilfe der Ribosomen. Die Informationen über die Synthese der Ribosomen selbst hingegen sind bisher viel geringer. Z. B. ist noch unbekannt, ob das Eiweiß der Ribosomen auf demselben Wege synthetisiert wird, wie das lösliche Eiweiß oder aber ob hierbei spezielle Synthesewege von der Zelle eingeschlagen werden.

Unter anderem haben insbesondere die neueren Untersuchungen von BRITTEN und MCCARTHY (1962), BRITTEN *et al.* (1962), MCCARTHY und BRITTEN (1962) und MCCARTHY *et al.* (1962) Erkenntnisse über den Aufbau der Ribosomen in der Zelle gebracht.

Danach wird zunächst freie Ribosomen-RNS synthetisiert. Diese freie RNS oder das sogenannte Eosom wird in einem weiteren Schritt mit Eiweiß beladen und so zu einer Ribosomen-Vorstufe, genannt Neosom, umgebaut, die ca. 25% Eiweiß enthält. Ein weiterer Zusatz von Eiweiß ist erforderlich, damit die fertigen Ribosomen entstehen, die bei *E. coli* etwa 37% Eiweiß enthalten.

Chloramphenicol (ClA), das häufig benutzt wurde, um die Synthese der Ribosomen-RNS zu untersuchen, hemmt neben der Synthese der löslichen Eiweiße auch die Synthese fertiger Ribosomen. Die unvollkommenen Ribosomen, die unter ClA-Einfluß synthetisiert werden, enthalten nach KURLAND, NOMURA und WATSON (1962) ca. 25% Eiweiß. Diese Partikel, die gemäß dem Eiweißgehalt den Neosomen von BRITTEN und Mitarbeitern entsprechen (BRITTEN und MCCARTHY, 1962, BRITTEN *et al.*, 1962, MCCARTHY und BRITTEN, 1962 und MCCARTHY *et al.*, 1962), wurden von NOMURA und WATSON (1959) ClA-Partikel genannt.

MCCARTHY *et al.* (1962) fanden jedoch, daß unter ClA-Einwirkung ein Teil der Ribosomen-RNS in einer Form gebildet wird, die weitgehend eiweißfrei ist.

Bei den Diskussionen über die Rolle der Aminosäuren bei der Ribosomen-RNS-Synthese, die bisher nicht vollkommen verstanden wird, wurde meist nicht beachtet, daß zwei verschiedene Typen von Ribosomen-Vorstufen existieren, von denen nur die eine eiweißhaltig ist. Normalerweise ist die Synthese der Ribosomen-RNS in der Zelle von Aminosäuren abhängig. Das ist aus der Tatsache bekannt, daß Bakterienzellen, welche eine Aminosäure für ihr Wachstum benötigen, die RNS-Synthese stoppen, wenn im Medium diese Aminosäure fehlt. Bei Gegenwart von ClA können kleine Mengen der benötigten Aminosäure die RNS-Synthese wieder in Gang bringen, während die Synthese von Protein gehemmt bleibt. ARONSON und SPIEGELMAN (1961a, b) fanden, daß bei hohen Konzentrationen von ClA die RNS-Synthese von einem äußeren Aminosäureangebot unabhängig wird.

Da einerseits vorausgesetzt wurde, daß der größte Teil der ClA-RNS in Form von eiweißhaltigen Partikeln existiert, zum anderen aber bei hohen Konzentrationen von ClA Aminosäuren für die Ribosomen-RNS-Synthese nicht mehr benötigt werden, wurde von KURLAND und MAALØE (1962) angenommen, daß eine bestimmte Menge vorgebildetes Eiweiß in der Zelle existiert, das wahrscheinlich benutzt wird, um mit der ClA-RNS die eiweißhaltigen Ribo-

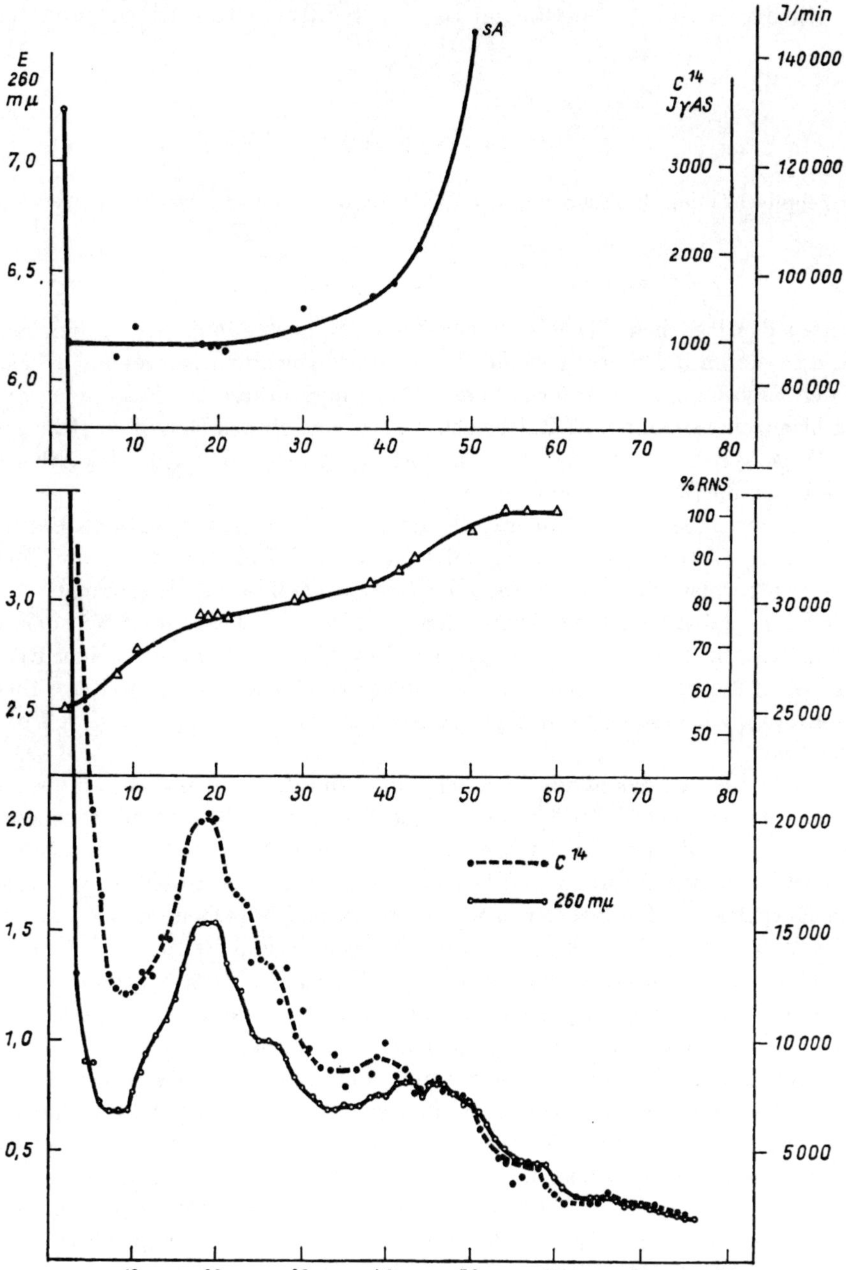

Abb. 1. Auftrennung der Ribosomenfraktion einer Methionin-Mangelmutante eines Stammes von *E. coli* — K 12 auf einer DEAE-Säule (Kap. O,7 mäq./g.)

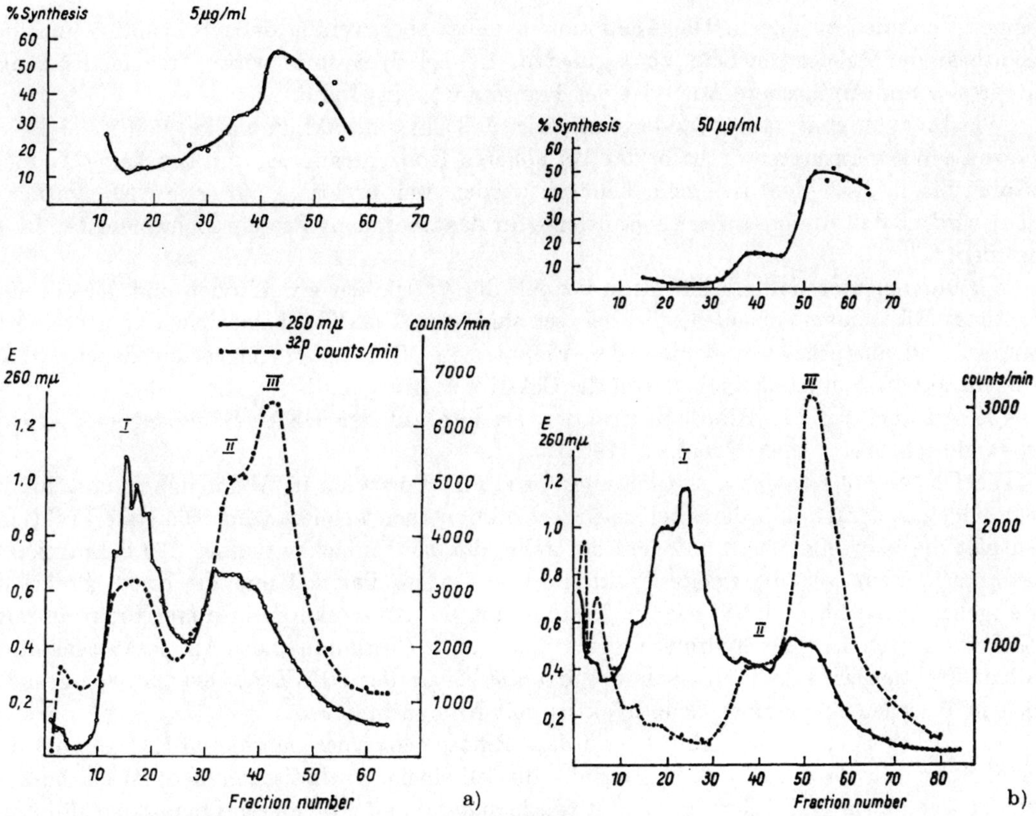

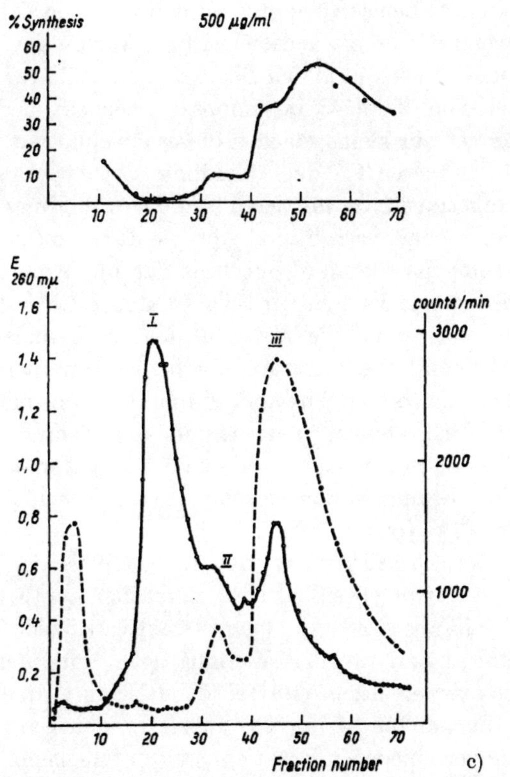

Abb. 2 (a, b, c). Der Effekt verschiedener ClA-Konzentrationen auf den Einbau von ^{32}P in Ribosomen. 60 Min. ClA-Einwirkung, Trennung auf der DEAE-Säule

Fraktion I: Vorgebildete Ribosomen (= „70 S-Fraktion")

II: Fraktion, die ca 25% Eiweiß enthält

III: Fraktion, die weitgehend eiweißfrei ist

somen-Vorstufen zu bilden. Die Aminosäuren selbst aber werden danach benötigt, um die Synthese der Ribosomen-RNS zu regulieren. In diesem System wirkt Transfer-RNS als Repressor und Aminosäure-Adenylat der Transfer-RNS als Induktor.

Wie BRITTEN *et al.* (1962) fanden auch wir, daß ClA eine Akkumulation von freier RNS bewirkt. Wir vermuteten deshalb, daß bei höheren Konzentrationen von ClA keine Aminosäuren für die RNS-Synthese mehr benötigt werden, weil praktisch nur freie RNS synthetisiert wird, so daß Aminosäuren als Bausteine für das ribosomale Protein nicht mehr benötigt werden.

Wir untersuchten deshalb mit Hilfe von ^{32}P die Anteile der eiweißfreien und der eiweißhaltigen Ribosomen-Vorstufen, die bei verschiedenen ClA-Konzentrationen synthetisiert werden und überprüften außerdem den Einbau von ^{14}C-Lysin in die verschiedenen Ribosomenfraktionen in Abhängigkeit von der ClA-Konzentration.

Die Auftrennung der Ribosomenfraktion erfolgte auf der DEAE-Säule in einer etwas veränderten Weise nach MIDGLEY (1962).

Die DEAE-Säule trennt die Ribosomen bzw. ihre Vorstufen in Abhängigkeit von ihrem Eiweißgehalt derart, daß die eiweißreichste Fraktion zuerst eluiert wird. Die erste Fraktion enthält die vorgebildeten Ribosomen der Zelle, die der Einfachheithalber „70 S-Fraktion" genannt werden soll, die zweite Fraktion eiweißärmere Partikel und die dritte Fraktion weitgehend eiweißfreie RNS, wie die Bestimmung der Aminosäuren in dieser Fraktion mit Ninhydrin nach der Säurehydrolyse ergab. Eine exakte Bestimmung des Aminosäuregehaltes dieser Fraktion wird dadurch erschwert, daß die Eluate der DEAE-Säule auch nach gründlichem Waschen eine geringe Grundreaktion mit Ninhydrin geben.

Im vorliegenden Falle (Abb. 1) wurden Ribosomen einer Methionin-Mangelmutante eines Stammes von *E. coli* – K 12 getrennt, die auf einem synthetischen Medium bei Zusatz von Methionin zur Nährlösung gezüchtet wurde und der in der mittleren Logphase 5 Minuten lang ^{14}C-Leucin zugesetzt worden war. Die Tatsache, daß die Bakterien in einem aminosäurearmen Medium wuchsen, erklärt, warum der Prozentsatz an eiweißarmen Ribosomen-Fraktionen unter normalen Bedingungen, d. h. bei Abwesenheit von ClA, so groß ist. Beim Züchten von *E. coli* B in aminosäurereichem Medium fanden wir unter normalen Bedingungen immer nur kleine Mengen dieser eiweißarmen Fraktionen.

Im oberen Teil der Abbildung ist die spezifische Aktivität in Impulsen pro μg Aminosäure aufgetragen. Im mittleren Teil der Abbildung ist der RNS-Gehalt in Beziehung zum Aminosäuregehalt nach Säurehydrolyse für verschiedene Fraktionen aufgetragen. (Glutaminsäure diente als Standard-Substanz für die Aminosäurebestimmung. Zur Umrechnung auf das ribosomale Protein wird der Faktor 1,7 benutzt. Im vorliegenden Falle wurde nicht umgerechnet, so daß die Werte für den prozentualen Anteil an RNS in der Abbildung zu hoch erscheinen.) Die Trennung der beiden eiweißarmen Fraktionen ist hier zwar nicht sehr gut, daß es sich aber einwandfrei um zwei verschiedenartige Fraktionen handelt, ist deutlich aus den Diagrammen zu ersehen, die die Trennung von ^{32}P-markierten Ribosomen zeigen.

Abbildung 2 zeigt den Einbau von ^{32}P und damit die Synthese der Ribosomen-RNS während einer Stunde in den verschiedenen Ribosomenfraktionen von *E. coli* B in Abhängigkeit von der ClA-Konzentration.

Bei 5 μg ClA/ml werden noch Ribosomen der „70 S-Fraktion" und auch ein größerer Anteil von eiweißhaltigen Vorstufen synthetisiert, außerdem erscheint auch weitgehend eiweißfreie RNS. Ab 50 μg ClA/ml wird keine ^{32}P-Aktivität mehr in der „70 S-Fraktion" gefunden und von den eiweißhaltigen Vorstufen werden nur noch geringe Mengen gebildet. Es existiert der größte Teil der RNS in weitgehend eiweißfreier Form.

Es war nun weiter von Interesse, den Einbau von ^{14}C-Aminosäuren unter ClA-Einfluß in die verschiedenen Fraktionen zu untersuchen.

Die nächste Abbildung (3a) zeigt einen 5 minütigen Einbau von ^{14}C-Lysin in die ribosomale Fraktion normaler Bakterien (*E. coli* B). Die Bakterien wuchsen in einem synthetischen Medium, welches Asparagin als N-Quelle enthielt. Das meiste der Radioaktivität erscheint in der „70 S-Fraktion". Es ist jedoch zu sehen, daß Radioaktivität auch in der RNS-Fraktion erscheint, in der wir mit Ninhydrin nur Spuren von Aminosäuren fanden.

Um klare Resultate zu erhalten, wurden bei den Versuchen, wo wir den Einfluß von ClA auf den Einbau von ^{14}C-Lysin in das ribosomale Protein untersuchten (Abb. 3b, c, d), die Bakterien vor Zusatz des ^{14}C-Lysins 5 Minuten mit ClA vorinkubiert. 10 Minuten nach Zusatz der radioaktiven Aminosäure wurde das Wachstum gestoppt. Die Menge des zugefügten radioaktiven Materials war für alle hier gezeigten Experimente die gleiche.

Bei 5 µg ClA/ml, unter Bedingungen also, wo die RNS-Synthese noch an Aminosäuren gebunden ist, wird ^{14}C-Lysin in alle Fraktionen der Ribosomen eingebaut, wenn auch in geringerem Maße als unter normalen Bedingungen. Jedoch ist die relative Hemmung des Einbaus in der „70 S-Fraktion" am größten. Das kann bedeuten, daß die Synthese des löslichen Proteins durch ClA stärker gehemmt wird als die des ribosomalen Proteins.

Bei 50 µg ClA/ml werden nur noch Spuren von ^{14}C-Lysin in die Ribosomenfraktionen eingebaut. In Abb. 3 (c und d) wurde die Skala, die die Impulse anzeigt, ausgedehnt, um den geringfügigen Einbau der Radioaktivität zeigen zu können. Die Tatsache, daß bei 50 µg ClA/ml nur noch Spuren von ^{14}C-Lysin in die Ribosomenvorstufen eingebaut werden, erklärt unserer Meinung nach die Befunde von Kurland und Maaløe (1962), daß ab dieser ClA-Konzentration keine extern zugefügten Aminosäuren mehr für die RNS-Synthese notwendig sind.

Wie die vorhergehende Abbildung über die ^{32}P-Einbau-Versuche gezeigt hatte, lag bereits bei dieser ClA -Konzentration der größte Teil der RNS weitgehend in eiweißfreier Form vor. Bei 500 µg ClA/ml ließ sich in keiner der Ribosomen-Fraktionen mehr ^{14}C-Lysin nachweisen.

Die Ergebnisse dieser Untersuchungen im Zusammenhang mit denen anderer Autoren erlauben unserer Meinung nach folgende Deutung:

Die Aminosäuren werden für die RNS-Synthese als Bausteine für das ribosomale Protein benötigt. Unter normalen Bedingungen enthält auch die RNS-Fraktion, die mit Ninhydrin nur Spuren von Aminosäuren anzeigt, kleine Mengen an Aminosäuren oder Peptiden. Bei Einwirkung hoher ClA-Konzentrationen auf die Bakterienzelle wird jedoch nach den Ergebnissen der Versuche mit ^{14}C-Lysin der Einbau von Aminosäuren oder Peptiden in diese RNS-Fraktion verhindert, so daß der Umbau zur nächsten eiweißhaltigen Ribosomen-Vorstufe nicht stattfinden kann.

Wir nehmen an, daß normalerweise die weitere Synthese von neuer Ribosomenvorstufen-RNS nur möglich ist, wenn ein adäquater Betrag dieser Ribosomen-Vorstufen-RNS in die Ribosomen eingebaut wird. Es sollte demnach also eine enge Koppelung zwischen Neusynthese von Ribosomen-RNS und Verwendung der vorher synthetisierten RNS für die Ribosomen-Synthese bestehen. Diese Koppelung könnte aber durch ClA gelockert werden.

Die Abhängigkeit der RNS-Synthese von Aminosäuren wird von einem Gen kontrolliert, dem sog. RC-Locus, wie Stent und Brenner (1961) zeigen konnten. Bei Ausschaltung dieses Gens durch Mutation wird die strenge Abhängigkeit der RNS-Synthese von Aminosäuren auch ohne Anwesenheit von ClA gelockert.

Weiterhin wäre zu diskutieren, in welcher Form die Aminosäuren bei diesen Prozessen beteiligt sind.

Im Zusammenhang mit der Hypothese, daß Aminosäureadenylat der Transfer-RNS als Induktor für die RNS-Synthese wirkt, wäre zu erwägen, ob die an Transfer-RNS gebundenen Aminosäuren Bausteine des Ribosomen-Proteins sind. Darauf kann bisher keine sichere Antwort gegeben werden. Aus den Untersuchungen von Rendi und Ochoa (1962) über den

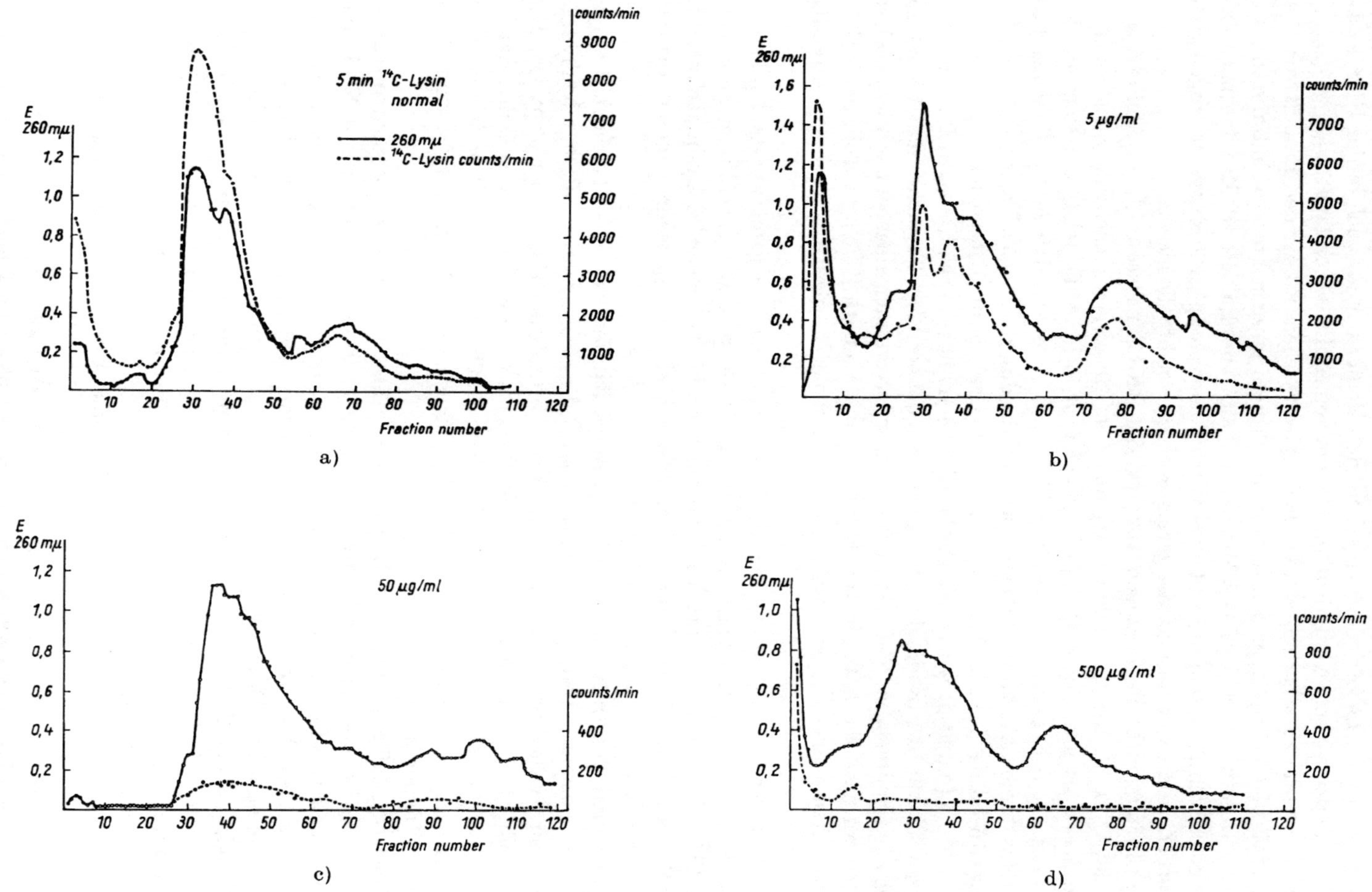

Abb. 3 (a, b, c, d). Der Effekt verschiedener ClA-Konzentrationen auf den Einbau von ^{14}C-Lysin in die Ribosomen. 10 Min. Einwirkung von ^{14}C-Lysin bei Gegenwart von ClA auf die Bakterien. Trennung auf der DEAE-Säule

Effekt von ClA auf die Proteinsynthese in zellfreien Präparationen von *E. coli* geht hervor, daß die Aufnahme von freien Aminosäuren durch Transfer-RNS bei Gegenwart von ClA nicht gehemmt ist.

Hingegen fanden HUNTER und GOODSALL (1961), daß die Synthese von Lipo-Aminosäure-Komplexen bei Gegenwart von ClA vermindert wird. Danach besteht die Möglichkeit, daß solche Komplexe an der Synthese des ribosomalen Eiweißes beteiligt sind.

Wir glauben, daß weiterer Aufschluß über die Bedeutung der Aminosäuren für die ribosomale RNS-Synthese erhalten werden kann, wenn mehr über die Synthese des ribosomalen Eiweißes bekannt ist.

Literatur

ARONSON, A. T., and S. SPIEGELMAN, 1961a: Biochim. biophysica Acta **53**, 70.
ARONSON, A. T., and S. SPIEGELMAN, 1961b: Biochim. biophysica Acta **53**, 84.
BRITTEN, R. J., and B. J. MCCARTHY, 1962: Biophys. Journ. **2**, 49.
BRITTEN, R. J., R. B. ROBERTS, and B. J. MCCARTHY, 1962: Biophys. Journ. **2**, 83.
HUNTER, G. D., and R. A. GOODSALL, 1961: Biochem. Journ. **78**, 564.
KURLAND, C. G., and O. MAALØE, 1962: J. Mol. Biol. **4**, 193.
KURLAND, C. G., M. NOMURA, and J. D. WATSON, 1962: J. Mol. Biol. **4**, 388.
MCCARTHY, B. J., and R. J. BRITTEN, 1962: Biophys. Journ. **2**, 35.
MCCARTHY, B. J., R. J. BRITTEN, and R. B. ROBERTS, 1962: Biophys. Journ. **2**, 57.
MIDGLEY, J. E. M., 1962: Biochim. biophysica Acta **61**, 513.
NOMURA, M., and J. D. WATSON, 1959: J. Mol. Biol. **1**, 204.
RENDI, R., and S. OCHOA, 1962: J. Biol. Chem. **237**, 3711.

Einige Probleme in der Sequenzanalyse von Ribonukleinsäuren

H. G. Zachau

Institut für Genetik der Universität zu Köln

Die Entdeckung der zentralen Rolle der Ribonukleinsäuren in der Proteinsynthese hatte im Gefolge, daß sich in den letzten Jahren zahlreiche Forscher der Arbeit an der Primär- und Sekundärstruktur der Ribonukleinsäuren zuwandten. Vereinfachend sagt man heute, daß in der Proteinsynthese die genetische Information aus einer Desoxyribonukleotid-„Schrift" über Ribonukleotid-„Schriften" in die Aminosäure-„Schrift" der Proteine übersetzt wird; die Desoxyribonukleinsäure des genetischen Materials steuert über Ribonukleinsäuren mit ganz oder teilweise komplementärer Nukleotidsequenz den Aufbau der Aminosäuresequenz eines spezifischen Proteins (Zusammenfassungen z. B. Chantrenne, 1961, Crick, 1963). Hypothetische Teile dieses Bildes, wie der Adaptor-Mechanismus, sollten sich durch Sequenzanalyse der beteiligten Ribonukleinsäuren klären lassen.

Die Analyse der Nukleotidsequenz von Ribonukleinsäuren befindet sich noch in den Anfängen. Bei hochmolekularen Ribonukleinsäuren, wie der Matrizen-RNA*), der Ribosomen-RNA oder der RNA einiger Viren, lassen sich bisher nur statistische Aussagen über die Verteilung der Bausteine in der Kette machen. Am ehesten einer Sequenzanalyse zugänglich dürften die relativ niedermolekularen Transfer-Ribonukleinsäuren (Mol. Gew. 20000–30000, 60–90 Nukleotide) sein, die von mehreren Arbeitskreisen untersucht werden (Zusammenfassungen z. B. Holley, Ingram, Cantoni, 1963, Zachau, 1962). Bei einigen Transfer-Ribonukleinsäuren kennt man bereits längere Stücke der Nukleotidkette, von der Kenntnis einer Gesamtsequenz ist man allerdings noch weit entfernt.

Für die meisten Methoden der Sequenzanalyse ist das Vorliegen einer reinen und molekular einheitlichen RNA die Voraussetzung. Einige Virus-Ribonukleinsäuren sind nach physikalischen und biologischen Kriterien einheitlich, und es besteht bisher kein Grund anzunehmen, daß sie nicht auch nach chemischen Kriterien einheitlich sind. Schwieriger liegen die Verhältnisse bei den anderen erwähnten Ribonukleinsäuren. Hier können die vorhandenen physikalischen und biologischen Methoden der Reinheitsprüfung nur als Anhaltspunkte dienen. Z. B. kann man nicht sicher sein, daß eine Transfer-RNA, die physikalisch einheitlich erscheint und im enzymatischen Test nur mit einer Aminosäure reagiert, auch molekular einheitlich ist. Mehr als einmal hat es sich herausgestellt, daß in derartigen Präparaten zwei oder drei Nukleinsäuren enthalten sind, deren Verhalten bei physikalischen Untersuchungen ähnlich, deren Aminosäure-Spezifität gleich, deren Nukleotidsequenz aber verschieden ist.

---

*) Die folgenden Abkürzungen werden verwendet: RNA = Ribonukleinsäure, s-RNA = lösliche Ribonukleinsäure, UMP = Uridinmonophosphat.

Ob eine Nukleinsäure auch im chemischen Sinne einheitlich ist, erweist sich erst bei der Sequenzanalyse. Strenggenommen kann man daher keine RNA – ausgenommen die erwähnten Virus-Nukleinsäuren, bei denen die physikalischen und biologischen Reinheitskriterien stärker sind – für einheitlich erklären, da noch in keinem Fall die Sequenzanalyse zu Ende geführt wurde.

Der klassische, bei der Strukturaufklärung von Proteinen vielfach beschrittene Weg der Sequenzanalyse benutzt die spezifische enzymatische Spaltung der Kette. In den Bruchstücken der Kette läßt sich die Reihenfolge der Bausteine durch Abbau vom Ende her ermitteln. Verwendet man zur Gewinnung der Bruchstücke zwei Enzyme, die in der Kette neben verschiedenen Bausteinen spalten, so kann man überlappende Sequenzen und schließlich die gesamte Bausteinsequenz der Kette erhalten (Zusammenfassung z. B. BRAUNITZER, 1961). Dieses Prinzip der Sequenzanalyse wird auch auf dem Ribonukleinsäuregebiet angewendet. Jedoch führt die Spaltung einer Ribonukleinsäure mit spezifischen Enzymen zu Mononukleotiden und zu einer großen Zahl kleinerer Oligonukleotide. Während in der Sequenzanalyse der Proteine bei statistischer Verteilung der Bausteine in der Kette ein neben zwei von zwanzig Aminosäuren spaltendes Enzym im Durchschnitt Dekapeptide liefert, ergibt ein Enzym, das neben einem oder zwei der vier Hauptnukleotide einer Nukleinsäure spaltet, im Durchschnitt Tetra- bzw. Dinukleotide. Aus so kleinen Bruchstücken eine Nukleotidkette zu rekonstruieren, dürfte schwierig sein, zumal man bisher erst zwei RNA-spaltende Enzyme kennt, die eine für die Sequenzanalyse ausreichende Spezifität besitzen. Erwünscht sind daher Methoden, die definierte größere Bruchstücke der Kette liefern.

Es gibt mehrere Denkmöglichkeiten für die Gewinnung größerer Oligonukleotidbruchstücke: Enzymatische Spaltung unter Bedingungen, bei denen nur wenige besonders leicht „zugängliche“ Bindungen angegriffen werden, Spaltung neben den sogenannten seltenen Nukleotiden usw. Diese Möglichkeiten werden in mehreren Laboratorien erprobt, bisher hat sich jedoch keine zu einer praktisch anwendbaren Methode entwickeln lassen.

Hier soll über den Versuch berichtet werden, die UV-induzierte Uracil-Dimerisierung zur Gewinnung größerer Oligonukleotidbruchstücke zu verwenden (ZACHAU, 1964). – Pankreas-Ribonuklease, die eine Nukleotidkette der Sequenz . . . XpUpUpXp . . . in drei Bruchstücke zerlegt, sollte neben keinem der beiden UMP-Moleküle spalten, wenn Dimerisierung eingetreten ist (vgl. Schema Abb. 1). Man würde ein höheres Oligonukleotid isolieren, das in seine

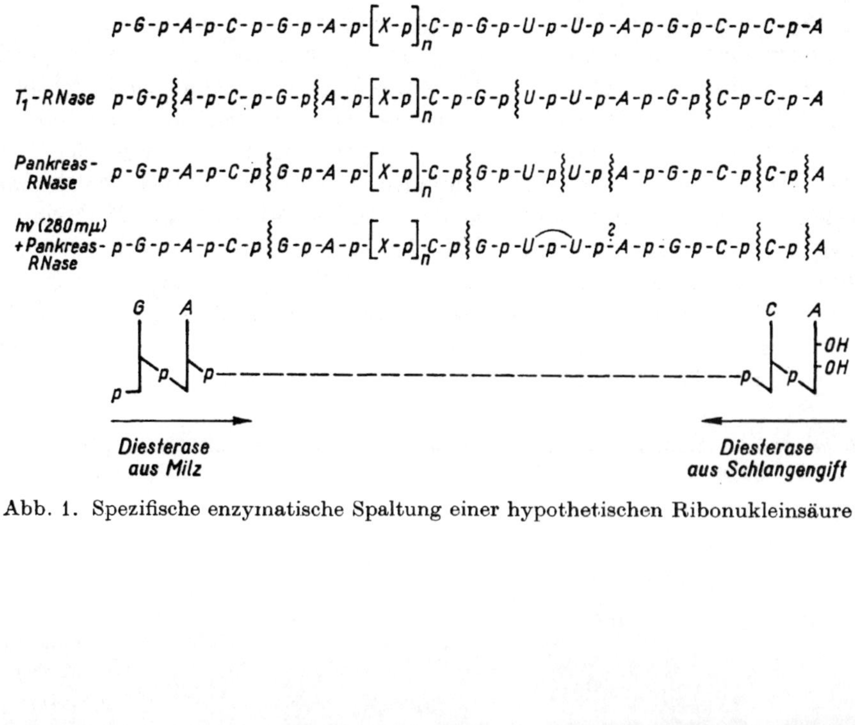

Abb. 1. Spezifische enzymatische Spaltung einer hypothetischen Ribonukleinsäure

Bestandteile zerlegt werden kann (s. unten) und damit eine längere Nukleotidsequenz erkennen läßt.

Aus Uracil entstehen bei UV-Bestrahlung das 4-Hydroxy-4.5-dihydro-uracil und ein Uracil-Dimeres (Abb. 2) (Zusammenfassungen: Shugar, 1960, Wacker, 1963, Smith, 1963). Zwischen Uracil und seinem Dimeren stellt sich ein photochemisches Gleichgewicht ein, doch wird aus dem Gleichgewicht durch die photochemisch irreversible Wasseranlagerung ständig Monomeres abgezogen. Die Lage dieses „Pseudogleichgewichts" der Dimerisierung ist stark abhängig von der Wellenlänge des eingestrahlten UV-Lichts und von der Konzentration sowie vom Aggregatzustand der bestrahlten Lösung. Bei Bestrahlung mit 275–285 mμ-Licht überwiegt die Dimerisierung, da in diesem Wellenlängenbereich die Absorption des Uracils um Größenordnungen höher ist als die des Dimeren und damit der Unterschied in der Quantenausbeute (Abb. 2) überkompensiert wird. Bei 240 mμ herrscht die Monomerisierung des gebildeten Dimeren vor, mit einer anschließenden langsameren Hydratisierung der Uracilmoleküle. Diese bisher an Uracil, Uridin, Di- und Polyuridylsäure untersuchten Reaktionen sollten bei UMP-UMP-Sequenzen in der RNA-Kette im Prinzip ähnlich verlaufen. Mit Sicherheit lassen sich weder die Dimerisierung noch die Dimerspaltung durch Bestrahlung zur Vollständigkeit führen, eine hundertprozentige Ausbeute ist aber bei der Zuordnung einer Reihenfolge von Oligonukleotiden in der Sequenzanalyse auch nicht notwendig.

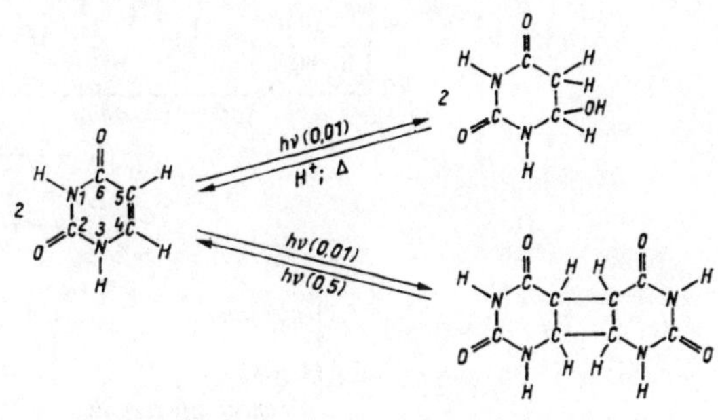

Abb. 2. Reaktionen des Uracils, in Klammern sind ungefähre Quantenausbeuten angegeben

Um das bisher nicht bekannte UMP-Dimere zu erhalten und in seinen Eigenschaften zu studieren, wurden konzentrierte wäßrige Lösungen von 2'/3'-UMP mit UV-Licht verschiedener Wellenlängen bestrahlt und verschiedene Isolierungsmethoden für das UMP-Dimere erprobt (Zachau, 1964). Nach Bestrahlung mit dem 254 mμ-Licht einer Sterilisierlampe ließen sich 21% des eingesetzten UMP als Dimeres isolieren. Bessere Ausbeuten ließen sich durch 280 mμ-Bestrahlung erhalten. Auch aus 280 mμ-bestrahlter Polyuridylsäure konnten nach alkalischer Hydrolyse UMP-Dimere isoliert werden. Dieser Versuch und alle anderen 280 mμ- und 240 mμ-Bestrahlungen wurden mit einem unter Leitung von M. Delbrück gebauten UV-Monochromator ausgeführt, der von H. E. Johns konstruiert wurde und demnächst beschrieben werden soll.

Aus s-RNA, die mit 280 mμ-Licht bestrahlt war, bis die Akzeptoraktivität für Phenylalanin auf 58% und für Lysin auf 25% der Anfangsaktivität abgesunken war, wurde nach alkalischer Hydrolyse UMP-Dimeres isoliert. Aus dem Vergleich mit der Menge an terminalem Guanosindiphosphat konnte geschätzt werden, daß unter diesen Bedingungen im Durchschnitt jede zweite RNA-Kette ein UMP-Dimeres enthielt. Ein kleiner Teil des UMP im Dimeren könnte durch Desaminierung von Cytidylsäure entstanden sein, die Hauptmenge stammte jedoch wahrscheinlich aus UMP-UMP-Sequenzen.

Um zu prüfen, ob sich die UMP-Dimeren im oben angedeuteten Sinne zur Sequenzanalyse verwenden lassen, wurde 280 mμ-bestrahlte s-RNA (das Gemisch aller Transfer-Ribonukleinsäuren) mit Pankreas-Ribonuklease zu Mono- und Oligonukleotiden gespalten (Abb. 3). Bei Chromatographie des Gemischs an Diäthylaminoäthyl-Cellulose in 7 m-Harnstofflösung (Tomlinson and Tener, 1962) wurden zunächst die Mono- und dann die Dinukleotide eluiert und dann die höheren Oligonukleotide jeweils in Gruppen gleicher Kettenlänge. Die untersuchte

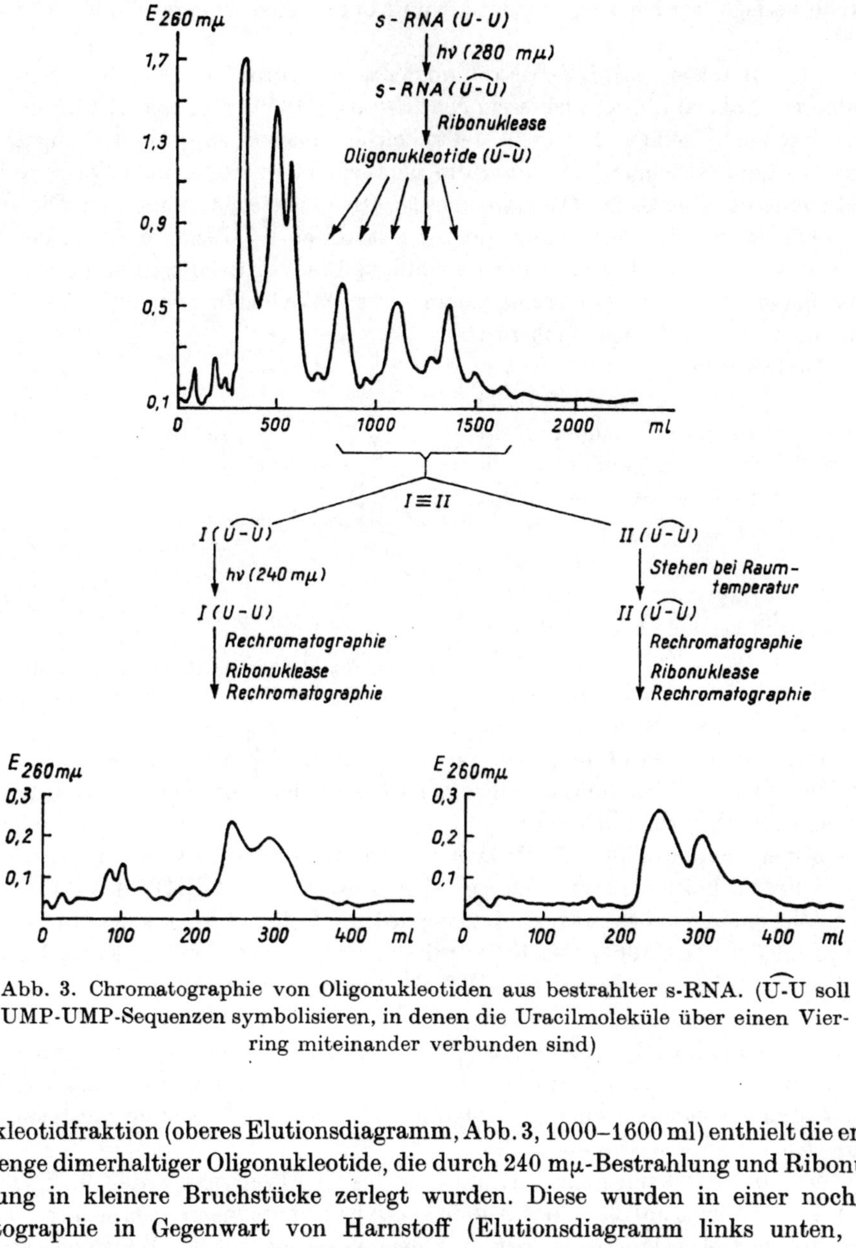

Abb. 3. Chromatographie von Oligonukleotiden aus bestrahlter s-RNA. (U͡-U soll UMP-UMP-Sequenzen symbolisieren, in denen die Uracilmoleküle über einen Vierring miteinander verbunden sind)

Oligonukleotidfraktion (oberes Elutionsdiagramm, Abb. 3, 1000–1600 ml) enthielt die erwartete kleine Menge dimerhaltiger Oligonukleotide, die durch 240 mμ-Bestrahlung und Ribonukleasebehandlung in kleinere Bruchstücke zerlegt wurden. Diese wurden in einer nochmaligen Chromatographie in Gegenwart von Harnstoff (Elutionsdiagramm links unten, Abb. 3) vor der Hauptfraktion eluiert. Da die kleineren Bruchstücke bei Weglassen der 240 mμ-Bestrahlung (Elutionsdiagramm rechts unten, Abb. 3) und unter anderen Kontrollbedingungen nicht erschienen, läßt sich der Versuch in der erwähnten Weise deuten: Wird RNA vor der Ribonuklease-Spaltung mit 280 mμ-Licht bestrahlt, so lassen sich große Oligonukleotidbruchstücke isolieren, die durch 240 mμ-Bestrahlung in kleinere Bruchstücke übergehen.

Weitere Versuche mit einheitlichen Nukleinsäuren, z. B. reinen Transfer-Ribonukleinsäuren, sind notwendig. Aber bereits auf Grund der beschriebenen Versuche ist es wahrscheinlich, daß die UV-induzierte UMP-Dimerisierung zur Analyse bestimmter Nukleotidsequenzen in RNA verwendet werden kann.

Literatur

BRAUNITZER, G., 1961: Die Ermittlung der Konstitution einer klassischen Peptidkette, Z. analyt. Chemie **181**, 514—526.

CANTONI, G. L., H. ISHIKURA, H. H. RICHARDS, and K. TANAKA, 1963: A model for the base sequence of serine-s-RNA. Cold Spring Harbor Symposia on Quant. Biol. **28**, 123—132.

CHANTRENNE, H., 1961: The biosynthesis of proteins. Pergamon Press, Oxford.

CRICK, F. H. C., 1963: The recent excitement in the coding problem. In: Progress in nucleic acid research (Editors: J. N. Davidson, and W. E. Cohn), Vol. I, 164—217, Academic Press, New York.

HOLLEY, R. W., J. APGAR, G. A. EVERETT, J. T. MADISON, S. H. MERRILL, and A. ZAMIR, 1963: Chemistry of aminocacid-specific ribonucleic acids. Cold Spring Harbor Symposia on Quant. Biol. **28**, 117—121.

INGRAM, V. M., and J. A. SJÖKVIST, 1963: Studies on purified alanine-specific transfer RNA. Cold Spring Harbor Symposia on Quant. Biol. **28**, 133—138.

SHUGAR, D., 1960: Photochemistry of nucleic acids and their constituents. In: The nucleic acids (Editors: E. Chargaff, and J. N. Davidson), Vol. III, 39—104, Academic Press, New York.

SMITH, K. C., 1963: Photochemistry of the nucleic acids. In: Photobiology: Action of light on living materials (Editor: A. C. Giese), Academic Press, New York, im Druck.

TOMLINSON, E. V., and G. M. TENER, 1962: The use of urea to eliminate the secondary binding forces in ion exchange chromatography of polynucleotides. J. Amer. chem. Soc. **84**, 2644—2645.

WACKER, A., 1963: Molecular mechanisms of radiation effects. In: Progress in nucleic acid research (Editors: J. N. Davidson, and W. E. Cohn), Vol. I., 369—399, Academic Press. New York.

ZACHAU, H. G., 1962: Aspekte der Nucleinsäure-Biochemie. In: Symposium über funktionelle und morphologische Organisation der Zelle (Herausgeber: P. Karlson), S. 40—55. Springer-Verlag, Heidelberg.

ZACHAU, H. G., 1964: UV-induzierte Uracil-Dimerisierung in löslicher Ribonucleinsäure. Hoppe Seyler's Z. Physiol. Chemie. **336**, 176—188.

Experiments and Speculations on the Mechanism of Inter-allelic Complementation

J. R. S. Fincham

John Innes Institute, Bayfordbury, Hertford, England

Many cases are now known in micro-organisms where, among a series of strains apparently mutant in the same structural gene and defective in the same enzyme, some pair-wise combinations show complementation, with formation of active enzyme, when the two mutant genomes are brought into the same cell. After a period in which this phenomenon caused much perplexity the stage has now been reached where most workers in the field are prepared to accept the following explanation. It is supposed that the normal enzyme is a homopolymer, that is composed of a fixed number of identical sub-units (polypeptide chains). The active product formed as a result of bringing the two mutant genomes into a common cytoplasm is taken to be a heteropolymer, containing sub-units of *both* mutant types. Through one requirement for enzyme activity being supplied by one kind of mutant sub-unit and another requirement supplied by the other, enzyme activity may be possible in such a heteropolymer even though neither type of homopolymer is active. These requirements for activity may be the presence of specific amino acid side-chains necessary for the functioning of the active centre of the enzyme, or structural features necessary for the correct conformation of the protein, or, as I shall argue later, a combination of both. In this paper I shall present the results of some experiments on complementing mutants of *Neurospora crassa* defective in the enzyme NADP*)-linked glutamate dehydrogenase (GDH).

Properties of Neurospora NADP-linked GDH

The NADP-linked GDH is fairly easy to obtain in a state of near purity (Fincham and Coddington, 1963; Barratt and Strickland, 1963). Recent determinations of the molecular weight by sedimentation and diffusion measurements, carried out by my colleagues A. Coddington and A. Rodgers, at our Institute gave a value of 260.000–270.000 in agreement with Barratt and Strickland. However, in the presence of sodium dodecyl sulphate at a concentration of 2 mg./ml. the protein dissociates completely to give an apparently homogeneous material of molecular weight ca. 50.000. Amino acid analysis, together with estimates by the ,,fingerprinting "technique of the numbers of tryptic and chymotryptic pep-

*) NADP = nicotinamide-adenine nucleotide phosphate.

tides containing specific amino acids, suggests that the protein is constructed out of identical polypeptide chains each of molecular weight 27.000—28.000. These data lead us to believe that the enzyme is an aggregate of identical sub-units (a homopolymer), the number of subunits being probably ten. It seems likely that sodium dodecyl sulphate causes dissociation into dimers, and that the two chains in each dimer are held together by bonds not easily disrupted by this agent.

Properties of Neurospora mutants defective in NADP-GDH

Mutants defective in NADP-linked GDH are all located genetically within a short segment of the fifth linkage group, the *am* locus. This locus is extremely short in terms of the recombination frequency between its known end; the prototroph frequency observed from intercrosses of the most widely separated mutants is only about 10^{-4}. Nevertheless, with the exceptions of two examples of apparent recurrent mutation at the same site, all the known *am* mutants map at different points within the *am* locus (PATEMAN, personal communication – in preparation). All the mutants show a long lag in growth from conidial inocula on minimal medium and this lag is eliminated by supplementation of the medium with L-glutamate, L-aspartate, L-alanine, or any one of the other L-α-amino acids which serve as a ready source of α-amino groups through transamination reactions. The fact that the mutants grow at all on minimal medium is thought to be due to the presence in *Neurospora* of a NAD-linked GDH which is not affected by the *am* mutations (SANWAL and LATA, 1960). Probably because of their ability to grow slowly on minimal medium *am* mutants are not easy to select in large numbers by the standard methods, and only some 20 primary *am* alleles (as opposed to alleles derived secondarily by revertant selection) are known. A recent mutant hunt by DAVID STADLER using nitrous acid as a mutagen resulted in the isolation of am^{14}–am^{19}, which have added considerably to our knowledge of the locus.

Complementation relationships

When combined in heterocaryons the majority of pairs of mutants grow no better on minimal medium than mutant homocaryons. Indeed, most of the mutants do not complement with any other mutant of the series. However, some pairs do show complementation as revealed by growth without lag on minimal medium and formation of GDH superficially resembling the wild type enzyme. The pattern of complementation is shown in Figure 1.

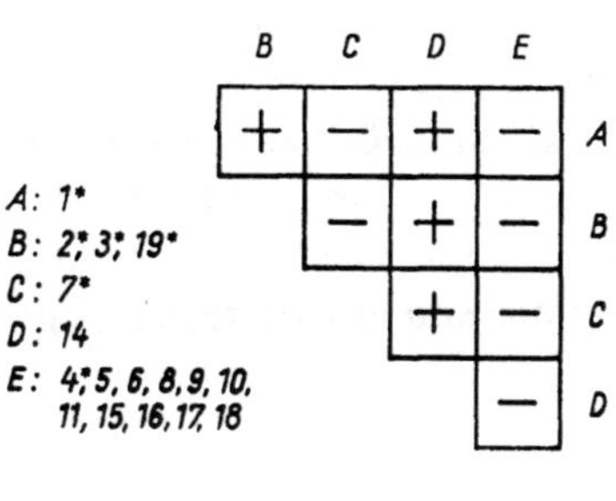

Fig. 1. Chart showing the complementation relationships of *am* mutants; + shows complementation and – no complementation. The mutants are divided into five classes A—E, and the numbers of the mutants falling into each class are shown. Asterisks indicate the formation of cross reacting material (CRM). The data on mutants 14 to 19 are by courtesy of D. R. STADLER, and the data on CRM were kindly supplied by D. B. ROBERTS

The enzyme formed as a result of complementation of *am* mutants seems never to be identical to wild type GDH. Not only is the *level* of enzyme activity relatively low in complementing heterocaryons; the *kind* of enzyme is also different. The property which we have used more than any other to distinguish complementation enzymes is heat stability. All the complementary combinations of mutants produce enzyme which is less stable than wild, but the degree of instability is different in each case. Combinations involving am^1 give, in general, relatively stable products, although the enzyme formed by am^1 and am^2 is more highly unstable. Combinations involving am^{14} with any allele other than am^1 give extremely unstable varieties of GDH. It was this kind of observation which first led to the proposal that interallelic complementation did not involve the regeneration of a wild-type enzyme-forming apparatus by some kind of recombination process, but rather that protein elements of mutant types were still present in the complementation product (FINCHAM, 1959). In most kinetic constants and in electrophoretic mobility in starch or polyacrylamide gel the enzyme varieties formed by complementation are very similar or identical to wild type GDH. The band of enzyme activity was located in the gels by an adaptation of the method of MARKERT and MØLLER (1959). Since the electrophoresis gels show a strong sieving effect in the molecular size range in question, the electrophoretic evidence is taken to mean that complementation enzyme must contain a normal number of polypeptide sub-units. This conclusion has been checked by ultracentrifuge analysis in the case of $am^1 + am^3$.

Properties of mutant forms of the protein in relation to complementing ability

The same fractionation procedure as is used for the isolation of wild type enzyme results in the isolation of proteins, obviously related to GDH, from several of the mutants (FINCHAM, 1962). These mutant proteins are (with the exception of the one produced by am^{19}) identical to wild type enzyme in their electrophoretic mobility in polyacrylamide gel. In one case, that of am^1, the mutant protein appears to be totally devoid of enzymic activity. In three other cases, am^2, am^3, and am^{19}, some enzymic activity can be demonstrated. As has been shown in detail in a previous publication (FINCHAM, 1962) the am^2 and am^3 proteins, although almost inactive in the standard assay system involving glutamate synthesis, can be activated for glutamate oxidation in reaction mixtures containing NADP and a high concentration of glutamate. I have recently found that good activation of am^3 protein can equally well be obtained in mixtures containing NADP with high concentrations of some other ions such as succinate. Having been activated in such a mixture the protein will catalyse glutamate synthesis when introduced into the standard assay system although the reaction is very short lived; it seems that the presence of reduced NADP causes deactivation of the mutant enzyme. In general the am^2 and am^3 proteins have similar properties except that the am^2 variety is less readily activated. The am^{19} protein, which has only very recently been isolated, is of a much more extreme mutant type. It gives only very low activity even under the most favourable conditions, although it is clear that a slow and very incomplete activation does occur when it is incubated with NADP and high glutamate. None of these three activable proteins seems to be at all effective *in vivo*, since the mutants which produce them show just as extreme an auxotrophy as any others of the *am* series.

There remains am^{14} which has exceptionally interesting properties. As will be seen from Fig. 1 it is more versatile in its complementation than any other mutant of the series. However, repeated attempts to isolate a GDH-like protein from this mutant failed. We were confirmed in our conclusion that am^{14} produces no such protein by some immunological results kindly communicated to us by Mr. DAVID ROBERTS, working in Dr. PATEMAN's laboratory in Cambridge (ROBERTS, in the press). ROBERTS has used three criteria for the detection of immunologically related protein in mutants: neutralisation of anti-GDH antibodies by mutant extracts, detection of a precipitin band corresponding to that due to GDH on OUCHTERLONY double diffusion plates, and the more rigorous identification of such a band by the immunoelectrophoresis technique. The three methods gave completely consonant results. Protein related to GDH was clearly present in am^1, am^2, am^3, am^4, am^7 and am^{19} (note that of these only am^4 is not known to complement with another mutant) but it was as clearly absent in am^{14}.

At this point I will present a hypothesis of complementation which seems likely to apply to this system and perhaps to others. One can imagine two kinds of reason why a mutant protein fails to show normal enzymic activity. First it may have lost one of the essential amino acid side-chains comprising the active centre of the enzyme, but its three-dimensional folding structure (conformation) may be normal and just as stable as that of the normal enzyme. The defect in am^1 could be of this type. Second, all the components of the active centre may still be present, but the activity is not exhibited because the groups are in the wrong spatial relationship due to a conformational abnormality perhaps originating in some distant part of the polypeptide chain. It seems very likely that the defects in am^2, am^3 and am^{19} are of this type, since the mutant protein has potential activity in each case, and the reversible activation which has been most clearly demonstrated for the am^3 protein is suggestive of a switch between active and inactive conformations with the inactive favoured under physiological conditions. Now if, in a heterocaryon, GDH molecules are formed containing some sub-units of a conformationally normal but irreparably inactive type, and others of a potentially active but conformationally abnormal variety, it seems very likely that the former will tend to stabilize the latter in the „correct" conformation. This will perhaps be particularly likely to happen if the heteropolymer contains a predominance (perhaps 4 dimers out of 5) of the conformationally stable sub-unit. Such a heteropolymer would presumably be subject to some degree of internal strain, which would account for the relative thermolability of the complementation enzymes.

On this hypothesis the apparently anomalous mutant am^{14} is best explained by saying that it produces a mutant GDH subunit which, left to itself, folds up in such an abnormal way that it will not form polymers and consequently form no protein recognisable as related to GDH. In a cell which is also producing GDH sub-units which *are* capable of polymerisation some of the am^{14} sub-units may be „rescued" and incorporated into polymers, their folding being forced into a more normal form by the constraints imposed by neighbouring sub-units.

In the case of the combinations $am^2 + am^{14}$ and $am^3 + am^{14}$ one must suppose that some mutual correction of conformation occurs, the am^{14} sub-unit causing some beneficial adjustment in the folding of the am^2 or am^3 sub-units. Such an arrangement with, so to speak, two unstable structures propping each other up, could well be a very precarious one, and on this view it is not surprising that the enzyme formed in the heterocaryons in question is so extremely sensitive to heat.

Evidence from reversions

Another kind of evidence encourages belief that the foregoing argument is on the right lines. PATEMAN has isolated many prototrophic revertants from am^3 following UV treatment (PATEMAN and FINCHAM, 1963). Some of these are not distinguishable enzymically from standard wild type. However many others, which fall into at least six distinguishable types, produce GDH which, though somewhat active under physiological conditions, is clearly different from wild type enzyme. These abnormal revertants from am^3 tend to show a certain family resemblance between the GDH varieties which they produce in that nearly all show some degree of activation on incubation with substrate mixtures, and most of them have an abnormally high MICHAELIS constant for ammonium ion. It has been demonstrated that all these revertants are due to further mutation in the *am* region, but available techniques have not been sensitive enough to permit us to say whether a further mutation at the original site or a „suppressor" mutation at a second site is the explanation of the restored enzyme activity. On other grounds however it is virtually certain that most or all of the abnormal revertants must be due to mutation at a second site, since there are far too many different classes of revertant for a single site to be involved, if we equate a site with a DNA nucleotide pair. Thus it seems very likely that the original am^3 defect is still present in the polypeptide chain of each abnormal revertant enzyme, but that its effect has been made much less extreme by a compensating modification elsewhere in the chain. This conclusion implies that the am^3 defect must have been of a conformational character.

Results of a rather similar nature have recently been obtained with am^{14} by D. R. STADLER working in my laboratory. In this case reversions to the true wild type condition have not yet been demonstrated. Instead many secondary mutants with abnormally heat-sensitive GDH have been obtained. The degree of heat sensitivity varies from one revertant to another, and there seem to be several different classes. The abnormal GDH varieties in the am^{14} revertants, like those from the am^3 revertants, show a family resemblance, in this case in their common sensitivity to heat. Here again it seems likely that the original mutational abnormality of the am^{14} polypeptide chain is still present but its effect has been ameliorated through a second change in the molecule. Here again, then, it seems reasonable to suppose that the essential groups of the active centre must all have been present in the am^{14} defective sub-unit.

The general argument is supported by older information of a less extensive character on revertants from am^1 and am^2 (PATEMAN, 1957). From am^1, all the revertants seem similar to true wild type, so far as they were tested. This would naturally be the case if the defect in the am^1 protein were of an irreparable kind such as could only be cured by a true reverse mutation. Among a limited sample of revertants from am^2, on the other hand, at least one was quite different from wild type and produced GDH with properties consistent with the idea that the enzyme had acquired a secondary modification rendering it much more easily activated.

Experiments on in vitro complementation

The hypothesis that enzyme formed by complementation is heteropolymeric, composed of sub-units of two mutant types, was greatly strengthened by the demonstration that active enzyme can be formed from mixtures of purified mutant proteins *in vitro*. The experiments on mixtures of *am*[1] and *am*[2], and of *am*[1] and *am*[13] proteins have been reported elsewhere (Fincham and Coddington, 1963, a, b) and will not be described again in detail here. Briefly, the procedure consists in mixing the mutant proteins in phosphate buffer at pH 5.8 and, after a period of incubation, adjusting the pH to 7.4. Both at pH 5.8 and pH 7.4 the reaction is very fast, being half-maximal within seconds and essentially finished in half an hour. The mechanism of the *in vitro* complementation reaction is still obscure. Naturally our first thought was that at pH 5.8 the proteins dissociated into sub-units and that at pH 7.4 reassociation with hybrid formation occurred. However, ultracentrifuge studies, recently extended to cover a wide range of protein concentrations, offer no evidence that the proteins dissociates at pH 5.8; in fact the s values were slightly higher at the lower pH. It seems possible that hybrid aggregates might be formed as the result of *exchange* of sub-units, without the sub-units ever being free in solution, if there was at pH 5.8 an equilibrium between the normal protein and a small proportion of a higher order aggregate.

I have recently shown that *am*[1] and *am*[19] proteins will also show complementation *in vitro*, and that the best conditions for the reaction are those already worked out for the *am*[1] + *am*[3] combination. Thus we now have three systems in which the reaction can be demonstrated, one component being the *am*[1] protein in each case. Some generalisations can be made which are true for all three systems:

1. For a constant total amount of protein the optimal ratio of the two components is of the order of 5–10 to 1 in favour of the *am*[1] component. This result is quite consistent with the idea, mentioned above, that the *am*[1] protein sub-unit is the component conferring conformational stability on the heteropolymer, and that stabilisation, with full expression of the latent activity of the other component, can only occur when the *am*[1] sub-units are in the majority.
2. With a variable concentration of *am*[1] protein and a constant concentration of the other component the yield of active enzyme increases linearly, or with *am*[2] or *am*[19] protein more than linearly, with *am*[1] protein concentration up to a several-fold excess of *am*[1]. With a large excess of the *am*[1] concentration a maximum yield is approached.
3. With a constant concentration of *am*[1] protein and increasing concentrations of the other component the yield of activity increases very steeply at first but at a rapidly decreasing rate. The yield of activity actually declines when the concentration of the variable component is increased beyond about a 2-fold excess over the *am*[1] protein. This effect of an *optimum* concentration of the second component for a constant concentration of *am*[1] protein is very marked with *am*[2] and *am*[19] and less so, though still definite, with *am*[3].

These last two observations suggest that more than one kind of hybrid protein can be formed as a result of the exchange of sub-units and that, as higher concentrations of the *am*[2], *am*[3] or *am*[19] protein are added, an increasing proportion of the *am*[1] protein becomes combined in hybrids which are inactive because they do not have a high enough proportion of the *am*[1] component to stabilise the active conformation. The finding of a plateau region of the curve rather than a definite optimum in the reciprocal experiment suggests that the highest possible ratio of *am*[1] sub-units to those of the other component gives the best activity. It may be that one *am*[3] (or *am*[2] or *am*[19]) dimer is sufficient to supply the active centre and that the other 4 dimers are best supplied by *am*[1], if there are indeed 10 sub-units arranged in 5 firmly bound pairs.

Are hybrids really formed in the in vitro reaction?

In view of the mystery surrounding the mechanism of the *in vitro* complementation reaction it is more than ever necessary to demonstrate that hybrids actually are formed. There are, indeed, strong reasons for supposing that they must be. The only conceivable alternative is for one protein component to somehow activate the other without permanently binding to it or exchanging any material. This would be an improbably novel type of protein-interaction. Any such activation is evidently not catalytic in nature since it is apparent, from the experiments on varying the concentrations of the different components, that both interacting proteins are somehow used up in the reaction. It would, nevertheless, be much more satisfying to have some direct physical or chemical demonstration of the hybrid nature of the product.

Information relevant to this question has been obtained in two of the three *in vitro* complementation systems. Different approaches were used in the two cases. The first approach was made possible by the observation, which has been repeatedly confirmed but not yet explained, that the *am*³ protein emerges earlier than wild type GDH from a column of diethylaminoethyl-cellulose in a gradient of increasing pH 7.4 phosphate buffer concentration. The *am*¹ protein resembles wild type in this respect. Thus it is possible to carry out a chromatographic fractionation of a mixture of *am*¹ and *am*³ proteins with and without a previous treatment at pH 5.8 to bring about the complementation reaction. Such experiments have been reported elsewhere (Fincham and Coddington, 1963, a, b). To summarize the results, when the mixture was chromatographed on the column without prior reaction at pH 5.8 there was a clear separation of two peaks of protein, though with a partial overlap, and all the enzymic activity characteristic of *am*³ protein was in the first peak. When the same protein mixture was reacted at pH 5.8, readjusted to pH 7.4, and subjected to the identical column fractionation, the resolution into two peaks was found to be less definite, with some protein running between the *am*³ and *am*¹ components and obscuring their separation. In this intermediate region there was a very well defined peak of enzyme activity due to complementation. The complementation enzyme peak came out of the column well behind the peak of remaining *am*³-like activity. It is certainly tempting to assume that the complementation peak consists of hybrid protein because of its intermediate position. Such a conclusion does not, however, really follow from the evidence, since the physical basis of the chromatographic difference between the two proteins is not known. There seems to be no difference in electrical charge between the proteins, and if the fractionation is due to a shape difference one must reckon with the perhaps far-fetched possibility that the chromatograph'cally intermediate fractions may simply consist of one of the two components with a permanently altered shape as a result of transient contact with the other component. Studies on the stoichiometry of the reaction, which in principle would solve the problem, are technically difficult because of the incomplete separation of the various components of the reaction mixture. The available data do suggest that *both* mutant proteins contribute materially to the product.

The second approach to the analysis of complementation reaction mixtures was opened up very recently when we found that *am*¹⁹ protein migrates slightly faster than the other proteins of the series in polyacrylamide gel electrophoresis (Ornstein and Davis, 1962). Only preliminary results are so far available but they seem of sufficient interest to be mentioned here. When *am*¹ and *am*¹⁹ proteins are mixed at pH 7.4 and subjected to electrophoresis at pH 8.7 there is a clear separation of two protein bands, as expected. Staining the gels for GDH activity shows no active band. When the two proteins are mixed at pH 5.8, readjusted to pH 7.4 and then fractionated by exactly the same electrophoretic procedure, what appear to be the same two protein bands are *still* visible. There is no obvious hybrid band. What is more, when one half of a gel from such an experiment is stained for protein and the other half for GDH activity, the activity band, which has appeared as a result of complementation, coincides with the protein band in the position expected for am^1 protein.

There are two ways of explaining this rather disconcerting result. First, we might discard our whole hypothesis and admit that am^1 protein can be activated by contact with am^3 protein *without* hybridisation. Or we can say that the electrophoretic separation is not due to a charge difference at all but rather to a shape difference. Since the gel has a very stringent sieving effect in the 200.000 + molecular weight range, it is quite likely that a small difference in shape could cause a difference in the ability of the molecule to penetrate the pores in the gel. The experiment can then be interpreted in conformity with our previous discussion, as follows. The am^1 protein is the ,,right" shape, as is wild type protein and (as nearly as makes no difference to migration rate in the gel) the am^3 protein. The am^{14} protein is, however, very much the ,,wrong" shape. The active hybrid, notwithstanding the fact that it contains some am^{14} sub-units, probably in a small minority, is the ,,right" shape. Consequently it moves as am^1 protein or wild type GDH in the gel. Naturally, I prefer this second explanation.

Fortunately there are several obvious ways in which these alternative interpretations of the $am^1 + am^{19}$ system can be discriminated, and we hope soon to have a clear answer to the question of whether hybrid aggregates are formed or not.

Summary and conclusions

1. Mutants of the *am* series in *Neurospora crassa* are deficient in NADP-linked glutamate dehydrogenase (GDH). Though most *am* mutants do not complement with any of the others, several pairwise combinations do, in heterocaryons, show complementation with formation of active enzyme.
2. With one exception, the complementing mutants produce protein closely related immunologically and in other properties to the normal enzyme, and, again with one exception, the non-complementing mutants do not. The complementing mutant which appears to form no related protein complements effectively in more combinations than any other mutant of the series.
3. In three instances, one member of a complementing pair of mutants produces related protein which can be induced to show GDH activity under appropriate conditions of incubation, while the other produces a totally inactive protein variety. In each of these cases the proteins can be isolated from the individual mutants and made to react together *in vitro* to form active enzyme. There is a well defined optimum ratio of the reacting protein varieties. In each case the totally inactive variety has to be in considerable excess over the potentially active variety for optimum specific activity.
4. The normal GDH appears to be an aggregate of 8 or 10 identical sub-units, as are all the mutant varieties examined. The complementation products, formed either *in vitro* or *in vivo*, resemble normal GDH in molecular weight but are always less stable to heat. The available evidence suggests that the complementation product is, in each case, a mixed aggregate containing sub-units of both mutant types.

5. It is suggested that in the cases considered the complementation is due to the stable activation of a potentially active but conformationally unstable mutant sub-unit through its becoming incorporated in an aggregate composed predominantly of a mutant sub-unit which is conformationally normal but inactive. The complementing mutant which apparently forms no protein may also belong to the potentially active but conformationally unstable category; the folding error in this case may be of so extreme a nature that the mutant sub-units, in a homocaryon, do not aggregate and are so not recognisable as GDH.

References

BARRATT, R. W., and W. N. STRICKLAND, 1963: Purification and characteristics of a TPN — specific glutamic dehydrogenase from *Neurospora crassa*. Arch. Biochem. & Biophys., **102**, 66—76.

FINCHAM, J. R. S., 1959: On the nature of the glutamic dehydrogenase formed by inter-allelic complementation at the *am* locus of *Neurospora crassa*. J. Gen. Microbiol., **21**, 600—611.

FINCHAM, J. R. S., 1962: Genetically determined multiple forms of glutamic dehydrogenase in *Neurospora crassa*. J. Mol. Biol., **4**, 257—274.

FINCHAM, J. R. S., and A. CODDINGTON, 1963 a: Complementation at the *am* locus of *Neurospora crassa*: a reaction between different mutant forms of glutamate dehydrogenase. J. Mol. Biol., **77**, 96—105.

FINCHAM, J. R. S., and A. CODDINGTON, 1963b: The mechanism of complementation between *am* mutants of *Neurospora crassa*. Cold Spring Harb. Symp. Quant. Biol., **28**, 517—527.

MARKERT, C. L., and F. Møller, 1959: Multiple forms of enzymes: tissue ontogenetic, and species specific patterns. Proc. Nat. Acad. Sci., Wash., **45**, 753—763.

ORNSTEIN, L., and B. J. DAVIS, Disc Electrophoresis, preprint distributed by Kodak Ltd., Kirkby, Liverpool, U. K.

PATEMAN, J. A., 1957: Back-mutation studies at the *am* locus in *Neurospora crassa*. J. Genetics, **55**, 444—455.

PATEMAN, J. A., and J. R. S. FINCHAM, 1963: (abstract). Partial revertants at the *am* locus in *Neurospora crassa*. Heredity, **18**, 382.

ROBERTS, D. B., and J. A. PATEMAN, 1964: Immunological studies of amination deficient strains of *Neurospora crassa*. J. Gen. Microbiol., **34**, 295—305.

SANWAL, B. D., and M. LATA, 1961: The occurrence of two different glutamic dehydrogenases in *Neurospora*. Canad. J. Microbiol., **7**, 319—28.

Tissue Specificity and the Control of Gene Action[1]

Drew Schwartz

Department of Biology, Western Reserve University[2] and Biology Division, Oak Ridge National Laboratory[3]

Seven alleles of the E gene which specifies the pH 7.5 esterase have been found segregating in populations of maize and its close relative, teosinte. These alleles specify different forms of the enzyme which differ in their electrophoretic migration rates. Most of the analyses have been done by starch gel electrophoresis, but the differences are also found in electrophoresis on paper, cellulose acetate, agar, and acrylamide gels. The enzyme occurs in all tissues of the plant, but is found in highest concentration in those regions which are actively growing, e. g. the plumule of the young seedling, immature endosperm, base of the leaf blade and leaf sheath, and in the root tips. This distribution of the enzyme in the actively growing regions is best illustrated by the following experiment. A corn root is frozen and thawed, cut in two longitudinally (an aerial root is used because of its large size), and a strip of filter paper is inserted in the cut so that the filter paper is wetted along its length, essentially mapping the root longitudinally from the tip back to the region of maturation and differentiation. The strip of filter paper is then inserted in the starch gel and electrophoresed. The pH 7.5 esterase, which migrates to the negative pole, is concentrated in the region of the root tip.

All of the seven alleles form hybrid enzymes when two alleles exist in the same plant in heterozygous condition. In each case the F_1 heterozygote contains three enzyme bands, the two parental forms as well as the hybrid, and the hybrid enzyme shows a migration rate intermediate between those of the parental forms, a fact consistent with the notion that the enzyme is a dimer composed of two identical or homologous subunits (Schwartz, 1960).

In addition to the structural alleles, which specify enzymes that differ in charge, a number of ,,regulatory mutants“ designated as ,,prime“ alleles have also been found (Schwartz, 1962). The ,,prime“ alleles represent alterations at or very close to the site of the structural gene. No recombination has been found between the structural gene and the factor responsible for the ,,prime“ mutant effect in 3700 tested progeny. These mutants do not cause any detectable modification in the form of the enzyme, but alter the timing of gene action, the rate of enzyme synthesis, or both. ,,Prime“ mutants have been found for four of the seven structural alleles: E^F, E^N, E^S, E^T. As yet ,,prime“ mutants have not been found for the alleles E^L, E^R, E^W. The ,,non-prime“ alleles are designated as the standard types. When the ,,prime“ allele is active, the enzyme produced cannot be differentiated from the enzyme produced

1) This work was supported in part by National Science Foundation Grant number GB-302.

2) Present address.

3) Operated by Union Carbide Corporation for the United States Atomic Energy Commission.

by the corresponding standard allele, by the criteria of electrophoretic migration rate and inactivation studies. Thus, four of the seven structural alleles exist in two forms, standard and „prime", and both forms produce enzymes with the same charge and size.

The prime alleles fall into two classes as regards their behavior in developing endosperm tissue. In all of these studies the level of gene action is determined by developing the zymograms after electrophoresis and comparing the intensities of the enzyme bands produced by two alleles in heterozygous tissue, one of the alleles being of the standard type. The standard alleles are active throughout the development of the endosperm up to the time at which the kernels mature and start to dry. One type of the „prime" allele shows an altered timing of gene action so that enzyme synthesis is cut-off precociously after ten to fourteen days from pollination, depending on the temperature at which the plant is grown. This cut-off is limited to the „prime" allele. In heterozygotes consisting of one „prime" allele and one standard allele, the activity of the standard allele persists unaltered even after the „prime" allele becomes inactive. For example, in $E^{F'}/E^{F'}/E^{N}$ heterozygous endosperm, only the NN type enzyme is found in sixteen day old material.

The second type of „prime" allele also shows normal activity in the young endosperm, but in the older tissue the activity of the gene is much reduced, rather than being completely cut off. Thus in the young heterozygotes of a standard and a „prime" allele, say $E^{F}/E^{N'}/E^{N'}$, the intensities of the three pH 7. 5 esterase bands are as expected for equal activity of both alleles. However, by sixteen days from pollination the intensity of the NN and NF bands are much reduced as compared with the FF band, with the greatest reduction observed in the intensity of the NN band.

The „prime" alleles show about normal activity in the seedlings. Some are slightly more active and others less active than the standard alleles. In F_1 heterozygotes containing a standard and a „prime" allele, the hybrid band is heavier than either of the parental bands. However, in the aerial roots two of the prime alleles – $E^{N'220}$ and $E^{N'469}$ show a marked divergence from the behavior of the standard alleles. $E^{N'469}$ is of the type which causes a complete cessation of gene activity early in the development of the endosperm while $E^{N'220}$ only reduces the level of gene action. In the aerial roots both of these alleles show a striking increase in activity as compared with the standard alleles. In heterozygotes such as $E^{N'220}/E^{S}$, the NN band is most intense, the NS hybrid band weaker, and the SS band very light. Thus we see that the relative activity of the same two alleles can differ markedly in different tissues of the plant. In the endosperm tissue the „prime" allele shows much reduced activity as compared with the standard allele; in the plumule of the seedling the two show about equal activity, whereas in the aerial root the „prime" allele is much more active than the standard. The increased activity of $E^{N'220}$ and $E^{N'469}$ appears to be limited to the aerial roots. In the other roots of the plant and in leaf tissue the relative activities of these alleles are similar to that of the plumules.

These results have an important bearing on the problem of differentiation and suggest that different controlling systems or elements may be functioning in different tissues of the same plant to regulate the action of a particular gene. On the basis of the inducer hypothesis for control of gene action proposed by PARDEE, JACOB and MONOD (1959), one would have to postulate three different inducers acting in the three tissues. The prime allele would be more responsive to the aerial root inducer than the standard allele in the same nucleus; both allelic types about equally responsive to the inducer of the plumule; and the „prime" allele less responsive to the endosperm inducer than the standard allele. However, other regulatory systems are possible, and one of these is presented in another paper (SCHWARTZ 1964). These results indicate that whatever the controlling system involved, regulation is not an all or none process which merely turns genes on or off, but can also regulate the level of gene activity. Tissue specificity may also depend upon enzyme balance or the relative concentrations of a group of enzymes as determined by differential gene activity in addition to the occurrence of completely different enzymes in these tissues.

Differential turnover rates can be ruled out as the explanation for these results. Synthesis of the pH 7.5 esterase is limited to the meristematic region of the root. Enzyme concentration drops off in the region behind the root tip. However, the relative concentrations of the enzyme bands in the heterozygotes of $E^{N'220}$ and $E^{N'469}$ with the standard alleles remain constant throughout. If the enzymes specified by the prime alleles are less labile than those of the standard alleles, the differences in intensities of the enzyme bands should increase along the root from the meristematic region to the region of maturation.

The difference in relative activities of the prime and standard alleles in the aerial roots appears to be under genetic control. In some genetic backgrounds this difference disappears, but these studies are still inclomplete.

Literature cited

PARDEE, A. B., F. JACOB, and J. MONOD, 1959: The genetic control and cytoplasmic expression of „inducibility" in the synthesis of β-galactosidase in E. coli. J. Mol. Biol. **1**, 165–178.

SCHWARTZ, D., 1960: Genetic studies on mutant enzymes in maize: Synthesis of hybrid enzymes by heterozygotes. Proc. Nat. Acad. Sci. U. S. **46**, 1210–1216.

SCHWARTZ, D., 1962: Genetic studies on mutant enzymes in maize. III. Control of gene action in the synthesis of pH 7.5 esterase. Geneties **47**, 1609–1615.

SCHWARTZ, D., 1964: Genetic studies on mutant enzymes in maize. IV. Comparison of pH 7.5 esterases sythesyzed in seedling and endosperm. Genetics **49**, 373–377.

Regulatory Function of Sorbose on Sugar Metabolism in *Neurospora*

W. Klingmüller

Max-Planck-Institut für Erbbiologie, Berlin-Dahlem

I should like to give you a short report on work that is still in progress. This work is dealing with genetic regulation mechanisms in *Neurospora crassa*, the well known mould. In this mould we are investigating certain steps of sugar metabolism and the possible regulation of sugar metabolism by structural and functional genes.

I wish to state clearly from the beginning that our data are not conclusive yet, nor are our theoretical considerations the only ones possible. However, since the topic of genetic regulation mechanisms is discussed here, we feel we should mention our findings, preliminary as they are, to add certain new aspects to the general picture, and to stimulate further work.

Let me start with some general facts.

Neurospora normally grows as a large, irregular mycelium. This is the wildtype trait. There are, however, mutants that grow in small, dense clusters, like little colonies. They have the colonial trait.

Even the wildtype mould can be forced into colonial growth, if a certain chemical substance is added to the growth medium. This substance is sorbose, a sugar. Sorbose is used widely by all people working with *Neurospora*, to produce colonial growth, that is to facilitate handling of the mould.

Sorbose, apart from inducing colonial growth, has a second effect on *Neurospora*. Under certain conditions it reduces viability very strongly. This has been found recently by de Serres *et al.* (1962). The strong effect of sorbose on viability of *Neurospora* is what I shall be talking about now. Later on, some remarks shall be added concerning the phenomenon of colony formation.

What is it, de Serres and co-workers found? Let me explain briefly the first slide, taken from their paper (Fig. 1). The normal medium for growth of *Neurospora* contains sucrose and sorbose in certain amounts. Sucrose serves as carbon source, and sorbose serves to induce colonial growth. Such media were autoclaved for different periods of time. Conidia were then added to the media, and germination was checked after several days. In media autoclaved for a long time, viability was high, but with shorter autoclaving times, lower viabilities resulted. If filteristerlized sucrose was used in combination with sorbose, viability was at a minimum. On filtersterilized sucrose free of sorbose, viability was high. With media, the sucrose of which had been replaced by filtersterilized glucose plus fructose, no effect of added sorbose on viability was found.

The authors did not propose an explanation in terms of basic mechanisms. However, we became interested in such an explanation. We started work with the following question:

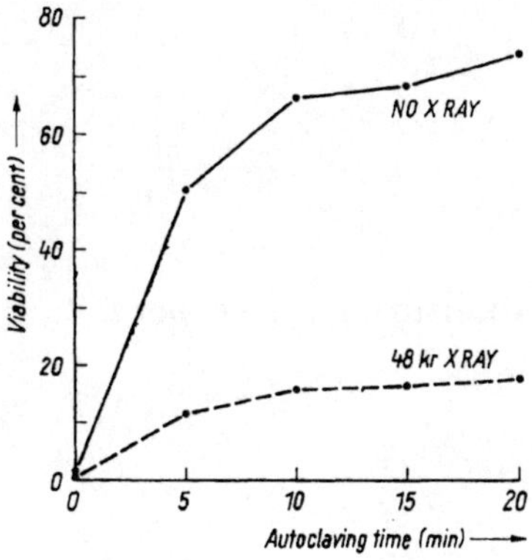

If the wildtype does not grow on filtersterilized sucrose in presence of sorbose, is it possible to produce mutants that do grow? The answer is yes.

By treating conidia of the mould with nitrous acid in suitable concentrations, and pouring high amounts of the treated conidia into agar with high sorbose content, it was possible to select strains that do grow in spite of sorbose. The trait is called S^- operationally, and we are talking about S-mutants.

Fig. 1. Viability of wildtype conidia in Westergaard's medium containing 1.0% sorbose and 0.1% sucrose autoclaved for the indicated times. From de Serres *et al.* (1962)

The growth features of these mutants are given in the next three figures. The mutants grow well on sucrose, if sorbose is present; the wildtype is strongly inhibited (Fig. 2). The mutants grow on fructose, if sorbose is present; the wildtype does not (Fig. 3). The mutants grow on glucose, if sorbose is present; the wildtype grows as well (Fig. 4).

By treating S-mutants with nitrous acid once more, mutants of still better growth in presence of sorbose have been produced. They will be called S-doubles operationally. Growth features of these mutants as compared to wildtype and S-mutants are shown in Fig. 5.

All mutants analyzed so far are of true chromosomal origin. The S- and S-double traits segregate normally if mutants are back-crossed to wildtype. Recently we have been able to localize the S-factor more specifically. This was done by crossing the S-mutants with a set of tester strains with markers covering all linkage groups. The results for 4 S-mutants analyzed so far show that the S-factor in all of them is localized in the left arm of linkage groop VI, close to the yellow marker.

From our results a provisional working hypothesis has been formed, which is depicted in Fig. 6. The heavy lines indicate facts that are already known, the thin lines indicate, whatis still hypothetical.

Ac cording to this hypothesis, sucrose is split by invertase into glucose and fructose. The locus for invertase and possible other substances involved in this reaction is indicated in Fig. 6 as Sucr.-Abbau. Fructose is transformed by fructokinase into fructose-1-phosphate. The locus for fructokinase and further enzymes involved in fructose decomposition is indicated as Fruct.-Abbau. Sorbose, in the wildtype, is supposed to act on a repressor locus. It stimulates the repressor locus to form a repressor substance, which acts via an operator locus. From the operator locus both the loci for sucrose decomposition and fructose decomposition are blocked at the same time.

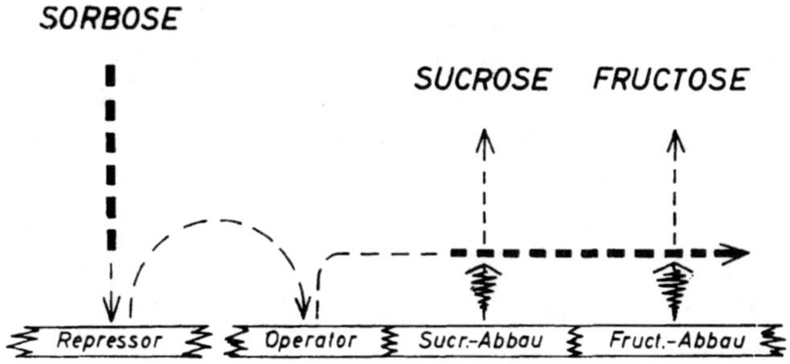

Fig. 6. Scheme of provisional working hypothesis on sorbose action. The heavy lines indicate facts that are already known, the thin lines indicate, what is still hypothetical

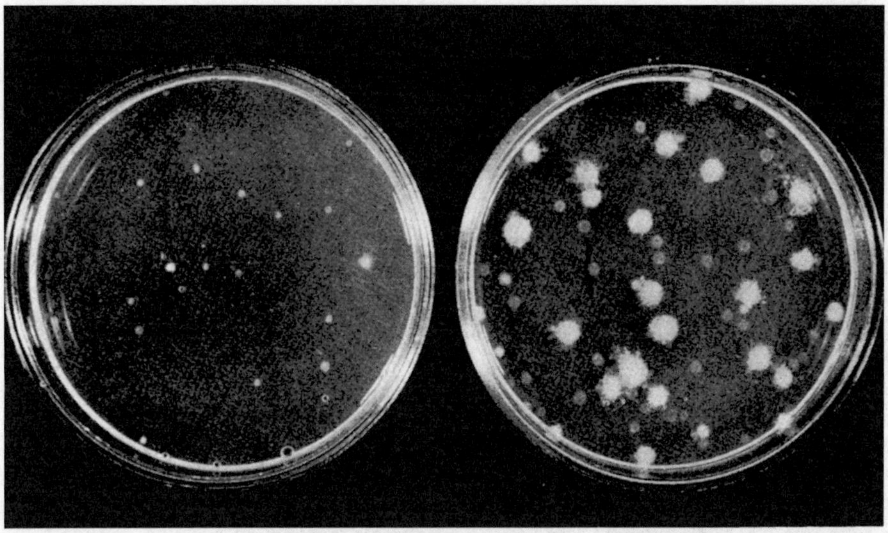

Fig. 2. Growth of wildtype (left) and *S*-strain (right) on FRIES' minimal agar containing 0.01% sucrose and 0.1% sorbose, both filtersterilized. Age of cultures 6 days

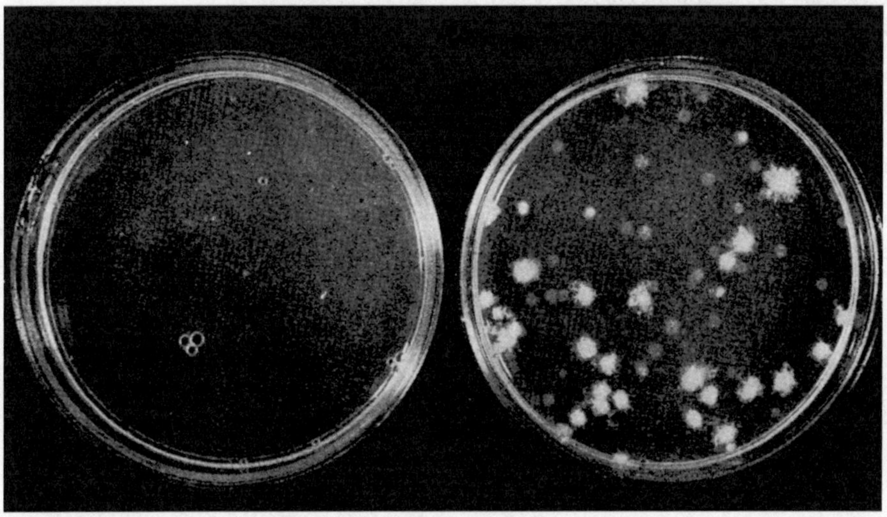

Fig. 3. Same as above, but 0.01% fructose instead of sucrose

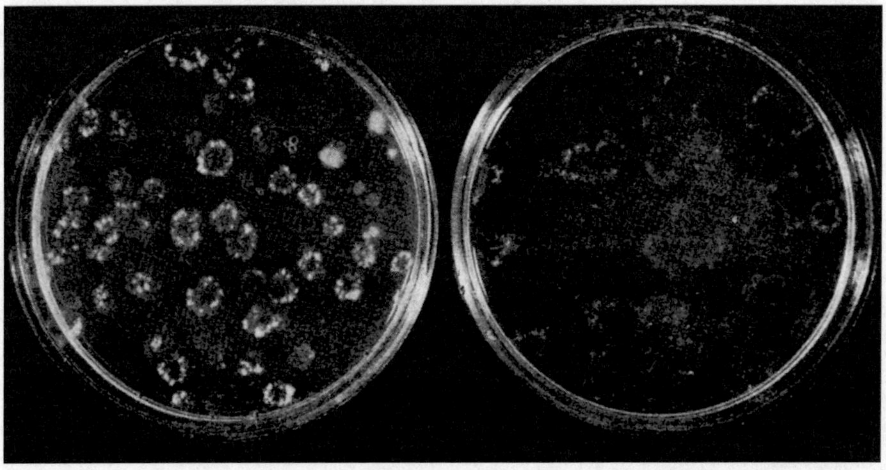

Fig. 4. Same as above, but 0.01% glucose instead of sucrose. Age of cultures 3 days

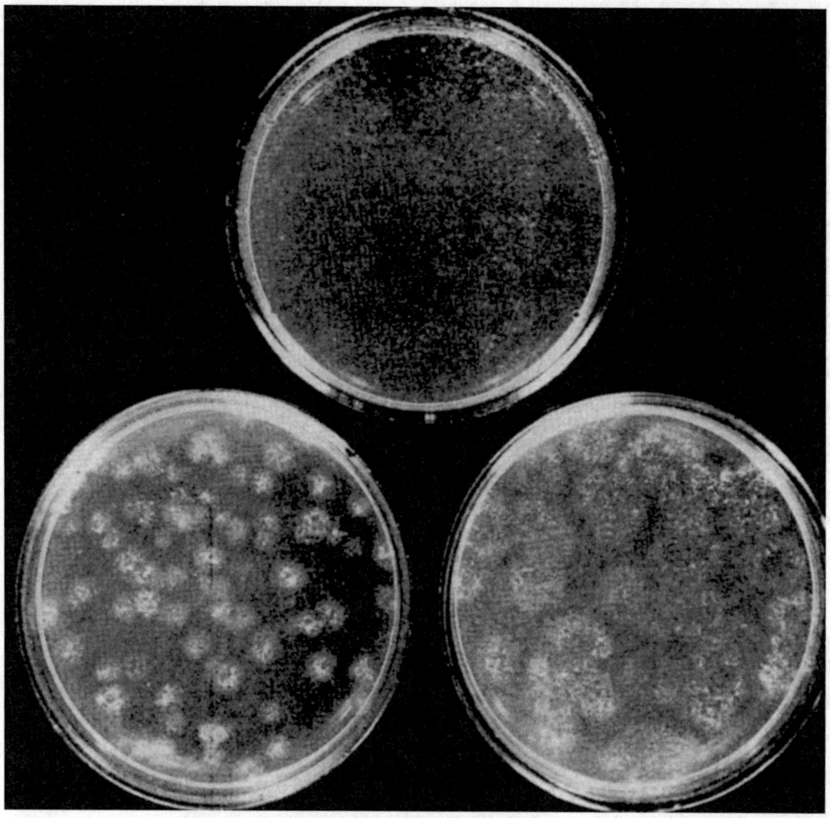

Fig. 5. Growth of wildtype (top), *S*-strain (bottom left) and *S*-double strain (bottom right) on FRIES' minimal, containing 0.025% filtersterilized sorbose. Age of cultures 4 days

In the mutants, either the repressor locus or the operator locus is knocked out or partly inactivated, depending on the *S*- or *S*-double characteristic. Therefore, the two loci under consideration can not be blocked by sorbose. The mutants should be constitutive for the respective enzymes. They grow on sucrose or fructose even if sorbose is present.

The details of the scheme suggested here are under investigation. Whether it is applicable or not will depend on the results. Since glucose is utilized in the presence of sorbose, the reduction of viability by sorbose in sucrose and fructose media seems to be of a rather specific nature. This is what makes us postulate a genetically controlled regulation mechanism. Reduction of viability should not be due to an overall growth inhibition of the mould by sorbose, and mutants should not be due to an overall increase in resistance against sorbose. That glucose is utilized in the presence of sorbose may however be due to another reason. We are considering at present the possibility that a second metabolic pathway is involved in glucose catabolism. This second pathway of direct oxydation of glucose via gluconolactone is known to exist in certain fungi. It might well be that this second possible pathway is not influenced by sorbose, whereas the main pathway is blocked, either in certain steps, or completely.

Thus far, I was concerned with the effect of sorbose on viability of *Neurospora*. In concluding my report, I should now like to add briefly certain findings on the phenomenon of colony formation. Is there any connection between the sorbose effect on viability, the sorbose effect inducing colony formation, and the genetic factor for colony formation?

At present we have checked one aspect of this question: What happens, when the *S*-trait is crossed into the *col*-mutants? Will the *col*-trait be relieved, in the same manner as the viability reducing effect of sorbose is relieved by the *S*-factor? The answer is, these crosses do not work. This fact is shown in Fig. 7. Crosses of several S^+-isolates, the wildtype reisolates from 4 *S*-mutants, with *col* were all fertile. But crosses of several isolates of S^- with *col*

S-mutant nr.

1			2			3			5		
a	b	c	a	b	c	a	b	c	a	b	c
Ascospore isolate nr.	Growth with sorbose	Fertility with col									
4	–	+	4	+	–	1	–	+	4	–	+
9	–	+				4	–	+	15	–	+
11	–	+				6	–	+	20	–	+
20	–	+				7	–	+	7	+	–
13	–	–				10	–	+	9	+	–
15	?	?				12	–	+	10	+	–
1	+	–				27	–	+	17	+	–
6	+	–				3	+	–			
7	+	–				26	+	–			
12	+	–									
18	+	–									
19	+	–									
21	+	–									

Fig. 7. Correlation between *S*-characteristic and fertility in crosses with a colonial mutant. Wildtype reisolates of strain 74 A as well as *S*-isolates were crossed with *col* K 3/17 a ad 38701 (courtesy of Dr. H. G. Kølmark)

were sterile, with only one exception. The implications of this finding are not clear at present. However, the result does indicate a correlation between the different genetic factors. This fact may finally become important for interpretation of the action of the *S*-locus.

I should like to repeat that our data are still of a rather preliminary nature. In spite of this we think they are suggestive of a genetically controlled regulatory mechanism in sugar metabolism of *Neurospora*. Whether this regulatory mechanism is similar to those found in bacteria, or whether it has some original features, will be a task for further work.

Reference

Serres, F. J. de, H. G. Kølmark, and H. E. Brockman, 1962: Nature **193**, 556–557.

Mutationen zur Resistenz gegen katabolische Repression der Enzymsynthese bei *E. coli*

JOSEPH LENGELER und PETER STARLINGER

Institut für Genetik der Universität zu Köln

Seit längerer Zeit ist bekannt, daß die Synthese einer Reihe von induzierbaren Enzymen auch in Gegenwart eines geeigneten Induktors durch Glukose gehemmt wird (EPPS und GALE, 1942; MONOD, 1942). Diese Hemmung der induzierbaren Enzymsynthese ist aber nicht auf Glukose beschränkt. Unter gewissen Stoffwechselbedingungen können auch andere energieliefernde Stoffe, z. B. Glycerin, die induzierbare Enzymsynthese hemmen.

MAGASANIK untersuchte die Hemmung der induzierbaren Enzymsynthese genauer und stellte auf Grund dieser Untersuchungen die folgende Hypothese auf: Nicht Glukose selbst, sondern ein unbekanntes Abbauprodukt dieses Zuckers hemmt die Enzymsynthese. Dieses Abbauprodukt, wie auch andere Zwischenprodukte des Intermediärstoffwechsels, häuft sich an, wenn die Zellen in Glukose wachsen. Glukose wird nämlich schnell umgesetzt, und die biosynthetischen Reaktionen können die anfallenden Spaltprodukte nicht schnell genug entfernen. Andere Energiequellen, wie Glycerin, werden im allgemeinen nicht so schnell verarbeitet, so daß es nicht zu einer Anhäufung von Zwischenprodukten kommen kann. Hemmt man aber den Abfluß der Intermediärprodukte durch eine Beeinträchtigung der biosynthetischen Reaktionen, so kann auch in Gegenwart von Glycerin so viel von dem unbekannten Zwischenprodukt aufgehäuft werden, daß es zu einer Hemmung der Enzymsynthese kommt.

Aufgrund dieser Annahmen führte MAGASANIK für den erwähnten Hemmeffekt den Namen „Kataboliten-Repression" ein (MAGASANIK, 1961).

Von verschiedenen Autoren wurden Mutanten isoliert, die keine Kataboliten-Repression mehr zeigen (ENGLESBERG, 1959; NEIDHARDT, 1960). In beiden Fällen war der Glukose-Stoffwechsel gestört, so daß die Mutanten auf Glukose als einziger Kohlenstoffquelle ein verringertes Wachstum zeigten. Diese Beobachtung paßt zu der Hypothese von MAGASANIK, nach der es bei einer Störung des Glukose-Stoffwechsels nicht zu einer Anhäufung von Zwischenprodukten und demnach auch nicht zu einer Hemmung der Enzymsynthese kommen sollte. In Übereinstimmung mit dieser Hypothese waren die beobachteten Fälle der Resistenz gegen Kataboliten-Repression unspezifisch. Die Synthese verschiedener untersuchter Enzyme erwies sich in gleichem Maße unempfindlich gegen Glukose.

Nach den heutigen Vorstellungen über die Synthese der Enzyme und über die Regulation dieser Synthese ist es aber nicht sehr wahrscheinlich, daß kleine Moleküle wie die Intermediärprodukte des Zuckerstoffwechsels für sich allein eine Hemmung der Enzymsynthese bewirken können. Ein Zusammenwirken dieser kleinen Moleküle mit spezifischen, genabhängigen Repressoren erschiene befriedigender (JACOB und MONOD, 1961).

Um die Beteiligung spezifischer Repressoren an der Kataboliten-Repression nachzuweisen, suchten wir nach Mutanten, die keine Beeinträchtigung ihres Glukosestoffwechsels zeigen, und bei denen nur die Synthese bestimmter Enzyme gegen Glukose unempfindlich geworden ist, während andere Enzyme noch der Kataboliten-Repression unterliegen.

Wir lassen zu diesem Zweck Zellen des Wildstammes in einem synthetischen Medium wachsen, das Galaktose und Glukose als Kohlenstoffquelle enthält. In diesem Medium bilden die meisten Zellen keine Enzyme des Galaktoseabbaues, weil die Glukose hemmend wirkt. Nur solche Zellen, die keine Kataboliten-Repression der Galaktose-Enzyme besitzen, werden auch unter diesen Bedingungen Galaktose-Enzyme herstellen. Die Zellen werden nun gewaschen und in ein Medium gebracht, das Galaktose als einzige Kohlenstoffquelle enthält. Die Mutanten, die gegen Glukose resistent sind und daher bereits Galaktose-Enzyme besitzen, haben in diesem Medium einen Wachstumsvorteil. Wiederholte Anwendung dieses Wachstumszyklus führt zu einer Anreicherung der Mutanten.

Zwei derartige Mutanten wurden bisher untersucht und zeigten die folgenden Eigenschaften:

1. Sie wachsen auf Glukose als einziger Kohlenstoffquelle ebensogut wie der Wildtyp.
2. Sie bilden in Gegenwart von Glukose größere Mengen von Galaktoseenzymen, während im Wildtyp in Gegenwart von Glukose weniger als $^1/_{10}$ der durch Induktion erreichbaren Menge gebildet wird.
3. Die Bildung von Tryptophanase und d-Serin-Desaminase ist in gleicher Weise durch Glukose gehemmt wie im Wildstamm.
4. Die Bildung von β-Galaktosidase ist in beiden Stämmen konstitutiv. In Gegenwart von Glukose werden etwa 40% der in Abwesenheit dieses Zuckers erreichten Enzymsynthese gefunden. Dies entspricht dem Ausmaß des Glukose-Effektes, das auch sonst in konstitutiven Stämmen bei der Bildung von β-Galaktosidase beobachtet wird.

Wir sehen in diesen Beobachtungen ein Anzeichen dafür, daß außer den niedermolekularen Abbauprodukten des Glukosestoffwechsels noch andere, genabhängige Faktoren eine Rolle bei der Kataboliten-Repression spielen. Wir hoffen, durch weitere Versuche klären zu können, ob es sich bei diesen genabhängigen Faktoren um Repressoren handelt, die durch einen Co-Repressor aus dem Glukosestoffwechsel aktiviert werden müssen.

Literatur

EPPS, H. M. R., and E. F. GALE, 1942: The influence of the presence of glucose during growth on the enzyme activities of *Escherichia coli.* Biochem. J. **36**, 619.

MONOD, J., 1942: Recherches sur la croissance des cultures bacteriennes. Paris: Hermann et Cie.

MAGASANIK, B., 1961: Catabolite Repression. Cold Spring Harbor Symp. Quant. Biol. XXVI, 249.

ENGLESBERG, E., 1959: Glucose inhibition and the diauxie phenomena. Proc. Nat. Acad. Sci. U. S. **45**, 1494.

NEIDHARDT, F. C., 1960: Mutant of aerobacter aerogenes lacking glucose repression. J. Bacteriol. **80**, 536.

JACOB, F., and J. MONOD, 1961: Genetic regulatory mechanisms in the synthesis of proteins. J. Mol. Biol. **3**, 318.

Kontrollierte RNS-Synthese in Riesenchromosomen

W. Beermann, Tübingen

Die zentrale Rolle, die die Ribonukleinsäure in ihren verschiedenen Formen als Mittler der genetischen Information, als Substrat und als Werkzeug in der Proteinsynthese der Zelle spielt, setzt die Existenz von Kontrollmechanismen, die die Produktion der einzelnen RNS-Typen regulieren, fast notwendigerweise voraus. Einen solchen Kontrollmechanismus glauben z. B. Jacob und Monod (1961) für die DNS-abhängige Synthese von *messenger*-RNS am Genom der Bakterien entdeckt zu haben (vgl. Attardi *et al.*, 1963). Er würde hier die Grundlage für die außerordentlich wirkungsvolle adaptive Regulation der Synthese bestimmter Enzyme bilden. Ein anderer Kontrollmechanismus, der die Höhe der Proteinsynthese in der Bakterienzelle nicht selektiv, sondern ganz allgemein beeinflußt und auf das Angebot der freien Aminosäuren anspricht, scheint ebenfalls in die DNS-abhängige RNS-Synthese – in diesem Fall die Synthese aller RNS-Typen – einzugreifen (vgl. Stent, dieses Symp.). Schon bei der Arbeit an Mikroorganismen ist es schwierig, den Nachweis zu führen, daß die untersuchten Regulationserscheinungen wirklich, wie es gefordert wird, auf einer Kontrolle der gen-abhängigen RNS-Synthese beruhen, insbesondere, wenn es sich um die Frage einer differentiellen Kontrolle jedes einzelnen „Operons" handelt. Die Prüfung der gleichen Fragen an komplexen, vielzelligen Organismen muß um ein vielfaches schwieriger sein, obwohl die Tatsache der Zelldifferenzierung – mehr als alle Adaptionsleistungen der Bakterien – zu der Annahme der spezifischen Induktion oder Repression bestimmter Komponenten der genetischen Information bei der intrazellulären Informationsübertragung, d. h. der DNS-abhängigen RNS-Synthese, geradezu herausfordert. Sicher enthält beispielsweise ein Retikulozyt vorwiegend messenger-RNS zur Codierung von Globin-Molekülen, und wahrscheinlich gilt Entsprechendes für den Gehalt von *messenger*-Molekülen für Muskelproteine in Myoblasten, oder von *messenger*-Molekülen für Trypsin in Pankreas-Zellen, usf.; aber der Beweis, daß diese Anhäufung bestimmter *messenger*-Typen in bestimmten Zelltypen, sofern sie nachgewiesen ist, auf differentieller Synthese beruht, müßte erst noch geführt werden. Man hätte etwa zu zeigen, daß die isolierten Kerne oder Chromosomen der differenzierten Zellen in vitro das für ihren Zelltyp charakteristische *messenger*-„Spektrum" produzieren. Die technischen Schwierigkeiten der biochemischen Identifizierung von *messenger*-RNS oder gar von mehreren *messenger*-Typen nebeneinander in in-vitro-Systemen liegen auf der Hand; zur Zeit muß es als nahezu unmöglich gelten, dem Problem der differentiellen Kontrolle der RNS-Synthese in den Kernen höherer Organismen auf diese Weise, d. h. mit rein biochemischen Methoden näherzukommen. Wir haben uns bemüht, das Problem zunächst von der cytologischen und genetischen Seite her in Angriff zu nehmen, und zwar an einem System, das die morphologische Definition von genetisch und operativ selbständigen Einheiten des Genoms[1]) gestattet: den mit polytänen Riesenchromosomen ausgestatteten Riesenzellen einiger Organe von Dipterenlarven, speziell von Larven der Arten *Chironomus tentans* und *Chironomus pallidivittatus*. Die folgenden Fragen waren zu beantworten: (1) Gibt es überhaupt Unterschiede in der Höhe der RNS-Synthese von Chromosomenort zu Chromosomenort? (2) Wird die Höhe der RNS-Synthese an jedem Chromosomenort individuell und autonom eingestellt, welcher Art ist die Kontrolle, und welches sind die individuell kontrollierten Einheiten? (3) Läßt sich die produzierte RNS als *messenger* für zellspezifische Proteinsynthesen identifizieren? (4) Welcher Kontroll-Mechanismus liegt der lokalen Regulation der RNS-Synthese in Interphase-Chromosomen zu Grunde? Diese Fragen sollen im folgenden im Zusammenhang mit einem Überblick über unsere bisherigen Ergebnisse besprochen werden.

1. Das Spektrum der RNS-Synthese in den Riesenchromosomen der Speicheldrüsen-Zellen von Chironomus

Hier seien zunächst einige allgemeine Bemerkungen über die Struktur und die genetische Gliederung der Riesenchromosomen vorausgeschickt. Riesenchromosomen findet man in den Zellkernen verschiedener larvaler und imaginaler Organe von Dipteren. Die larvalen Organe sind bei Abschluß der Embryonalentwicklung voll differenziert und funktionsfähig. Ihr weiteres Wachstum beruht allein auf Zellwachstum, nicht auf Zellvermehrung, so daß z. B. die Speicheldrüsen von *Chironomus* zu Ende des 4. Larvenstadiums aus nur etwa 50 Zellen riesiger Größe (bis $^1/_2$ mm Durchmesser) bestehen. Im Zuge des Wachstums der differenzierten Zellen entwickeln sich als Folge rhythmischer Verdoppelungen der Längselemente der Chromosomen oder Chromatiden – ohne Chromosomenteilung – die riesigen „polytänen" Chromosomen, d. h. kabelartige Verbände von tausenden homologer Einzelchromatiden, die sich zudem stark in die Länge strecken. Dieser Wachstumsprozeß enthüllt nach und nach immer mehr Einzelheiten der Feingliederung des Interphase-Chromosoms, deren wesentliches Merkmal das Chromomeren- oder Querscheibenmuster darstellt. Dieses Muster ist für jedes Chromosom charakteristisch und ist in allen Zellen eines Tieres, die überhaupt analysierbare Polytän-Chromosomen besitzen, praktisch gleich. Es muß deshalb eine genetisch festliegende Diskontinuität in den letzten Elementen oder Chromatiden darstellen, aus welchen sich das polytäne Chromosom aufbaut. Wir konnten zeigen (Beermann, 1952), daß alle scheinbaren Unstimmigkeiten in dem Querscheibenmuster homologer Chromosomen verschiedener Zellen auf technische Schwierigkeiten zurückführbar sind, wie z. B. die scheinbare oder tatsächliche Verschmelzung zweier benachbarter Querscheiben, die scheinbare Abwesenheit besonders feiner Querscheiben als Folge mangelhafter Auflösung, und endlich Unterschiede in der Färbungsintensität und den Abstandsbeziehungen einzelner Querscheiben, die durch das *puffing* verursacht sind.

Im wesentlichen ist die Chromomerengliederung der polytänen Chromosomen gekennzeichnet durch das abrupte Alternieren von DNS-reichen und DNS-armen Abschnitten, also den Chromomeren und den Interchromomeren. In Analogie mit den Lampenbürstenchromosomen und nach Daten von Swift (1963) darf man annehmen, daß auch die Interchromomeren DNS enthalten. Auch die Daten von Steffensen (1963) schließen diese Möglichkeit nicht aus. Die Länge der DNS-reichen Abschnitte, d. h. die Dicke der Quer-

[1]) Es sind nicht „operons" im Sinne von Jacob und Monod gemeint, s. w. u.!

scheiben, wechselt zwischen 0,05 μ und 0,5 μ, während die Größe der Interchromomeren nicht so stark zu variieren scheint. Der scheinbare Unterschied in der DNS-Konzentration zwischen Chromomeren und Interchromomeren ist wohl ausschließlich dem Unterschied in der Massendichte zuzuschreiben, der sich sowohl aus Untersuchungen über die Röntgenstrahlenabsorption wie auch aus elektronenmikroskopischen Daten ergibt. Er ist wahrscheinlich zurückzuführen auf ein Abwechseln zwischen stark aufgefalteten und nicht gefalteten Abschnitten des diskontinuierlichen DNS - Histon - Fadens, den jede einzelne Chromatide vermutlich darstellt.

Für die Frage nach der Verteilung der RNS-Syntheseaktivität ist es zunächst interessant, das Vorkommen und die Verteilung von RNS in den Riesenchromosomen zu untersuchen. Die RNS wird im mikroskopischen Präparat mit metachromatisch färbenden basischen Farbstoffen, wie dem Toluidinblau, am besten nachgewiesen (Pelling, 1959); die Spezifität der Reaktion wird mit Ribonuklease kontrolliert. Die Untersuchungen von Pelling (1964) zeigen, daß hochmolekulare RNS in den Riesenchromosomen der Speicheldrüsen vorkommt, aber sehr ungleichmäßig auf die verschiedenen Chromosomenorte verteilt ist. RNS läßt sich nur an solchen Stellen finden, die morphologisch als *puffs* charakterisiert sind, d. h. in Querscheiben, deren Struktur mehr oder minder aufgelockert und aufgebläht erscheint. Der subjektiv abschätzbare RNS-Gehalt dieser Chromosomenorte geht dabei etwa dem Grade der Auflockerung parallel (Abb. 1). Auf diese Weise ist also dem Verteilungsmuster der DNS und des Histons in den Riesenchromosomen ein von diesem deutlich verschiedenes Verteilungsmuster der RNS überlagert. Ein Vergleich der Daten von Pelling mit denen von Clever (1961), der die Verteilung der *puffs* mit einer Lichtgrün-Färbung studiert hat, zeigt, daß die RNS-reichen Orte zugleich auch immer reich an höheren Proteinen sind, die sich mit der Lichtgrün-Reaktion bei pH 4 anfärben. In den Speicheldrüsen sind es ungefähr 20% aller Querscheiben, die RNS enthalten und gleichzeitig aufgelockert erscheinen können; ihre Verteilung folgt keiner erkennbaren Regel, ist aber für die Chromosomen aller Speicheldrüsen-Zellen die gleiche (Abb. 2).

Wenn man annimmt, daß die RNS in den „RNS-Chromomeren" oder *puffs* (die gleichzeitig stets auch noch ihre DNS enthalten) nicht stationär als Strukturelement gebunden ist, sondern dort fortlaufend neu gebildet wird, – wenn man also diese Orte für Orte der chromosomalen RNS-Synthese hält –, so sollte man zunächst erwarten, daß der RNS-Gehalt und der Grad der Auflockerung dieser Orte als Ausdruck ihres dynamischen Charakters im Gegensatz zur DNS-Verteilung deutlich variiert. Dies ist auch der Fall. Clever und Pelling haben beide in ihren Untersuchungen gezeigt, daß nur etwa 50% aller nachweisbaren RNS-Orte in den Speicheldrüsenzellen von *Chironomus* in allen Tieren und unter allen Bedingungen tatsächlich *puffs* bilden; und auch diese in von Fall zu Fall deutlich verschiedenem Ausmaß (Abb. 3). Das könnte z. B. heißen, daß etwa die Hälfte aller RNS-Syntheseorte in den Speicheldrüsen-Chromosomen nur intermittierend tätig ist.

Diese Interpretation der RNS-Chromomeren als Syntheseort von RNS findet ihre Bestätigung in den autoradiographischen Bildern der Riesenchromosomen nach Einbau radioaktiv markierten Vorstufen der RNS. Injiziert oder verfüttert man Tritium- oder C^{14}-markierte Nucleoside (Uridin, Cytidin, Adenosin), oder inkubiert man die Speicheldrüsen mit diesen Stoffen in vitro, so entspricht das autoradiographisch nachweisbare Einbaumuster in die hochmolekulare RNS topographisch (und in der quantitativen Abstufung) genau dem Verteilungsmuster der RNS-Orte oder *puffs* (Tab. 1). Die enormen Dimensionen der Riesenchromosomen gestatten es, diese Aussage wirklich bis auf die einzelne Querscheibe zu präzisieren, wie es Pelling (1959) zuerst gezeigt hat (Abb. 4).

Daß der Einbau von Nukleosiden in die RNS der *puffs* nun tatsächlich den Ablauf einer RNS-Synthese an den gleichen Orten bedeutet, läßt sich auf verschiedene Weise wahrschein-

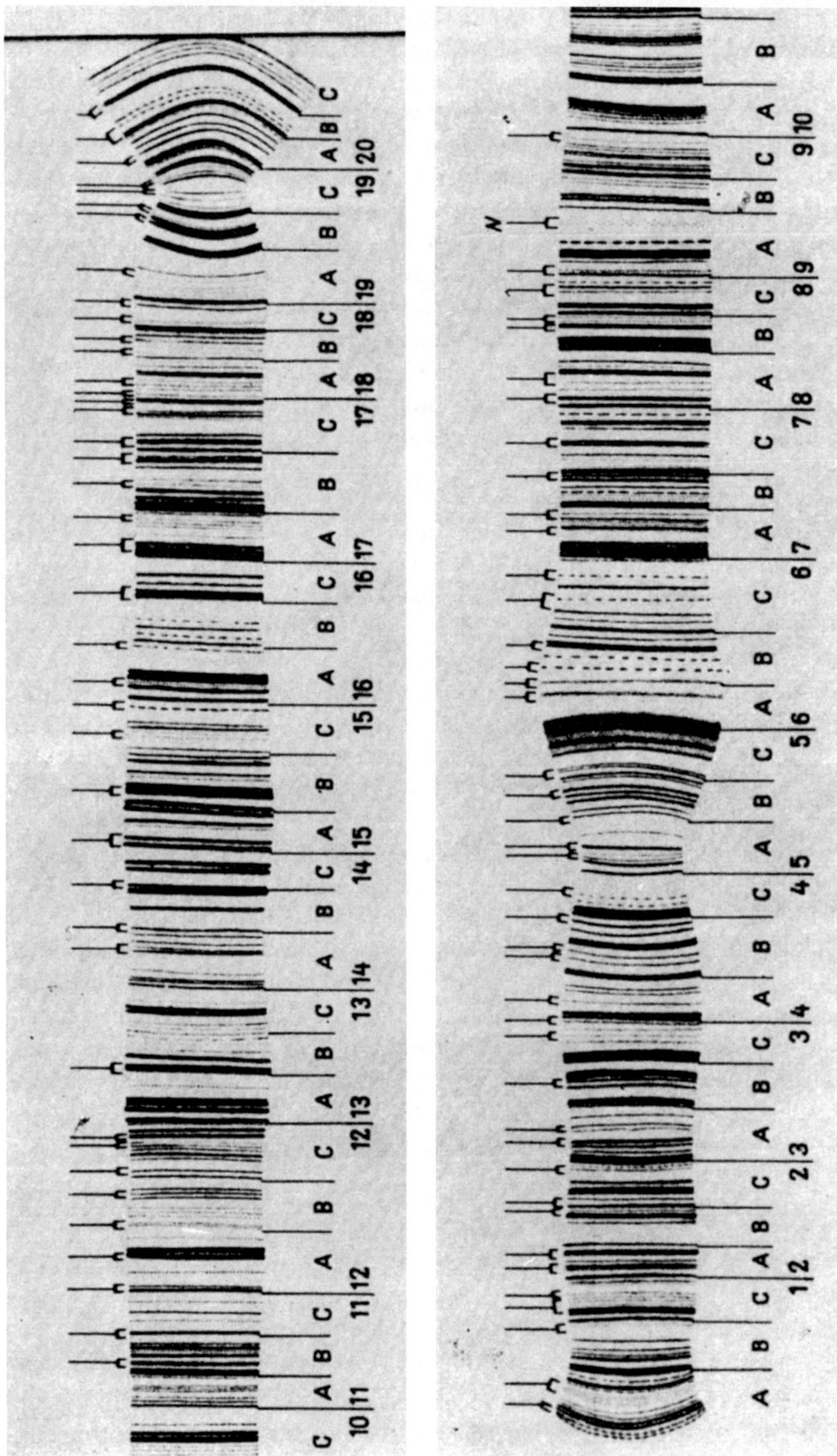

Abb. 2. Karte des Speicheldrüsen-Chromosoms II von *Chironomus tentans*, mit Markierung derjenigen Orte, die in den Speicheldrüsen regelmäßig oder intermittierend *puffs* bilden. Nach PELLING 1963

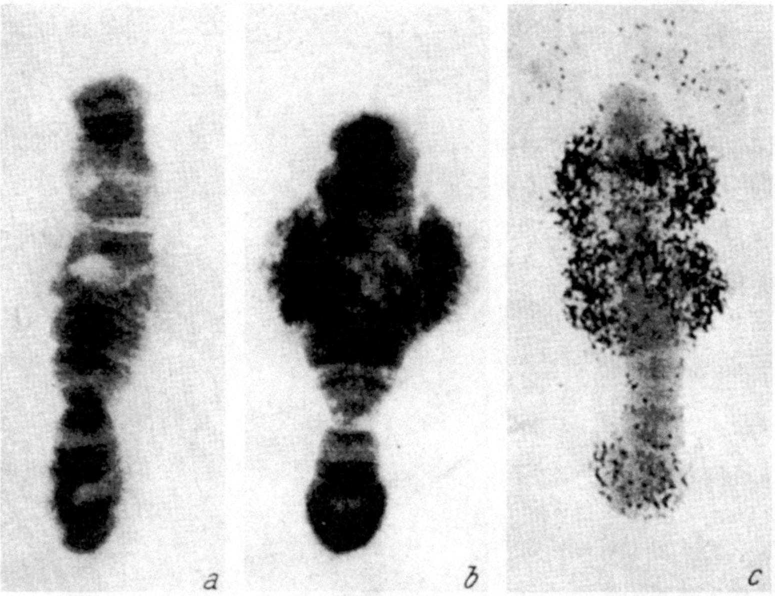

Abb. 1. Speicheldrüsen-Chromosom IV von *Chironomus tentans*
a) DNS-Verteilung nach Feulgen-Reaktion; b) Zusätzliche Darstellung der RNS-Verteilung mit Toluidinblau: Viele RNS in den Balbianiringen, aber auch in kleinen *puffs*; c) Inkorporation von H^3-Uridin in die 3 Balbiani-Ringe

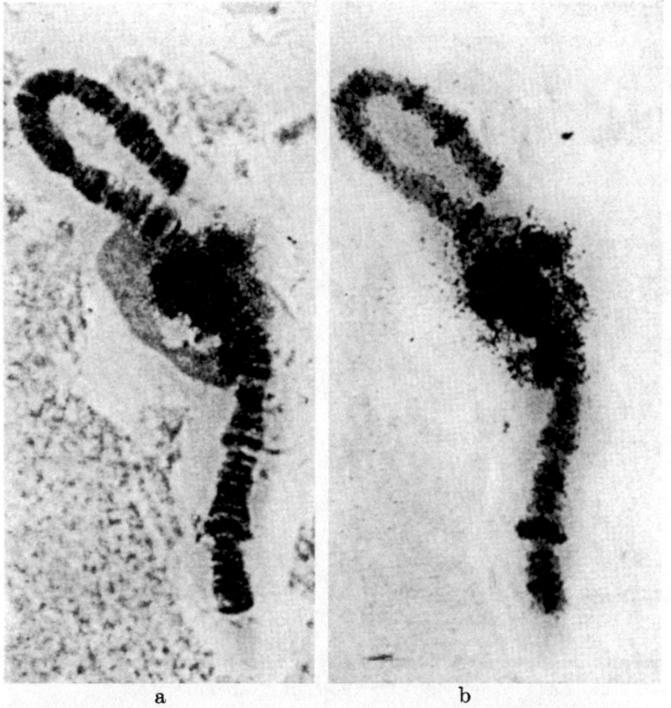

Abb. 4. Einbau von H^3-Uridin in das Speicheldrüsen-Chromosom II von *Chironomus pallidivitatus*. Autoradiographie: a) Fokus in der Ebene des Präparates, b) Fokus in der Filmschicht. Der Einbau ist in den *puffs* (und der Region des Nukleolenbildungsortes) lokalisiert. Cytoplasma fast unmarkiert

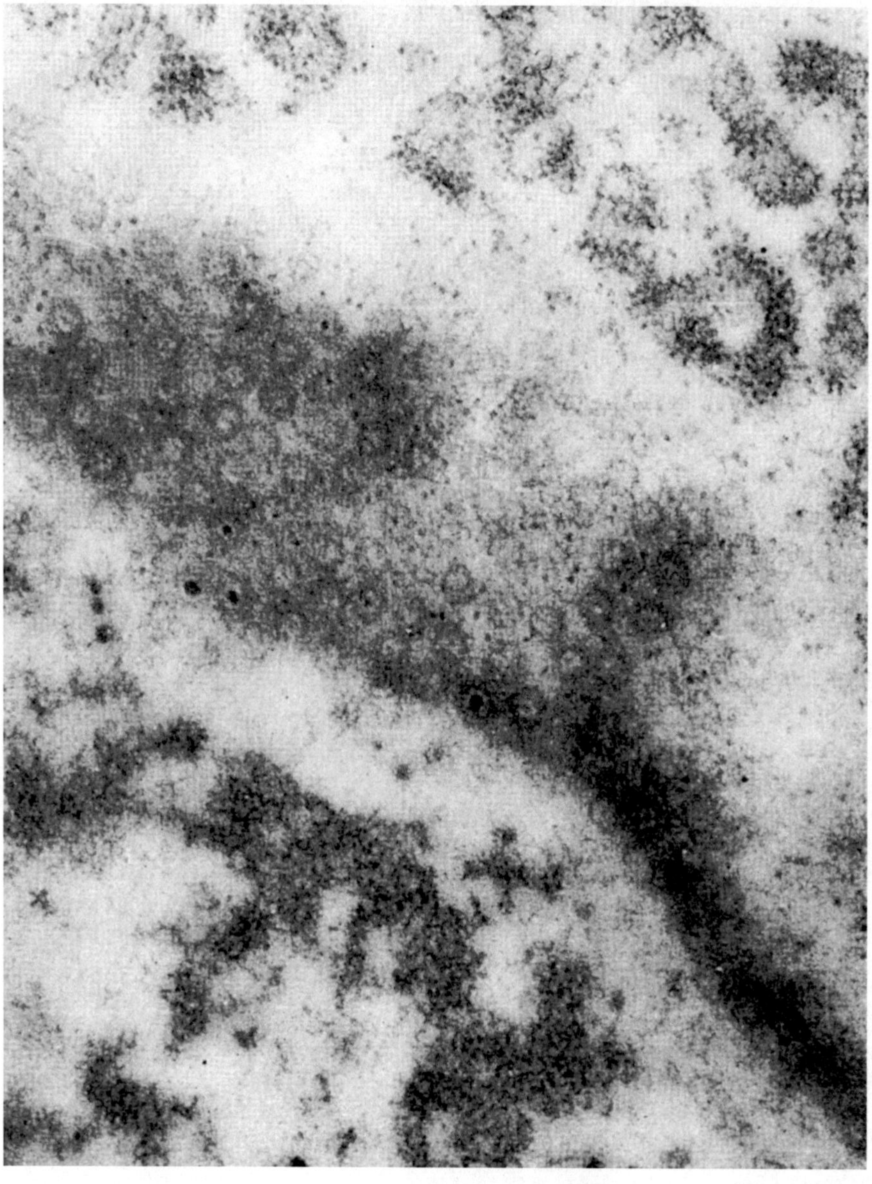

Abb. 5. Flachschnitt der Kernmembran eines Speicheldrüsen-Kernes im Elektronenmikroskop. Unten das Kern-Lumen mit chromosomalen Fibrillen und einzelnen großen RNP-Granula von den Balbianiringen BR 1 und BR 2. Oben Cytoplasma mit ergastoplasmatischen Strukturen und Ribosomen. Man beobachte das Eindringen der BR-Granula in die Poren der Kernmembran. 54000 ×

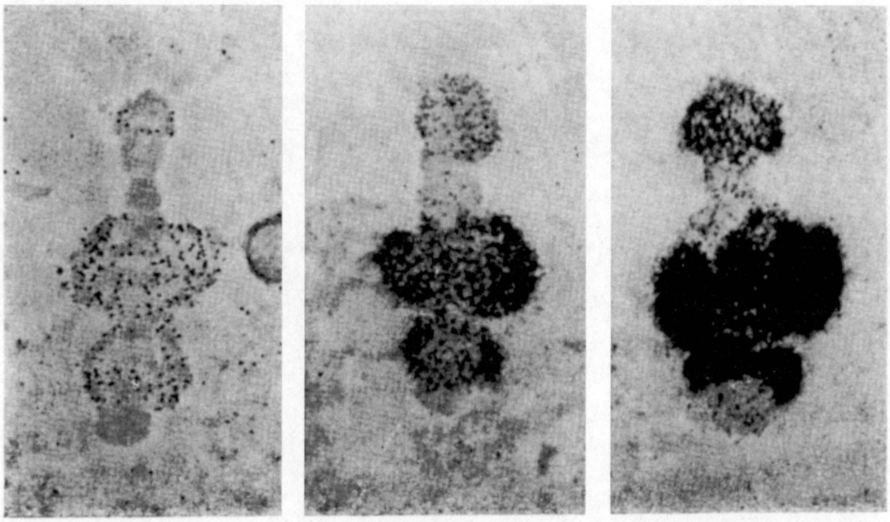

a b c

Abb. 6. Verschiedene Einbau-Intensitäten von H^3-Uridin in die Balbianiringe des IV. Chromosoms von *C. tentans*, bei gleichbleibender Größe dieser *puffs*. Vergr. 850 mal

a) 120 min nach Injektion fixiert, Expositionszeit 40 Tage; b) 30 min nach Injektion fixiert, Expositionszeit 45 Tage; c) 30 min nach Injektion fixiert, Expositionszeit 45 Tage

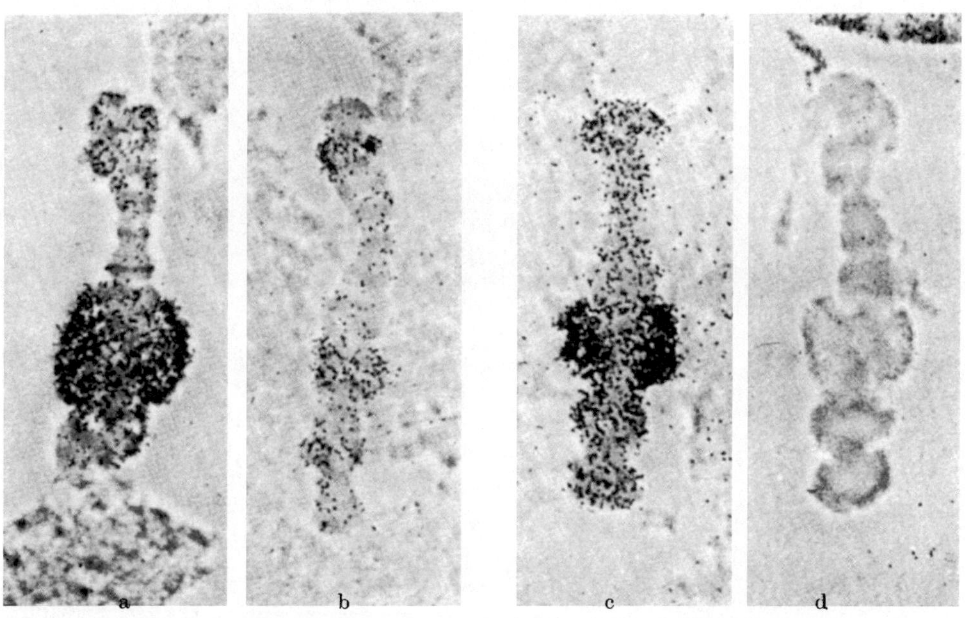

a b c d

Abb. 7. Wirkung von Actinomycin D auf die Größe der *puffs* (Balbianiringe BR 1 – BR3 des IV. Chromosoms) und auf den Einbau von H^3-Uridin. a, b und c, d repräsentieren jeweils die zwei Drüsen eines Tieres. a und c sind die in Standard-Rohrzuckerlösungen gehaltenen Kontrollen. b wurde 30 min in 0,04 γ/ml Actinomycin und danach 15 min in H^3-Uridin inkubiert. d wurde 60 min in 20 γ/ml Actinomycin und danach 30 min in H^3-Uridin inkubiert. Näheres im Text

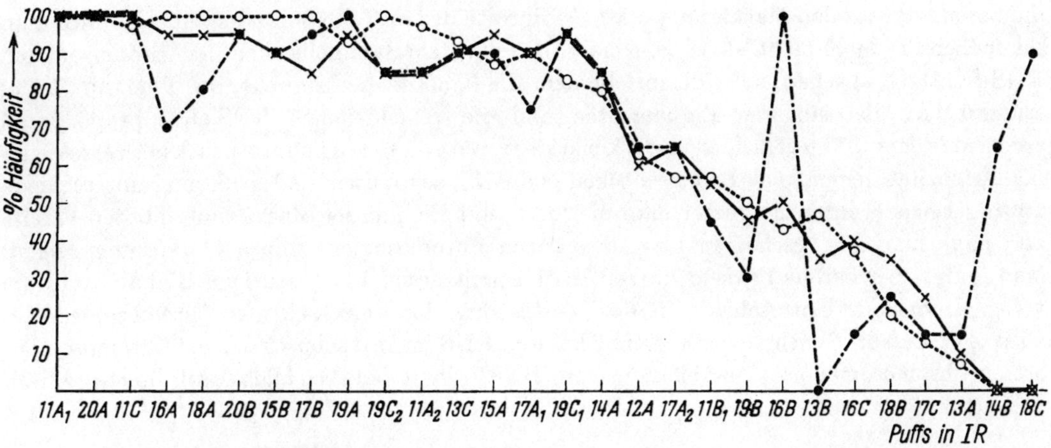

Abb. 3. Häufigkeit der *puffs* im Chromosomen-Arm IR der Speicheldrüsen von *Chironomus tentans* während des letzten Larvenstadiums. Die Larven wurden 0–1 Tag (●, n = 20), 7–8 Tage (×, n = 20) und 12–13 Tage (○, n = 30) nach der Häutung zum IV. Stadium fixiert. Nach CLEVER 1962

lich machen. Ein allgemeines Argument ergibt sich aus der Sequenz der RNS-Markierung der verschiedenen Zell-Orte und aus der Geschwindigkeit der Markierung: Stets sind die *puffs* (und die Nukleolen-Bildungsorte, auf die hier nicht eingegangen werden soll) zuerst markiert, obwohl die radioaktiven Nukleoside ja zunächst das sehr RNS-reiche Cytoplasma der Speicheldrüsen-Zellen passieren und wahrscheinlich dort auch phosphoryliert werden müssen, bevor sie in den Kern und an die Chromomeren gelangen. Die Markierung der *puffs* ist stets schon wenige Minuten nach der Zugabe der Nukleoside nachweisbar; die Markierung des Cytoplasma beginnt deutlich später und schreitet langsamer fort. Für die DNS-Abhängigkeit der RNS-Synthese, und damit für den chromosomalen Ursprung der markierten RNS, spricht auch die vollständige Hemmung des Nukleotid-Einbaus durch Actinomycin D (s. u.). Gegen die Möglichkeit, daß die Markierung der RNS nur durch das Anhängen der Nukleoside an bereits fertige RNS-Moleküle zustande kommt, läßt sich die hohe spezifische Aktivität der markierten *puff*-RNS ins Feld führen (PELLING 1964). In den am stärksten markierten Präparaten entspricht nämlich die Korndichte über den *puffs* einer spezifischen Aktivität,

Tabelle 1

Verteilung der RNS-Markierung in 3 Zellkernen einer Speicheldrüse 60 min nach Injektion von H^3-Uridin (Silberkornzahlen auf- bzw. abgerundet; mit * markierte Zahlen geschätzt) nach PELLING 1963

Strukturen		Kern 1 Aktivität (Silberkornanzahl)	Kern 2 Aktivität (Silberkornanzahl)	Kern 3 Aktivität (Silberkornanzahl)
1. Chromosom	(Puffs und Streuaktivität)	1250 (20,4%)	1200 (18,6%)	4100 (16,2%)
2. Chromosom	(Puffs und Streuaktivität)	1000 (16,4%)	1050 (16,3%)	3300 (13,0%)
	(Nukleolus)	500 (8,2%)	400 (6,2%)	4500 (17,8%)
3. Chromosom	(Puffs und Streuaktivität)	1050 (17,2%)	1100 (17,1%)	3400 (13,4%)
	(Nukleolus)	750 (12,3%)	550 (8,5%)	4800 (19,0%)
4. Chromosom	(Puffs und Streuaktivität)	85 (1,4%)	100 (1,6%)	300 (1,2%)
	(Balbianiring 1)	200 (3,3%)	200 (3,4%)	900* (3,6%)
	(Balbianiring 2)	1150 (18,8%)	1700* (26,4%)	3600* (14,2%)
	(Balbianiring 3)	120 (2,0%)	120 (1,9%)	400* (1,6%)

die bereits der totalen Markierung aller Uridinreste der *puff*-RNS nahe kommt. Wollte man schließlich die *puffs* nicht als Orte, sondern lediglich als Sammelbecken der chromosomalen RNS-Synthese ansehen, so widerspricht dem die Kinetik des Einbaus, die PELLING (1963) studiert hat. Bei längeren Einbauzeiten sind die verschiedenen RNS-Orte proportional zum Grade des *puffing* verschieden stark markiert; wäre dies lediglich Ausdruck der verschiedenen Kapazität der *puffs* als Sammelbecken von RNS, so müßten die Markierungsunterschiede umso geringer werden, je kürzer man markiert; mit Beginn der Markierung müßten bereits alle *puffs* markiert erscheinen bzw. die ganzen Chromosomen diffuse Markierung zeigen. Man findet aber bereits bei sehr kurzen Inkubationszeiten (bzw. niedrigen Einbauraten) die vollen Intensitäts-Unterschiede in der Markierung der verschiedenen Chromosomenorte. Dies zeigt, daß die Synthese der hochmolekularen RNS im Interphasekern von Chromosomenort zu Chromosomenort – unabhängig vom DNS-Gehalt – tatsächlich stark und spezifisch variiert.

2. Die Chromomeren als autonom kontrollierte Einheiten der RNS-Synthese: Differentielle Kontrolle der Synthese-Aktivität

Die Existenz bestimmter RNS-Synthese-Muster in den Riesenchromosomen wirft die Frage nach der Natur der reagierenden Einheiten auf, deren Verhalten die Art des Synthesemusters bestimmt. Welches ist ihre Ausdehnung, mit welchen genetischen Einheiten sind sie gleichzusetzen, und wie weit geht die Autonomie in der Kontrolle ihrer Syntheseaktivität? Da die RNS-Synthese-Aktivität der Chromosomenorte stets mit dem *puffing* einhergeht, das sich morphologisch und cytochemisch sehr verlässlich nachweisen läßt, können wir uns bei der Beantwortung dieser Fragen auf morphologische Befunde stützen. Studiert man ein- und denselben Chromosomenort in verschiedenen Zuständen des *puffing* (das ist bei besonders variablen *puffs* gelegentlich möglich, vgl. BEERMANN 1952), so erkennt man, daß der eigentliche Auflockerungsprozeß nur auf ein einzelnes Chromomer beschränkt ist (gelegentlich auch auf Doppel-Chromomeren). Benachbarte Chromomeren werden nur sekundär mit in die Auflockerung mit einbezogen, scheinen jedoch in ihrer Feinstruktur unbeeinträchtigt zu bleiben. Die Untersuchung von strahleninduzierten Umbauten (Translokationen, Inversionen) mit Bruchstellen im Bereich von *puffs* stützt diese Interpretation (BEERMANN, unveröff.). Die reagierende Einheit ist also höchstwahrscheinlich das Chromomer, zuweilen vielleicht 2 oder 3 zu einer höheren Einheit zusammengeschlossene Chromomeren. Diese Schlußfolgerung steht in gutem Einklang mit Daten und Überlegungen der *Drosophila*-Cytogenetik.

Die physische Lokalisation von „Genen“, also von durch den Komplementations-Test definierten funktionellen genetischen Einheiten, in den Speicheldrüsen-Chromosomen von *Drosophila* hat bisher stets zu dem Ergebnis geführt, diese Einheiten bestimmten einzelnen Querscheiben zuzuordnen, oder, wie im Falle der „komplexen“ Loci *white* und *bithorax*, einer Gruppe von 2 bis 3 eng benachbarten Querscheiben (vgl. GREEN 1963, LEWIS 1963). Es ist also wahrscheinlich, daß wir in den Chromomeren genetische Einheiten funktionellen, oder besser operativen Charakters vor uns haben, wie dies ja auch ihre operative Selbständigkeit bei der RNS-Synthese bezeugt. Wir können sie hypothetisch als Einheiten der „Transscription“ betrachten, wie im nächsten Absatz noch näher ausgeführt werden wird. Hier ist zunächst die weitere Frage nach dem tatsächlichen Ausmaß der operativen Selbständigkeit der Chromomeren von Interesse. Solange sich die Untersuchungen auf Zellen eines Organs und eines Entwicklungszustandes beschränken – die Zellen der larvalen Speicheldrüsen –, wird man sich mit der – allerdings fundamentalen – Aussage begnügen müssen, daß die

Chromomeren in ihrem Syntheseverhalten voneinander unabhängig sind: Einige produzieren viel, einige wenig, und einige vielleicht überhaupt keine RNS. Diese Selbständigkeit könnte aber eine prädeterminierte, früh in der Embryonalentwicklung fixierte oder gar „genetische" sein, die keiner stringenten Kontrolle mehr unterliegt. Die beobachteten Schwankungen in der Entfaltung einiger *puffs* ließen sich als zufällig oder als im Rahmen der Prädetermination erlaubte „Modulationen" abtun (vgl. KROEGER 1962). Ähnliche Gedanken liegen der Vorstellung eines „potentiellen" Aktivitätsmusters der Speicheldrüsen-Chromosomen zugrunde (CLEVER 1961). Gegen diese Interpretationen sprechen aber die Ergebnisse der vergleichenden Untersuchungen der Chromosomen und ihrer Aktivitätsmuster in verschiedenen Organen und Zelltypen sowie in verschiedenen Entwicklungszuständen.

Jedes Organ und jeder Zelltyp weist in seinen Chromosomen ein anderes, für ihn charakteristisches *puff*-Muster (RNS-Synthesemuster) auf: Parallel zur Zelldifferenzierung stellt man also auf der chromosomalen Ebene die Differenzierung verschiedener RNS-Synthesemuster fest; diese Muster können demnach nicht genetisch prädeterminiert sein (BEERMANN 1952). Daß sie auch nicht embryologisch (ontogenetisch) prädeterminiert sind, wird durch die folgenden Beobachtungen wahrscheinlich gemacht: Bestimmte Chromomeren sind in mehreren Organen zugleich „aktiv", aber in dem einen Organ durchschnittlich deutlich stärker als in dem anderen; dies würde einen Prägungs-Mechanismus voraussetzen, der die Chromomeren nicht bloß permanent an- oder abschaltet, sondern auch den mittleren Grad des Synthesevermögens vorherbestimmt. Entscheidender sind Beobachtungen, die man bei jeder Häutung und insbesondere bei der Metamorphose der Dipterenlarven machen kann (BEERMANN 1952, MECHELKE 1953, BREUER und PAVAN 1955, BECKER 1959, CLEVER 1961). In diesen Entwicklungsphasen ändert sich das RNS-Synthesemuster der Chromosomen rapide und charakteristisch, und es zeigt sich, daß selbst die größten *puffs* reversibel sind, d. h. zu ganz normal aussehenden inaktiven Querscheiben zusammenschrumpfen können, die keine RNS mehr synthetisieren. Andere, die vorher still gelegen haben, werden aktiv, zuweilen sind dies „quer" durch die verschiedensten Organe die gleichen Chromomeren (CLEVER 1961). Wir vertreten deshalb die Meinung, daß der Aktivitätszustand jedes einzelnen Chromomers (d. h. sein Vermögen, RNS zu produzieren) zu jeder Zeit einer rigorosen Kontrolle unterliegt. Die Chromomeren sind selbständige Einheiten der RNS-Synthese, deren Syntheseverhalten fortlaufend autonom reguliert wird. Bevor der Regulationsmechanismus selber besprochen wird, soll die Frage nach der Natur und den Funktionen der in den Chromomeren produzierten RNS gestellt werden, denn von ihrer Beantwortung hängt es natürlich ab, welchen biologischen Sinn die individuelle Regulation der RNS-Synthese auf der Ebene des Genoms haben könnte.

3. *Argumente für die messenger-Funktion der Puff-RNS*

Die Frage nach der Natur der RNS, deren Synthese in den Chromomeren individuell kontrolliert wird, läßt sich in allgemeiner und in spezieller Form angehen. Ist diese RNS *messenger*, oder enthält sie zumindest einen bestimmten Anteil von *messenger*-Molekülen, so würde man erwarten, daß diejenigen Chromomeren, die in einem bestimmten Zelltyp exklusiv und besonders stark synthetisch aktiv sind, genetische Information enthalten, die für diesen Zelltyp jedenfalls besonders relevant ist. Hieraus ergibt sich die Möglichkeit, die gestellte Frage für bestimmte einzelne Chromomeren mit genetischen Methoden speziell zu beantworten. In einem bestimmten, funktionell besonderen Sektor der Speicheldrüsen von

Chironomus pallidivittatus erscheint ein bestimmtes Chromomer, das in den anderen Sektoren der Speicheldrüsen oder in anderen Organen niemals aktiviert gefunden wurde, stets zu einem großen *puff* umgebildet. Zugleich mit dieser Besonderheit auf der chromosomalen Ebene zeichnen sich die „Sonderzellen“ durch die Fähigkeit aus, ein bestimmtes Sekretprotein zu produzieren, das morphologisch in der Form von spezifischen Mucoproteid-Granula erkannt wird und auch elektrophoretisch nachweisbar ist (Grossbach, unveröff.). Bei der nahe verwandten Spezies *Chironomus tentans* fehlt dieses Sekretprotein in den „Sonderzellen“ und zugleich bleibt auch die Aktivierung des genannten Chromomers aus: Es bildet also keinen *puff*. Der Unterschied zwischen beiden Spezies ist genetisch bedingt und spaltet wie ein Mendelfaktor, wobei sich die Unfähigkeit, das Sekretprotein zu produzieren, rezessiv verhält. Mit klassischen cytogenetischen Methoden läßt sich das „Gen“ leicht lokalisieren: Sein chromosomaler Locus fällt mit dem genannten Chromomer zusammen (Beermann 1961). Im heterozygoten Zustand ist das eine Allel aktiviert, d. h. das Chromosom des einen Elters bildet einen *puff*, und das andere bleibt inaktiv. Hieraus ergibt sich, daß das genannte Chromomer tatsächlich Information erhält, die für die Funktion des Zelltyps von besonderer Bedeutung ist, in welchem es RNS synthetisiert. Die RNS-Synthese scheint also mit der Übertragung dieser Information an die Zelle wesentlich zu tun zuhaben, – mit anderen Worten, sie kann als Transscriptions-Prozeß, d. h. als *messenger*-Synthese verstanden werden.

In allgemeiner Form führt die chemische Charakterisierung der *puff*-RNS ebenfalls zu einer Antwort auf unsere Frage. Beobachtungen von Pelling (1963) und eigene Befunde lassen es berechtigt erscheinen, den größten Teil der in einem *puff* in jedem Zeitpunkt nachweisbaren RNS-Moleküle als entweder gerade frisch synthetisiert oder als *in statu nascendi* befindlich anzusehen; die chemische Analyse dieser RNS kann demnach als repräsentativ für die neu-synthetisierte und rasch umgesetzte RNS angesehen werden, die in den Autoradiographien erfaßt wird und auf die es uns hier ankommt. Edström (1961) hat eine mikroelektrophoretische Methode entwickelt, die es erlaubt, RNS-Proben von 10^{-9} bis 10^{-10} g (100 µµg) auf ihre Basenzusammensetzung zu untersuchen. 10^{-9}g entsprechen größenordnungsmäßig etwa der RNS-Menge von 50 der größten *puffs* (Balbianiringe) der Speicheldrüsen-Chromosomen von *Chironomus*, oder von 5 Nukleolen, bzw. der Hälfte des Cytoplasmas der Speicheldrüsen-Zellen. Die Untersuchung dieser mit dem Mikromanipulator gesammelten Fraktionen (Edström und Beermann 1962) hatte folgendes Ergebnis: Die DNS von *Chironomus* gehört dem „AT-Typ“ an, mit im Durchschnitt etwa 30% G+C. Keine der untersuchten RNS-Fraktionen, auch nicht die *puff*-RNS, hat weniger als 40% G+C (nukleoläre und cytoplasmatische RNS 42%, einige chromosomale RNS-Fraktionen bis 48%). Da die Extraktionstechnik die Erfassung der löslichen Transfer-RNS ausschließt, bleibt eine Interpretation dieser Diskrepanz in den G+C-Werten anderen Untersuchungen überlassen. Vielleicht sind diejenigen Abschnitte der DNS, die die strukturelle Information für Proteine tragen, tatsächlich allgemein durch einen höheren G+C-Gehalt ausgezeichnet. Für unsere Frage sind andere Aspekte der Analysen-Daten von größerer Bedeutung: Während die nukleoläre und die cytoplasmatische RNS beide nahezu die gleiche und beide eine nahezu symmetrische Basenzusammensetzung aufweisen (A:U = 1, G:C = 1), sind die chromosomalen RNS-Fraktionen, insbesondere die aus den großen Balbiani-Ringen, alle in hohem Maße asymmetrisch zusammengesetzt, wobei in jedem Fall Adenin gegenüber Uracil und Cytosin gegenüber Guanin überwiegen (A:U = 2,2 für den Fall der RNS aus dem großen Balbiani-Ring BR 2). Hieraus geht zweierlei hervor: (1) die chromosomale RNS kann nicht der Vorläufer der nukleolären und der ribosomalen (cytoplasmatischen) RNS sein, und (2) die chromosomale, in den *puffs* synthetisierte RNS ist wahrscheinlich eine Kopie nur eines der beiden DNS-Stränge der Watson-Crick-Doppelhelix, und zwar immer desselben Stranges.

Diese letztere Schlußfolgerung, wie überhaupt die einzigartige Basenzusammensetzung, machen es wahrscheinlich, daß die Puff-RNS als *messenger* fungiert.

Als drittes Argument für die *messenger*-Funktion der puff-RNS läßt sich die folgende Beobachtung anführen: Im Bereich der zwei größten *puffs* in den Speicheldrüsenchromosomen von *Chironomus* (den Balbiani-Ringen BR 1 und BR 2), und nur hier, wird die RNS regelmäßig in Ribonucleoprotein-Granula eingebaut, die einen Durchmesser von ungefähr 300 Å erreichen. Wie man es von „Boten" (*messengers*) erwarten muß, diffundieren diese Granula in den Kernsaft ab und gelangen schließlich in die Poren der Kernmembran. Sie passieren diese Poren allerdings niemals als intakte Granula, sondern geben wahrscheinlich die *messenger*-Moleküle an die unmittelbar auf der anderen Seite der Poren nachweisbaren Ribosomen ab (Abb. 5). Man kann vielleicht annehmen, daß das Transportprotein bei diesem Vorgang im Kern zurückbleibt, um sich an den Balbiani-Ringen erneut mit RNS zu beladen, d. h. neue Granula zu bilden.

Die bisherigen Experimente und Analysen führen also zu dem Ergebnis, daß die RNS-Synthese in den Interphasenkernen differenzierter Zellen von Chromomer zu Chromomer individuell kontrolliert wird, und daß diese individuelle Regulation speziell die Synthese von *messenger*-Molekülen betrifft, also eine Kontrolle des genetischen Transscriptions-Prozesses darstellt. Die biologische Bedeutung dieses Befundes, speziell die Bedeutung für Fragen der Zelldifferenzierung, braucht nicht hervorgehoben zu werden. Ebenso interessant wird nunmehr die Frage nach dem molekularen Mechanismus, der die differentielle Aktivierung der Chromosomen kontrolliert.

4. Der Mechanismus der individuellen Kontrolle der RNS-Synthese in den Chromomeren

In seinen Untersuchungen über den Uridin-Einbau in die Speicheldrüsen-Chromosomen von *Chironomus* weist Pelling (1963) darauf hin, daß das generelle Synthese-Niveau des Kernes von Zelle zu Zelle und besonders von Individuum zu Individuum großen Schwankungen unterliegt (bis zur völligen „Abschaltung"), ohne daß sich dies in der Struktur der Chromosomen sichtbar manifestiert (Abb. 6, Tab. 2). Für diese generelle Regulation des RNS-Synthese-Niveaus lassen sich verhältnismäßig einfache chemische Mechanismen ausdenken – Kontrolle des Nucleosid-Triphosphat-Angebots, Kontrolle der Polymerase-Aktivität, oder ähnliches, die letzten Endes auf relativ unspezifische Faktoren ansprechen, z. B. Aminosäuren, pH, usw. („catholic inducer" nach Stent, dies Symp.). Für die individuelle Kontrolle der Synthese-Aktivität jedes einzelnen „Gens" sind die Bedingungen komplizierter: Sie setzt einmal die Existenz von spezifischen Schlüssel- bzw. Regulator-Substanzen (Repressoren, Induktoren) voraus und erfordert zum anderen einen Reaktionsmechanismus in der Molekularstruktur des Gens, der auf diese Regulatorsubstanzen spezifisch anspricht. Wir betrachten zunächst die zweite Forderung. Wie anfangs ausgeführt wurde, ist die Aktivierung der Chromomeren stets von bestimmten, drastischen Änderungen ihrer Feinstruktur und ihrer Proteinzusammensetzung begleitet. Diese Beobachtungen lassen sich morphologisch wie folgt interpretieren: Jede Querscheibe des Riesenchromosoms setzt sich aus tausenden homologer Elementar-Chromomeren zusammen. Im inaktiven Zustand bildet das dem Chromomer entsprechende Stück des DNS-Histon-Fadens ein in noch nicht bekannter Weise, aber wahrscheinlich geordnet zusammengefaltetes oder aufgewundenes Knäuel, in welchem zwar die DNS-Verdoppelung ungehindert ablaufen kann, die RNS-

Synthese aber blockiert ist. Im aktiven Zustand ist dieses Knäuel aufgelockert und im Extrem gänzlich zu einer langen Schleife entrollt bzw. entfaltet, wobei sich höheres Protein anlagert; die Hemmung der RNS-Synthese ist mehr oder minder aufgehoben. Im Fall der größten *puffs*, der Balbiani-Ringe, ist die Entfaltung der Elementar-Chromomeren in etwa 5 μ lange Schleifen elektronenoptisch direkt erkennbar (BEERMANN und BAHR 1954).

Tabelle 2

Markierungsunterschiede im Balbianiring BR 1 in den Speicheldrüsen eines Tieres. (Kornzahlen über einer Verzweigungshälfte des BR 1) nach PELLING 1963

Aktivitätsklassen (Silberkornanzahl über einer Verzweigungshälfte des Balbianirings 1)	Anzahl von Balbianiringen
unmarkiert	0
5– 25	4
25– 50	10
50– 75	10
75–100	9
100–125	2
125–150	6
150–175	5
175–200	2
200	2

Die quantitative Abstufung der RNS-Synthese in den *puffs*, wie sie parallel zu der Abstufung des *puffing* beobachtet wird, kann grundsätzlich auf dreierlei Weise zustandekommen: (1) durch die Regelung der molekularen Synthesegeschwindigkeit selber, (2) durch die Änderung des Taktes, in welchem die Synthese der RNS-Moleküle aufeinander folgt (z. B. Regelung der Distanz zwischen den starting points der an der DNS-Matrize nacheinander entstehenden RNS-Nukleotidketten), und (3) dadurch, daß ein veränderlicher Anteil der Elementar-Chromomeren innerhalb der aktivierten Querscheiben der polytänen Chromosomen inaktiv bleibt. Diese letzte Möglichkeit, die von PELLING (1963) in Betracht gezogen wird, würde also für das Elementar-Chromomer jede Regelung, die über das An- und Abschalten hinausgeht, ausschließen und damit dem polytänen Zustand eine Sonderstellung einräumen. Vorläufig ist es unmöglich, zwischen den aufgeführten Regelungs-Möglichkeiten zu entscheiden, doch muß jede Hypothese über den Regulationsmechanismus auch den Tatsachen des *puffing* Rechnung tragen. Ist das *puffing* selber ein wesentlicher Faktor in der Regulation der Synthesekapazität eines Locus, oder ist es nur eine notwendige Begleiterscheinung der Syntheseaktivität? Wir bevorzugen die erste Alternative, weil die absolute Höhe der RNS-Synthese in den *puffs* in weiten Grenzen schwankt und zeitweilig bis auf den Wert 0 absinkt, ohne daß dies in Größenschwankungen der *puffs* zum Ausdruck käme (PELLING 1964, Abb. 15); das *puffing* ist also ein Maß für die relative, nicht für die absolute, Syntheseleistung eines Locus, und wir glauben, daß es das Synthesevermögen kausal bestimmt.

Ungeklärt, wenn auch sicher bedeutsam ist die Rolle, die die Proteine in diesem Zusammenhang spielen: Die durch die Befunde von HUANG und BONNER (1962) nahegelegte Möglichkeit, daß die aktivierten Chromosomenorte kein Histon enthalten, ist nach den cytochemischen Untersuchungen von SWIFT (1962) für den Fall der *puffs* nicht unbedingt gegeben: zumindest lassen sich auch im Bereich der *puffs* geringe Mengen eines basischen Proteins nachweisen. Andererseits spricht das regelmäßige Vorkommen von höheren Proteinen entschieden für eine Beteiligung von Protein am Regulationsmechanismus. Wenn man nicht annehmen will, daß das gesamte *puff*-Protein als RNS-Polymerase oder als Transport-Protein fungiert, so könnte man sich beispielsweise vorstellen, daß dieses Protein die DNS zur Entfaltung bringt, indem es sich an bestimmten dafür vorgesehenen Stellen an die DNS anlagert; für die Anlagerung würde es der Aktivierung dieser Stellen durch die Induktor-Substanzen oder der Ablösung spezifischer Repressoren bedürfen. Die Entfaltung der DNS wäre in diesem Modell gleichbedeutend mit ihrer Aktivierung als RNS-Matrize. Von manchen Autoren (GALL 1962, SWIFT 1962) wird mit der Möglichkeit gerechnet, daß das Protein aktivierter Chromosomen-Orte an diesen Orten selbst synthetisiert wird, was u. a. für den Regulationsmechanismus weitere Deutungsmöglichkeiten zuließe. Jedoch ist der Aminosäure-Einbau in die *puff*-Proteine so schwach, daß er sich gut als Einbau fertiger Protein-Moleküle in die Chromosomen verstehen läßt.

Einen konkreten Einblick in den molekularen Mechanismus der Regulation der RNS-Synthese und des *puffing* sollten Experimente mit Substanzen geben, die die DNS abhängige RNS-Synthese hemmen. Wir haben Actinomycin D benutzt. Dazu wurden die Speicheldrüsen oder ganze Larven von *Chironomus* in Lösungen inkubiert, die Actinomycin D in Konzentrationen von 0,1 µg, 2 µg oder 20µg pro ml enthielten. CALLAN und GALL hatten in veröffentlichten Experimenten bereits gefunden, daß Actinomycin D die Chromomeren-Schleifen der Lampenbürsten-Chromosomen von Amphibien rapide zum Verschwinden bringt; IZAWA *et al.* (1963) erhalten das gleiche Ergebnis und schließen aus parallel durchgeführten Einbau-Versuchen, daß die Schleifen sich kontrahieren, weil das Actinomycin D die RNS-Synthese in den Schleifen hemmt. Unsere Versuche an den Riesenchromosomen zeigen, daß die Beziehungen zwischen RNS-Synthese und *puffing* nicht so einfach sind.

Bei der Anwendung von Actinomycin D in der Konzentration von 0,1 µg pro ml findet man bereits nach 30 Min. eine drastische Verkleinerung des großen Balbiani-Ringes BR2 auf weniger als die Hälfte seines ursprünglichen Durchmessers (Abb. 7b); bei längeren Inkubationszeiten wird eine nahezu vollständige Rückbildung erreicht. Erwartungsgemäß geht die RNS-Synthese in dem gleichen Maße zurück, wie die Größe der *puffs* reduziert wird. Obwohl sich alle anderen *puffs* im Prinzip ähnlich verhalten, zeigen sich doch deutliche Unterschiede in der Empfindlichkeit gegenüber Actinomycin. So ist z. B. der kleine Balbiani-Ring BR3 nach einer Stunde Inkubation noch fast so groß wie zu Beginn des Versuchs und inkorporiert radioaktives Uridin noch fast so intensiv wie in den Kontrollen. Dies mag auf einen geringeren Guanin-Gehalt der DNS dieses *puffs* hinweisen. Bis hierher sind die Experimente nicht im Widerspruch mit der Annahme, daß die Größenreduktion der *puffs* eine Folge der RNS-Synthese-Hemmung ist oder, daß die beiden Effekte zumindest eine gemeinsame Ursache haben und stets miteinander gekoppelt sind. Die Anwendung höherer Actinomycin-Konzentrationen widerspricht dieser Auffassung (Abb. 7d). Nach einer Stunde Inkubation in 20 µg pro ml Actinomycin D ist die RNS-Synthese in den Riesenchromosomen vollständig abgestoppt. Überraschenderweise wird jedoch bei dieser hohen Actinomycin-Konzentration die Größe der *puffs* nicht nennenswert reduziert; daß hier keine unspezifische Schädigung der Zellen vorliegt, wird dadurch wahrscheinlich gemacht, daß die zelluläre Proteinsynthese bei der verwendeten Actinomycin-Konzentration noch nach 2 Stunden unvermindert weiterläuft. Die Befunde lassen z. B. die folgenden zwei Deutungen zu: (1) Die Kontrolle des *puffing* ist ein komplexer Vorgang und erfordert die Mitwirkung mehrerer Faktoren, z. B. von Enzymen oder sogar spezifischen Ribonukleinsäuren; bei niederen Konzentrationen des Actinomycins bleibt der Kontrollmechanismus funktionsfähig, vielleicht weil die RNS-Synthese nicht vollständig blockiert ist; bei der hohen Konzentration des Actinomycins dagegen ist vielleicht der Kontrollmechanismus selbst ausgeschaltet, weil die Synthese der gesamten RNS augenblicklich blockiert wird. (2) Bei der hohen Konzentration werden womöglich alle Guanin-Reste der DNS augenblicklich mit Actinomycin besetzt, und es ließe sich vorstellen, daß damit eine Versteifung der Molekülstruktur verbunden ist, die ein Zusammenfalten unmöglich macht.

Mit dem Actinomycin D greifen wir in den molekularen Mechanismus des *puffing* gewissermaßen auf der niedrigsten, allen Chromomeren gemeinsamen Ebene ein. Wie oben bereits ausgeführt wurde, muß dieser Mechanismus aber auch Komponenten enthalten, die in der Lage sind, auf spezifische Signale anzusprechen, so daß das *puffing* in jedem einzelnen Chromomer individuell kontrolliert werden kann. In die im Anschluß an JACOB und MONOD

(1961) entwickelten Modellvorstellungen ließe sich denken, daß ein Teil des im Bereich der *puffs* nachweisbaren Proteins als Repressor oder Induktor funktioniert und nach der Verbindung mit spezifischen niedermolekularen Effektoren eine spezifische Affinität zu dem betreffenden Chromosomenort erwirbt (oder verliert). Auf der Suche nach spezifischen Effektoren hat Clever (1961) gefunden, daß das die Häutungen der Insekten auslösende Steroid-Hormon Ecdyson wahrscheinlich ein solcher Effektor ist. Schon 30 Min. nach der Injektion von physiologischen Dosen dieses Hormons in *Chironomus*-Larven beobachtet man die Entstehung eines *puff* an einer ganz bestimmten Stelle des Chromosoms I, und 30 Min. später geschieht das gleiche an einer anderen bestimmten Stelle des Chromosoms IV. Diese beiden Reaktionen auf das Hormon sind direkt konzentrationsabhängig. Der Schwellenwert der Konzentration, der gerade noch die Reaktion des *puffing* hervorruft, liegt bei dem ersten *puff* bei 10^{-7} µg/mg Larvengewicht und bei dem anderen bei 10^{-6} µg/mg Larvengewicht (Abb. 8). Diese Werte sind gleichbedeutend mit nur einigen hundert Molekülen Hormon pro Elementar-Chromomer in den Zellkernen der *Chironomus*-Larven. In der Normalentwicklung, wie im Experiment, folgt auf die Entstehung der beiden primären *puffs*, sofern sie lange genug aktiv waren, eine Kette von sekundären *puffing*-Reaktionen, die aber in verschiedenen Geweben verschieden sind und deren Amplitude nicht von der anfänglichen Konzentration des Hormons abhängt. Nur die beiden primären *puffs* scheinen also spezifische Rezeptoren des durch das Hormon dargestellten Entwicklungssignales zu sein. Für die sekundären *puffing*-Reaktionen wird man das Auftreten von Effektoren verantwortlich machen müssen, die in ihrem Vorkommen auf die einzelnen Zellen oder Organe beschränkt bleiben. Eine endgültige Klärung des molekularen Regulationsmechanismus der RNS-Synthese in Chromomeren ist erst dann zu erhoffen, wenn es gelingt, einige dieser intrazellulären Effektoren zu isolieren und zu identifizieren.

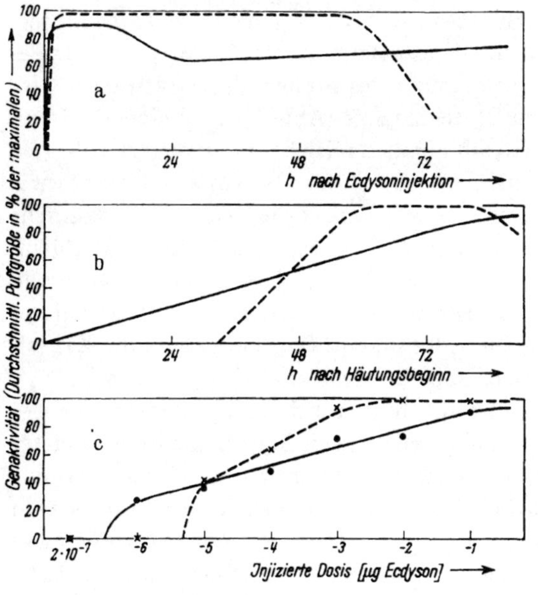

Abb. 8. Schema der Verhaltensweisen der *puffs* I-18-C und IV-2-B in der normalen und experimentell induzierten Häutung. (a) Zeitlicher Verlauf der Aktivitätsänderungen nach Häutungsauslösung durch Injektion von 45 CE Ecdyson. (b) Zeitlicher Verlauf der Aktivitätsänderungen in der normalen Puppenhäutung. (c) Abhängigkeit der Genaktivitäten von der Ecdysonkonzentration. Als Maß der Genaktivität ist die durchschnittliche *Puff*-Größe in % der maximalen genommen; Berechnung s. Clever (1961a). —— und ● *puff* I-18-C, ----- und × *puff* IV-2-B. Nach Clever 1963

Literatur

ATTARDI, G., S. NAONO, F. GROS, S. BRENNER, et F. JACOB, 1962: Effet de l'induction enzymatique sur la taux de synthèse d'un RNA messager spécifique chez *E. coli*. C. R. Acad. Sci., **255**, 2303.

BECKER, H. J., 1959: Die Puffs der Speicheldrüsenchromosomen von *Drosophila melanogaster*. 1. Mitteilung. Beobachtungen zum Verhalten des Puffmusters im Normalstamm und bei zwei Mutanten, Giant und Lethal-Giant-Larvae. Chromosoma (Berlin), **10**, 654–678.

BEERMANN, W., 1952: Chromomerenkonstanz und spezifische Modifikationen der Chromosomenstruktur in der Entwicklung und Organdifferenzierung von *Chironomus tentans*. Chromosoma (Berlin), **5**, 139–198.

BEERMANN, W., 1961: Ein Balbiani-Ring als Locus einer Speicheldrüsen-Mutation. Chromosoma (Berlin), **12**, 1–25.

BEERMANN, W., and G. F. BAHR, 1954: The submicroscopic structure of the Balbiani-Ring. Exper. Cell Res. **6**, 195–201.

BREUER, M. E., and C. PAVAN, 1955: Behavior of polytene chromosomes of *Rhynchosciara angelae* at different stages of larval development. Chromosoma (Berlin), **7**, 371–386.

CLEVER, U., 1961: Genaktivitäten in den Riesenchromosomen von *Chironomus tentans* und ihre Beziehung zur Entwicklung. I. Genaktivierungen durch Ecdyson. Chromosoma (Berlin), **12**, 607–675.

CLEVER, U., 1962: Genaktivitäten in den Riesenchromosomen von *Chironomus tentans* und ihre Beziehungen zur Entwicklung. II. Das Verhalten der Puffs während des letzten Larvenstadiums und der Puppenhäutung. Chromosoma (Berlin), **13**, 385–436.

CLEVER, U., 1963: Von der Ecdysonkonzentration abhängige Genaktivitätsmuster in den Speicheldrüsenchromosomen von *Chirononus tentans*. Developmental Biol. **6**, 73–98.

EDSTRÖM, J.-E., 1960: Extraction, hydrolysis, and electrophoretic analysis of ribonucleic acid from microscopic tissue units (microphoresis). J. Biophys. Biochem. Cytol., **8**, 39–43.

EDSTRÖM, J.-E., and W. BEERMANN, 1962: The base composition of nucleic acids in chromosomes, puffs, nucleoli, and cytoplasm of *Chironomus* salivary gland cells. J. Cell. Biology, **14**, 371–380.

GALL, J. G., 1962: Chromosomes and cytodifferentiation. In „Cytodifferentiation and macromolecular synthesis", ed. Locke, Academic Press, New York, pp. 119–143.

GREEN, M. M., 1963: Unequal crossing over and the genetical organization of the white locus of *Drosophila melanogaster*. Z. f. Vererbungslehre **94**, 200–214.

IZAWA, M., V. G. ALLFREY, and A. E. MIRSKY, 1963: The relationship between RNA synthesis and loop structure in lampbrush chromosomes. P. N. A. S., **49**, 544.

JACOB, F., and J. MONOD, 1961: Genetic regulatory mechanisms in the synthesis of proteins. J. Mol. Biol., **3**, 318–356.

KROEGER, H., 1963: Experiments on the extranuclear control of gene activity in Dipteran polytene chromosomes. J. Cellular Comp. Physiol. (Supplement), im Druck.

LEWIS, E. B., 1963: Genes and developmental pathways. Am. Zoologist, **3**, 33–56.

MECHELKE, F., 1953: Reversible Strukturmodifikationen der Speicheldrüsenchromosomen von *Acricotopus lucidus*. Chromosoma (Berlin), **5**, 511–543.

PELLING, C., 1959: Chromosomal synthesis of ribonucleic acid as shown by the incorporation of uridine labeled with Tritium. Nature (London) **184**, 655–656.

PELLING, C., 1964: Ribonukleinsäure-Synthese der Riesenchromosomen. Autoradiographische Untersuchungen an *Chironomus tentans* Fabr. Chromosoma (Berlin), **15**, 71–122.

STEFFENSEN, D. M., 1963: Localization of deoxyribonucleic acid exclusively in the bands of *Drosophila* salivary chromosomes. Proc. of the XI. International Congress of Genetics. **1**, 109.

SWIFT, H., 1962: Nucleic acids and cell morphology in Dipteran salivary gland. In: The molecular control of cellular activity, pp. 73–125, New York: McGraw-Hill Book Co., Inc.

Experimentell induzierte Inaktivierung Balbiani-Ring bildender Gen-Loci in Riesenchromosomen

R. Panitz

Institut für Kulturpflanzenforschung Gatersleben der Deutschen Akademie der Wissenschaften zu Berlin

Biochemische und genetische Untersuchungen der letzten Jahre haben wahrscheinlich gemacht, daß die Puffs und Balbiani-Ringe in den Riesenchromosomen der Dipteren-Larven Einheiten genetischer Information darstellen (Beermann 1962). So können wir heute mit großer Sicherheit annehmen, daß den unterschiedlichen Puffspektren in verschiedenen Zelltypen verschiedene Serien aktiver Gene entsprechen, die Funktion und Leistung der Zellen bestimmen. Unter dieser Voraussetzung ergibt sich die Möglichkeit, das Problem der Zelldifferenzierung als eine differentielle Aktivierung des in den Chromosomen lokalisierten genetischen Materials zu sehen, wobei zur Erklärung von Änderungen der Zellfunktion die Reversibilität des „puffing" herangezogen werden kann. Damit rücken zwei Fragen in den Vordergrund, deren Bearbeitung auf chromosomaler Ebene möglich ist: 1. wie entstehen Zellen unterschiedlicher Leistungen aus einem omnipotenten Ausgangsmaterial, und 2. wie erfolgt der Funktionswechsel spezialisierter Zellen während der Entwicklung.

Der Frage nach den Ursachen der zeitlichen Variation im Aktivitätsmuster der Gene wurde bei der Chironomide *Acricotopus lucidus* nachgegangen. Die Speicheldrüse von *Acricotopus* besteht aus drei Funktionsbereichen – dem Haupt-, Neben- und Vorderlappen-, die sich nach den Untersuchungen von Baudisch (1963a) in ihrer Syntheseleistung voneinander abgrenzen lassen. In Parallele dazu besitzt jeder Drüsenlappen ein charakteristisches Puffmuster, dessen Spezifität insbesondere durch die Ausbildung großer Balbiani-Ringe geprägt wird (Mechelke 1953, 1958). Die Aktivität der Balbiani-Ring bildenden Gen-Loci BR-3 und BR-4 im Vorderlappen der Speicheldrüse ist phasenspezifisch. Sie sind nur in der Larve aktiv und bilden ihre Funktionsstruktur im Vorpuppenstadium regelmäßig und vollständig zurück.

Ausgangspunkt der Untersuchungen war die Frage nach den Faktoren, die für die Inaktivierung dieser Loci verantwortlich sind. Um brauchbares Vergleichsmaterial für die Beurteilung experimenteller Befunde zu erhalten, wurde versucht, den normalen Rückbildungsverlauf der Balbiani-Ringe in vivo zu erfassen. Es wurden Tiere des IV. Häutungsstadiums, die aus Einzelzuchten stammten, mit zunehmendem Alter präpariert und der Grad der Rückbildung durch Auszählen der Balbiani-Ringe festgestellt. Die Klassifikation der Balbiani-Ringe erfolgte in drei Gruppen:

a) offene Balbiani-Ringe (+ Typen),

b) rückgebildete Balbiani-Ringe (– Typen),

c) in Rückbildung befindliche Balbiani-Ringe (± Typen).

Für die Beurteilung der Rückbildung des BR-4 ist von Wichtigkeit, daß nach den Untersuchungen von Mechelke (1961) die Zone seiner maximalen Aktivität während der Rückbildungsphase von distal zu proximal wandert. Der Einfachheit halber wurde hier auf die Aufstellung weiterer Klassifikationstypen verzichtet und alle Übergangsformen der ±Gruppe zugeordnet. Die Ergebnisse zeigen einen kontinuierlichen Rückbildungsverlauf und einen deutlichen Unterschied in der Reaktionsgeschwindigkeit beider Loci (Tab. 1).

Tabelle 1

Normalverhalten der Loci *BR*-3 und *BR*-4 im IV. Häutungsstadium bei 10° C. Angabe der Werte in Prozent. In Klammern Anzahl der Balbiani-Ringe, n = Anzahl der präparierten Tiere

Std.	n	Locus BR-3			Locus BR-4		
		+	+/–	–	+	+/–	–
125	4	100,– (64)	–	–	100,– (62)	–	–
150	4	91,3 (42)	8,7 (4)	–	97,7 (43)	2,3 (1)	–
175	4	89,3 (50)	7,1 (4)	3,6 (2)	89,6 (43)	10,4 (5)	–
200	5	76,3 (61)	15,– (12)	8,7 (7)	87,– (67)	13,– (10)	–
225	4	66,– (31)	17,– (8)	17,– (8)	77,8 (35)	20,– (9)	2,2 (1)
250	4	54,– (40)	25,7 (19)	20,3 (15)	74,7 (56)	22,6 (17)	2,7 (2)
275	5	43,1 (31)	30,5 (22)	26,4 (19)	64,4 (47)	31,5 (23)	4,1 (3)
300	3	20,– (7)	34,3 (12)	45,7 (16)	48,3 (14)	44,8 (13)	6,9 (2)
325	3	–	43,5 (20)	56,5 (26)	7,2 (3)	45,2 (19)	47,6 (20)
350	5	–	23,6 (17)	76,4 (55)	1,5 (1)	30,9 (21)	67,6 (46)
375	2	–	10,– (2)	90,– (18)	–	15,8 (3)	84,2 (16)
400	4	–	4,8 (2)	95,2 (40)	–	9,8 (4)	90,2 (37)

Wie schon eingangs erwähnt, lassen sich die Funktionsbereiche der Speicheldrüse auch hinsichtlich ihrer Syntheseleistungen stofflich unterscheiden. Das biochemische Charakteristikum des Vorderlappens ist entwicklungsbedingt. So tritt im Verlauf der Vorpuppenphase im Vorderlappen an der Spitze beginnend ein gelbes karotinhaltiges Sekret auf (Baudisch 1963b). Setzt man die Rückbildung der Balbiani-Ringe des Vorderlappens in Beziehung zum Auftreten der Karotinoide, dann ergibt sich eine auffällige Parallelität beider Prozesse (Abb. 1).

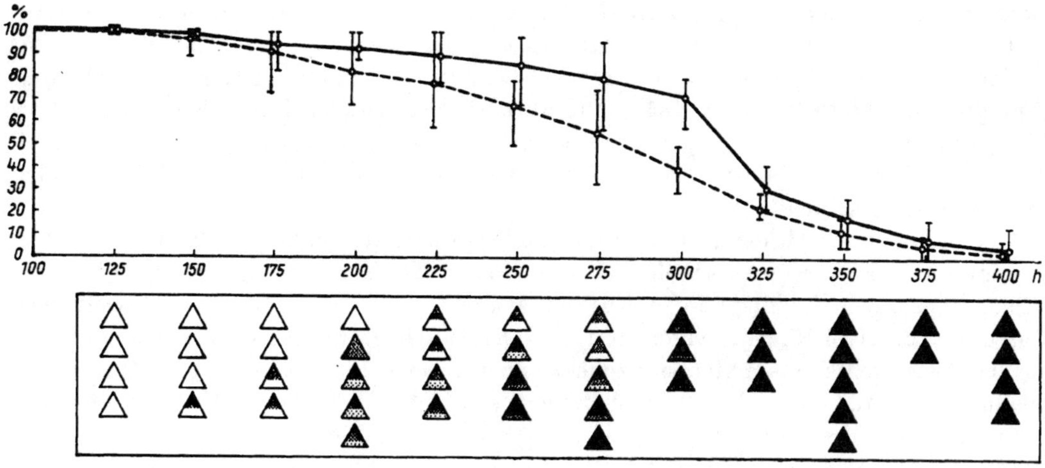

Abb. 1. Kurven der relativen Aktivitätsabnahme der Loci *BR-3* (unterbrochene Linie) und *BR-4* (durchgehende Linie) bei 10 °C im Vergleich zur Ausfärbung des Speicheldrüsenvorderlappens. Die relative Aktivität einer Zeitklasse ergibt sich aus der Summe des durchschnittlichen Prozentsatzes der ± Gruppe. Die Dreiecke zeigen den Grad der Karotineinlagerung in das Vorderlappensekret der untersuchten Tiere

Es wurde von der Annahme ausgegangen, daß die Rückbildung der Balbiani-Ringe nicht autonom erfolgt, sondern bestimmten Faktoren des inneren Milieus unterliegt. Um diese Annahme zu prüfen, wurden Transplantationen larvaler Speicheldrüsen in alte Vorpuppen durchgeführt. Die Ergebnisse bestätigen die Vermutung; die Balbiani-Ringe des Transplantats bilden sich im Wirt zurück, verhalten sich also milieubedingt. Das larvale Chromosom kann demnach die für die Vorpuppenphase charakteristischen Veränderungen wesentlich früher ausführen, wenn es vorzeitig dem entwicklungsbestimmenden Milieu ausgesetzt wird.

In cytologischer Hinsicht ergaben sich für die Rückbildung des *BR*-3 keinerlei Abweichungen vom normalen Bild (Abb. 2); dagegen blieb das für den *BR-4*-Locus typische Wandern seiner Aktivitätszone aus (Abb. 3). Anzeichen für eine schwache Aktivierung des proximalen Abschnitts sind vorhanden. So läßt sich in einigen Fällen ein mehr oder weniger starkes „puffing" dieser Region bemerken. Die Vermutung, daß diese Reaktion infolge der sehr kurzen Induktionszeit ausbleibt, ließ sich durch Versuche bei niedrigen Temperaturen unter Verwendung von Hämolymphe junger Vorpuppen nicht bestätigen.

Erwähnt sei, daß die Balbiani-Ringe des Haupt- und Nebenlappens ihre Struktur nicht zurückbilden. Das entspricht ihrem Verhalten während der Normalentwicklung. Nur nach längerer Kultivationsdauer werden sie welk, wobei allerdings so vollständige Rückbildungen wie beim *BR*-3 und *BR*-4 nicht zu beobachten sind (Abb. *4* und 5). Das Einschrumpfen ist kein Artefakt; dieser Vorgang läßt sich regelmäßig in alten Vorpuppen und jungen Puppen beobachten. Nach diesen Versuchen muß man annehmen, daß die Rückbildung durch einen Faktor ausgelöst wird, der in der Hämolymphe der Vorpuppe enthalten ist. Tatsächlich ließ sich auch die Rückbildung in vitro in präpupaler Hämolymphe induzieren, während die Kultivation von Larvendrüsen in larvaler Hämolymphe ohne Effekt blieb (Abb. 6).

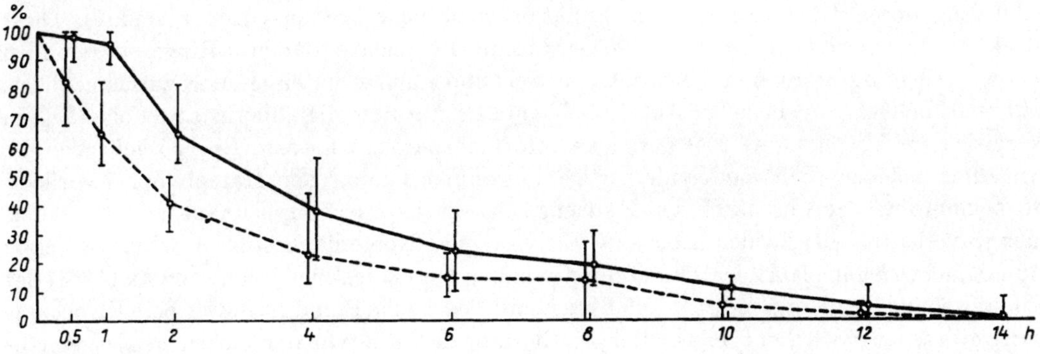

Abb. 6. Induzierte Inaktivierung der Loci *BR-3* (unterbrochene Linie) und *BR-4* (durchgehende Linie) durch Kultivation larvaler Speicheldrüsen in präpupaler-Hämolymphe bei 17° C. Angegeben ist jeweils die relative Aktivität

Die zeitliche Übereinstimmung zwischen dem Prozeß der Rückbildung und der Vorpuppenentwicklung ließ vermuten, daß die Metamorphosehormone für die Auslösung dieses Vorganges verantwortlich sind. Von uns früher in vitro durchgeführte Versuche hatten gezeigt, daß der die Rückbildung auslösende Faktor im Gehirnkomplex gebildet wird, demnach also unter den Metamorphose-Hormonen zu suchen ist (Panitz 1960). Diese Interpretation steht in Übereinstimmung mit den Befunden von Clever (Clever und Karlson 1960; Clever 1961) an *Chironomus*. Er konnte durch Injektion reinen Häutungshormons in Larven Puffveränderungen induzieren, die normalerweise erst in der Vorpuppe eintreten. Ebenso konnte Becker (1962) zeigen, daß die kurz vor der Pupariumbildung von *Droso-*

phila melanogaster gehäuft auftretenden Puffveränderungen in den Speicheldrüsenchromosomen durch ein Hormon der Ringdrüse ausgelöst werden.

Das Ziel weiterer Untersuchungen bestand darin, festzustellen, in welchem Teil des Gehirnkomplexes das Hormon gebildet wird. Zu diesem Zweck wurden Larven-Drüsen in larvaler Hämolymphe unter Zusatz verschiedener hormonbildender Teile des Gehirnkomplexes inkubiert. Wegen seiner Größe wurde ausschließlich mit dem Gehirnkomplex con *Calliphora*-Vorpuppen gearbeitet. Das ist auf Grund der Artunspezifität der Metamorphose-Hormone möglich. Wie Abb. 7 zeigt, wird die Rückbildung vornehmlich durch die Ringdrüse induziert; die Wirkung des Gehirns ist weitaus geringer. Da bekanntlich die Ringdrüse in der Vorpuppenphase fast nur Häutungshormon (Ecdyson) bildet, dürfte sicher sein, daß die Rückbildung durch dieses Hormon induziert wird. Die geringere Effektivität des Gehirns kann als Adsorptionseffekt angesehen werden.

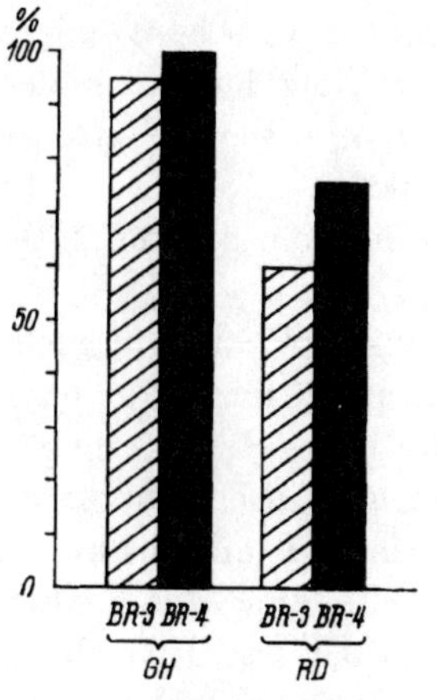

Abb. 7. Relative Aktivität von *BR-3* und *BR-4* nach 6-stündiger Inkubation der Speicheldrüsen von 7 Larven in larvaler Hämolymphe unter Zusatz von Gehirn (GH) oder Ringdrüse (RD). Die Drüsen jeder Larve wurden einzeln im Parallelversuch kultiviert

Eine eingehende Untersuchung der Ontogenese der Loci BR-3 und BR-4 erbrachte, daß diese Loci auch während der Häutung vom 3. zum 4. Larvenstadium auf die Hormonausschüttung durch Rückbildung ihrer Funktionsstruktur reagieren (Abb. 8 und 9). Diese Reaktion ist irreversibel, da im 4. Larvenstadium nur aktive Balbiani-Ringe vorgefunden werden. Allerdings werden im Gegensatz zur Vorpuppenphase nur einige Loci zurückgebildet, während die Mehrzahl in voller Aktivität bleibt. Es wäre möglich, hierin eine Folge des im Vergleich zur Vorpuppe weitaus geringeren Hormonspiegels zu sehen. Ebenso ließe sich die Annahme machen, daß eine andersartige Zusammensetzung der Hämolymphe vorliegt, da bekanntlich der Charakter der Häutungen (Larven- oder Puppenhäutung) durch das Mengenverhältnis der beiden Hormone Ecdyson und Neotenin bestimmt wird. Die erste Annahme erscheint plausibler, zumal durch jüngste Untersuchungen von Clever (1963) der Einfluß definierter Hormondosen auf Dauer und Grad von Puffaktivitäten bei *Chironomus* nachgewiesen werden konnte. Da sich die hormonale Situation der einzelnen Larvenhäutungen nicht voneinander unterscheidet, kann man annehmen, daß einzelne Balbiani-Ringe auch während der frühen Larvenhäutungen auf die Hormonausschüttung durch Rückbildung ihrer Struktur reagieren. Damit ergibt sich eine pulsierende Aktivität, die unter hormonaler Kontrolle steht.

Summary

The giant chromosomes of *Acricotopus lucidus* in each lobe of the tripartite salivary gland are characterized by a typical pattern of puffs. The specifity of these patterns is determined above all by especially large puffs, socalled balbiani-rings. Puffs and balbiani-rings are considered to be gene loci in the stage of full metabolic activity.

The spectrum of puffing changes during development. While some loci are always in full activity, others show alterations in activity going conform to development. The question raises, whether the temporal variation in gene activity undergoes autonomously, or is controlled by specific factors of the internal milieu.

Subject of our experiments were the loci *BR-3* and *BR-4*, which form large balbiani-rings only in the anterior lobe of the gland. These loci were chosen as being representative for showing a very strong relation to development, because they regress their functional structure during the prepupal stage of development always completely.

The experiments gave the following results: The inactivation of the loci *BR-3* and *BR-4* is inducable as well by transplantation of larval glands into a prepupa as by cultivation of larval glands in the hemolymph of a prepupa. The behaviour of balbiani-rings is according to that of normal development. On the other hand transplantation of salivary glands of the fourth instar larva into a larva and cultivation in larval hemolymph gave no effect.

These findings confirm the general conclusion, that the specifity of these gene reactions depends on the milieu of the host or the donor of hemolymph.

By simultaneous cultivation of the two salivary glands of a larva in larval hemolymph to which different parts of the brain complex were added the inactivating factor was found to be formed in a special part of the ring gland which is responsible for producing the moulting hormone (ecdysone) particularly.

This fact and also the observation that the period of activity of *BR-3* and *BR-4* is interrupted shortly during the last larval moult supports the conclusion, that the function of these loci is controlled by the moulting hormone of the ring gland.

Literatur

Baudisch, W., 1963: Aminosäurezusammensetzung der Speicheldrüsen von *Acricotopus lucidus*. Biol. Zbl. **82**, 351–361.

Baudisch, W., 1963: Chemisch-physiologische Untersuchungen an den Speicheldrüsen von *Acricotopus lucidus*. 100 Jahre Landwirtschaftl. Institute der Universität Halle, S. 152–159.

Becker, H. J., 1962: Stadienspezifische Genaktivierung in Speicheldrüsen nach Transplantation bei *Drosophila melanogaster*. Zool. Anz. Suppl. **25**, 92–101.

Becker, H. J., 1962: Die Puffs der Speicheldrüsenchromosomen von *Drosophila melanogaster*. II. Mitteilung. Die Auslösung der Puffbildung, ihre Spezifität und ihre Beziehung zur Funktion der Ringdrüse. Chromosoma (Berl.) **13**, 341–384.

Beermann, W., 1962: Genaktivität und Genaktivierung in Riesenchromosomen. Zool. Anz. Suppl. **25**, 44–75.

Clever, U., 1961: Genaktivitäten in den Riesenchromosomen von *Chironomus tentans* und ihre Beziehung zur Entwicklung. I. Genaktivierung durch Ecdyson. Chromosoma (Berl.) **12**, 607–657.

Clever, U., 1963: Von der Ecdysonkonzentration abhängige Genaktivitätsmuster in den Speicheldrüsenchromosomen von *Chironomus tentans*. Developmental Biology **6**, 73–98.

Clever, U., und P. Karlson, 1960: Induktion von Puffveränderungen in den Speicheldrüsenchromosomen von *Chironomus tentans* durch Ecdyson. Exp. Cell Res. **20**, 623–626.

Mechelke, F., 1953: Reversible Strukturmodifikationen der Speicheldrüsenchromosomen von *Acricotopus lucidus*. Chromosoma (Berl.) **5**, 511–543.

Mechelke, F., 1958: The timetable of physiological activity of several loci in the salivary gland chromosomes of *Acricotopus lucidus*. Proc. X. Int. Congr. Genetics II, 185.

Mechelke, F., 1961: Das Wandern des Aktivitätsmaximums im BR-4-Locus von *Acricotopus lucidus* als Modell für die Wirkungsweise eines komplexen Locus. Naturw. **48**, 29.

Panitz, R., 1960: Innersekretorische Wirkung auf Strukturmodifikationen der Speicheldrüsenchromosomen von *Acricotopus lucidus* (Chironomidae). Naturw. **47**, 359.

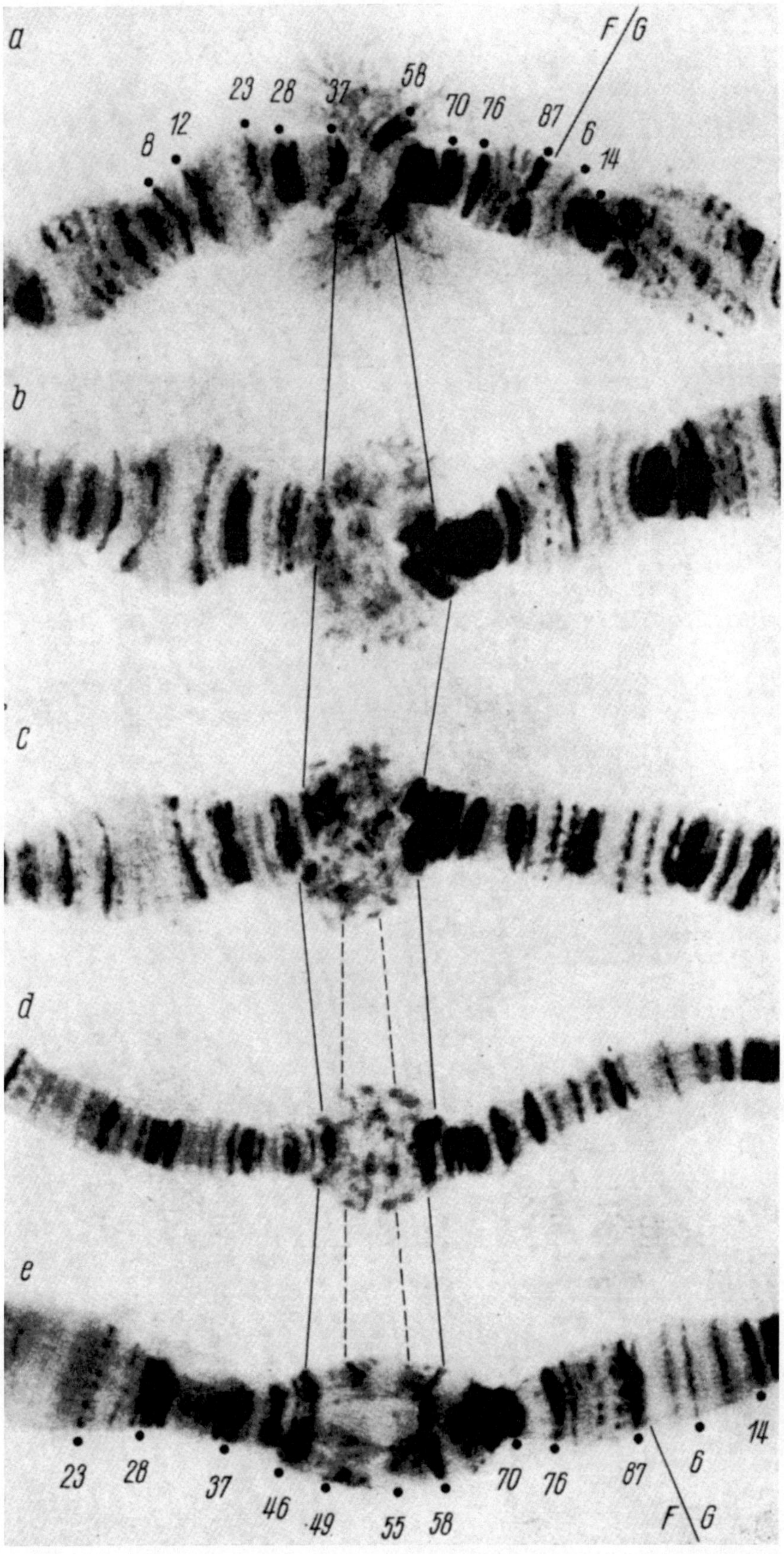

Abb. 2. Induzierte Rückbildung des Balbiani-Rings *BR-3*: a) offen, b—d) verschiedene Stadien der Rückbildung, e) vollständig zurückgebildet. Zusammengestellt aus verschiedenen Präparaten. Etwa 2200:1

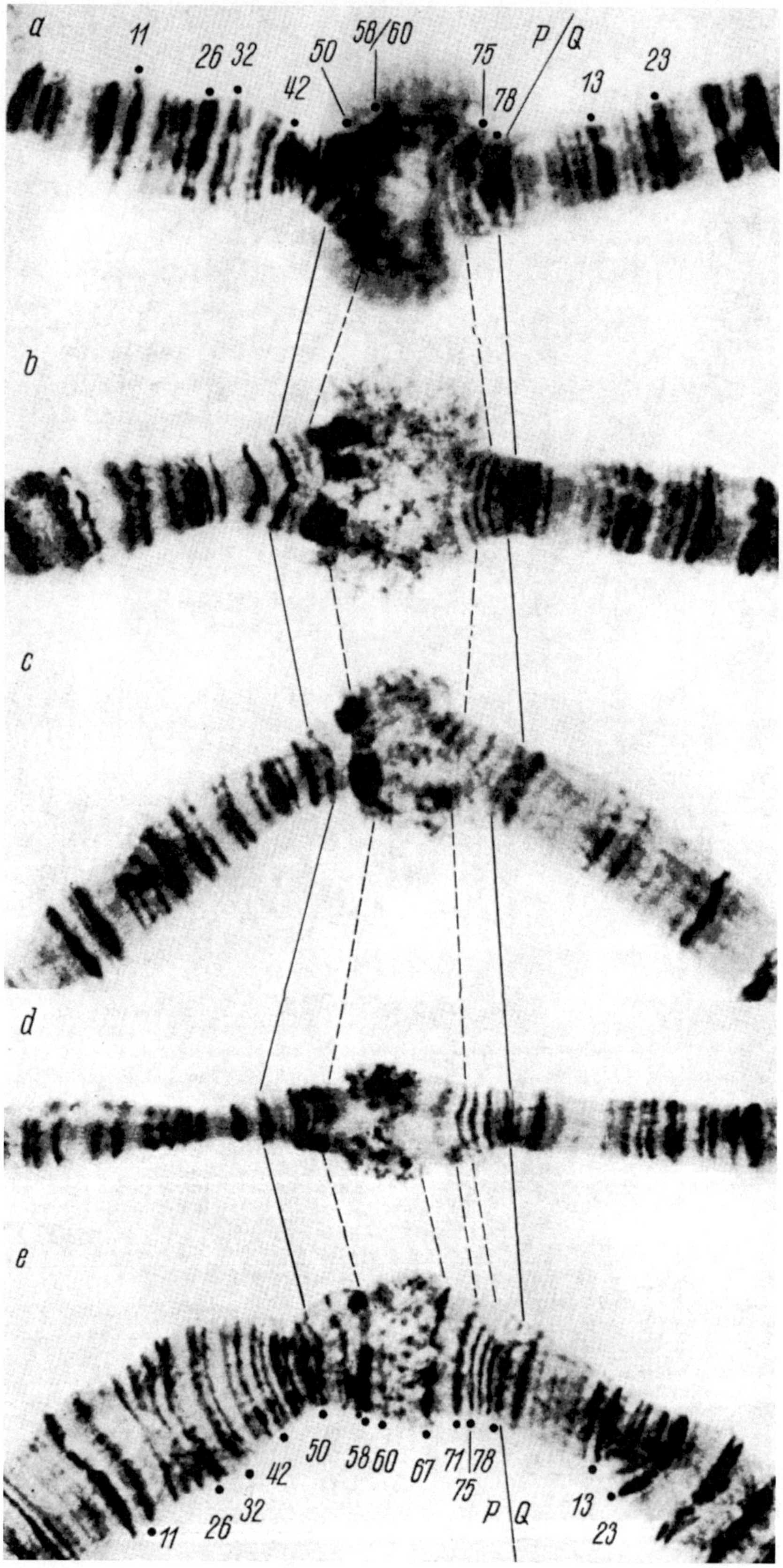

Abb. 3. Induzierte Rückbildung des Balbiani-Rings *BR-4*: a) offen, b—d) verschiedene Stadien der Rückbildung ohne Aktivierung der proximalen Region (P 50—60), e) vollständig zurückgebildet. Zusammengestellt aus verschiedenen Präparaten. Etwa 2200:1

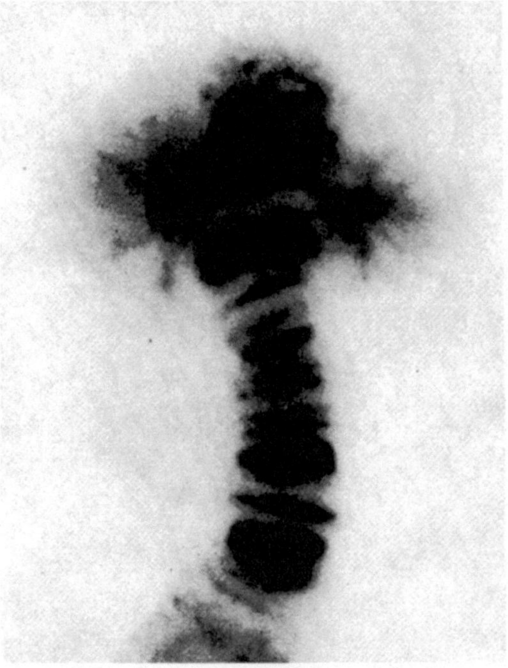

Abb. 4. Optimal ausgebildeter Balbiani-Ring *BR-1* aus dem I. Chromosom des Hauptlappens einer larvalen Speicheldrüse. 3750:1

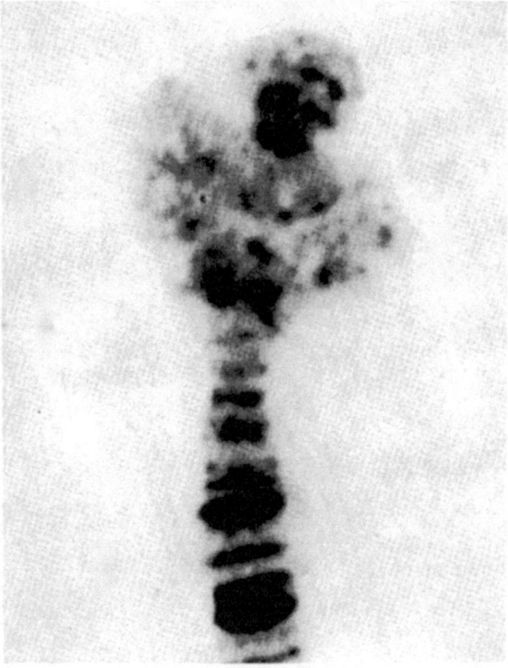

Abb. 5. Nach längerer Kultivationsdauer geschrumpfter BR-1. 3750:1

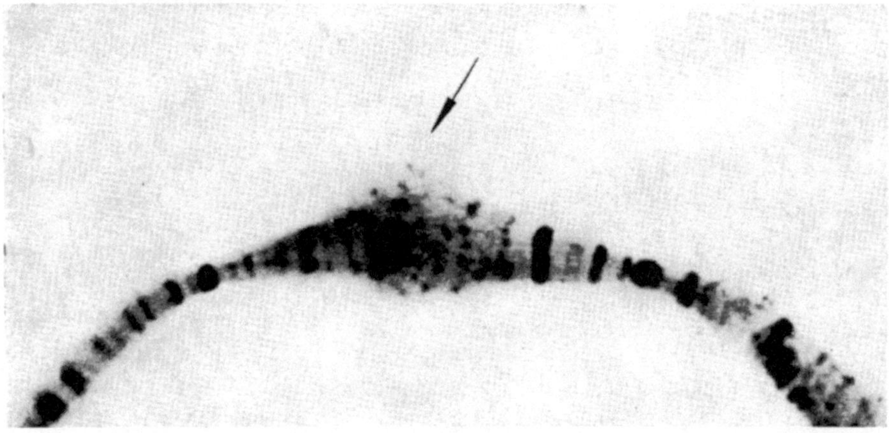

Abb. 8. Rückgebildeter Balbiani-Ring *BR-3* (Pfeil) aus einer Larve, die während der Häutung vom 3. zum 4. Larvenstadium präpariert wurde. 2000:1

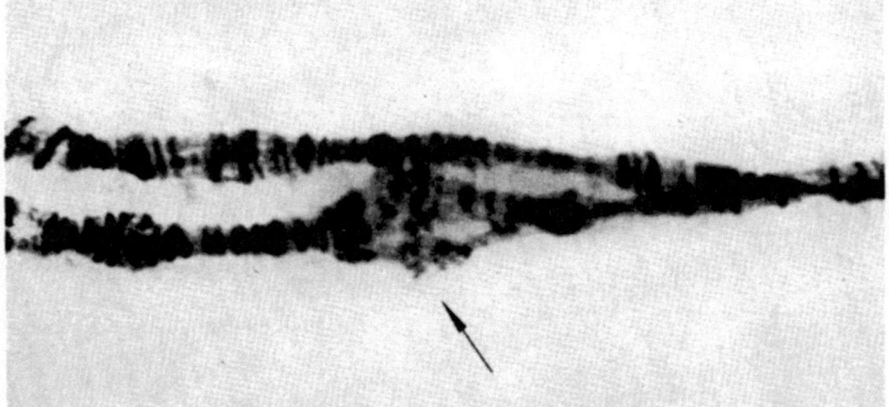

Abb. 9. Rückgebildeter *BR-4* (Pfeil) aus einem Häutungstier. 2000:1

Untersuchungen zur physiologischen Charakterisierung der einzelnen Speicheldrüsenlappen von *Acricotopus lucidus*

Walter Baudisch

Institut für Kulturpflanzenforschung Gatersleben der Deutschen Akademie der Wissenschaften zu Berlin und Institut für Genetik der Martin-Luther-Universität Halle

Cytologische Untersuchungen der Speicheldrüsenchromosomen von *Acricotopus lucidus* (Mechelke 1953) hatten ergeben, daß in den 3 voneinander abgrenzbaren Speicheldrüsenlappen der Acricotopuslarven und -vorpuppen ein unterschiedliches Strukturmuster der Riesenchromosomen festgestellt werden kann. Dazu kam die auffällige Beobachtung, daß in einem Teil der Speicheldrüsen, dem Vorderlappen, die Balbiani-Ringe beim Übergang vom Larven- zum Vorpuppenstadium eine entwicklungsbedingte Rückbildung erfahren.

Schon 1952 hatte Beermann nachgewiesen, daß in einzelnen Organen von *Chironomus*, wie Speicheldrüsen, Malpighigefäßen und den verschiedenen Darmabschnitten eine unterschiedliche Struktur der Riesenchromosomen vorhanden ist. Dem genetisch konstanten Querscheibenmuster bei den einzelnen Arten sind je nach Entwicklungs- oder Funktionszustand in den Organen verschiedene Strukturmodifikationen überlagert. Diese Befunde wurden als unterschiedliche Aktivität des genetischen Materials gedeutet. Die Puffs und Balbiani-Ringe wurden als Gene angesehen, durch deren Zusammenwirken der besondere Charakter der verschiedenen Zelltypen und die besonderen Funktionszustände kontrolliert und aufrechterhalten werden.

Wenn zwischen den Puffs und Balbiani-Ringen einerseits und dem Zellcharakter andererseits der geforderte genphysiologische Zusammenhang besteht, so muß die unterschiedliche Struktur der Riesenchromosomen in den einzelnen Speicheldrüsenlappen von *Acricotopus* eine unterschiedliche chemische Zusammensetzung der drei Drüsenlappen mit ihren Sekreten zur Folge haben. Papierchromatographische Untersuchungen der Aminosäurezusammensetzung zeigten nun, daß in Analogie zu der unterschiedlichen Chromosomenstruktur in den verschiedenen Speicheldrüsenlappen eine unterschiedliche Aminosäurezusammensetzung festzustellen ist.

Für die Aminosäureuntersuchungen wurden die einzelnen Drüsenlappen abgetrennt und in größerer Anzahl gesammelt. Zusammen mit ihren Sekreten wurden diese Speicheldrüsenlappen in 6 n Salzsäure hydrolysiert. Nach der papierchromatographischen Trennung der Hydrolysate konnten auf den Chromatogrammen mit verschiedenen Nachweisreagenzien charakteristische Unterschiede im Aminosäuregehalt der einzelnen Drüsenlappen festgestellt werden (Baudisch 1963b). Im Vorderlappen der Larven und Vorpuppen von *Acricotopus* ließen sich regelmäßig 16 Aminosäuren nachweisen.

Dieselben Aminosäuren wurden auch in Hydrolysaten des Haupt- und Nebenlappens der Speicheldrüsen gefunden. Zusätzlich wurde in diesen beiden Speicheldrüsenlappen sowohl in der Larve als auch in der Vorpuppe Hydroxyprolin nachgewiesen.

Im Körper der Tiere wurde Hydroxyprolin weder im Larven- noch im Vorpuppenstadium gefunden. Dagegen wurde diese Aminosäure in den von den Larven und Vorpuppen mit den Speicheldrüsensekreten gebauten Gehäusen nachgewiesen.

Die Larven von *Acricotopus* ernähren sich von fädigen Algen, meistens Spirogyra- und Oedogoniumarten. Um festzustellen, ob das Hydroxyprolin mit der Nahrung aufgenommen wird, wurden diese Nahrungsalgen ebenfalls papierchromatographisch untersucht. Hydroxyprolin konnte jedoch nicht nachgewiesen werden und es ist anzunehmen, daß es in den beiden Speicheldrüsenlappen synthetisiert wird.

Vor Beginn der Metamorphose durchläuft *Acricotopus lucidus* das Vorpuppenstadium. Die auffälligste Veränderung beim Übergang vom Larven- zum Vorpuppenstadium ist in den Sekreträumen des Vorderlappens der Speicheldrüsen zu beobachten. An der Spitze des Vorderlappens beginnend färbt sich das Drüsensekret allmählich gelb. Eine ebenso auffällige Veränderung erfährt zu diesem Zeitpunkt die Struktur der Balbiani-Ringe des Vorderlappens, die unter dem Einfluß des Ecdysons zurückgebildet werden (Panitz 1964).

Von Clever und Karlson (1960) wurden bei *Chironomus* unter dem Einfluß von Ecdyson ebenfalls Veränderungen des Strukturmusters der Riesenchromosomen beschrieben. Mit Beginn des Vorpuppenstadiums werden bei *Acricotopus* die beiden für den Vorderlappen spezifischen Balbiani-Ringe Br3 und Br4 (Mechelke 1953) und die nukleoläre Strukturmodifikation zurückgebildet. Die Rückbildung dieser spezifischen Strukturmodifikationen beginnt ebenso wie die Sekretfärbung an der Spitze des Vorderlappens, um allmählich zur Basis fortzuschreiten. Die Gelbfärbung des Vorderlappensekretes geht in auffälliger Weise parallel mit den sichtbaren Veränderungen der spezifischen Chromosomenstrukturen.

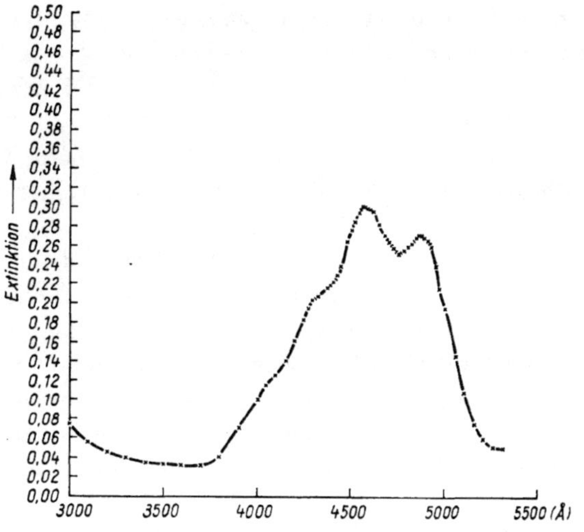

Abb. 5. Absorptionskurve einer Karotinoidfraktion (β-Karotin) aus dem Vorderlappensekret der Vorpuppenspeicheldrüsen

Für eine Analyse der Farbstoffe des Vorderlappensekretes wurde eine größere Anzahl von Speicheldrüsen gesammelt und die gelben Pigmente in Aceton gelöst, säulenchromatographisch getrennt und die Absorptionskurven in Hexan bestimmt. Das Vorderlappenpigment trennte sich an Calciumhydroxyd in drei Fraktionen, die sämtlich zur Gruppe der Karotinoide zu zählen sind (Baudisch 1963a). Die am stärksten vertretene Fraktion besteht aus β-Karotin. Die übrigen beiden Fraktionen konnten wegen der geringen zur Verfügung stehenden Substanzmengen nicht näher identifiziert werden.

Die an den Speicheldrüsenlappen von *Acricotopus* durchgeführten Aminosäureuntersuchungen und das Vorkommen von Karotinoiden im Vorderlappen während des Vorpuppenstadiums zeigen, daß in Analogie zu der unterschiedlichen Struktur der Riesenchromosomen in den einzelnen Speicheldrüsenlappen eine unterschiedliche physiologische Leistungsfähigkeit chemisch erfaßt werden kann. Die erhaltenen experimentellen Befunde unterstützen die Schlußfolgerungen, die Beermann (1952, 1961), Mechelke (1953, 1958) und andere bereits aus dem Vorhandensein unterschiedlicher Puffmuster der Riesenchromosomen in den verschiedenen Organen oder Organteilen gezogen haben.

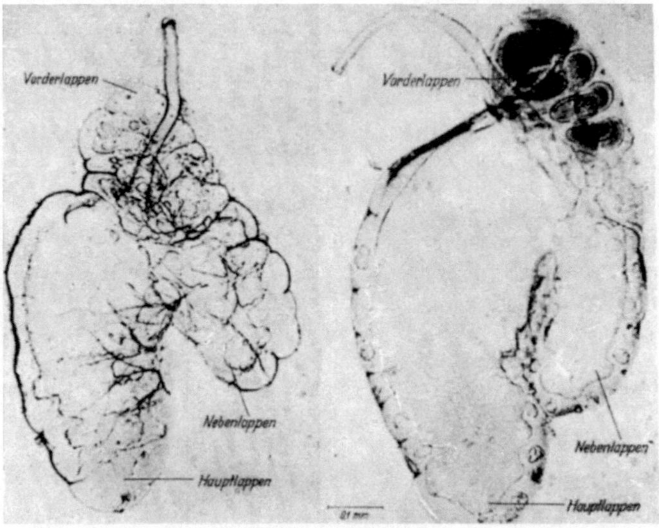

Abb. 1. Speicheldrüsen von *Acricotopus lucidus* (nach MECHELKE). Links: Speicheldrüse einer Altlarve. Rechts: Speicheldrüse einer Vorpuppe

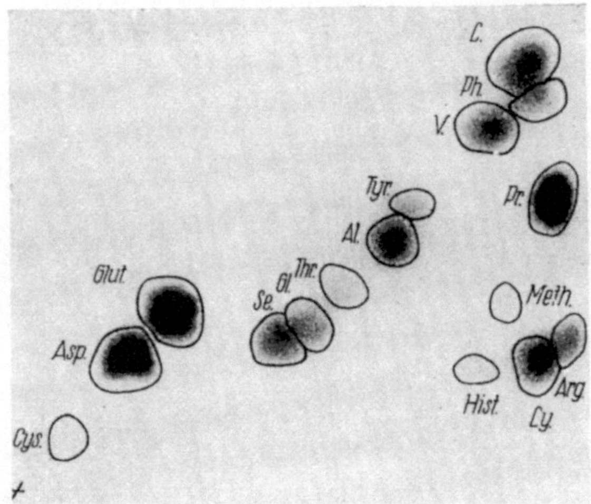

Abb. 2. Chromatogramm von Vorderlappenhydrolysaten. Nachweisreagens: Isatin in Äthanol

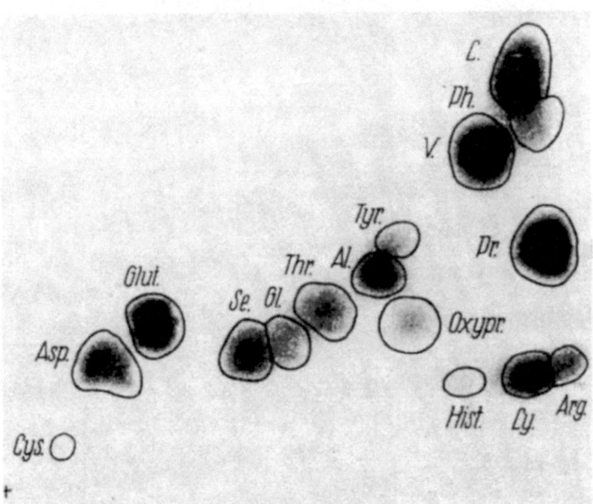

Abb. 3. Chromatogramm von Hauptlappenhydrolysaten. Nachweisreagens: Isatin in Äthanol

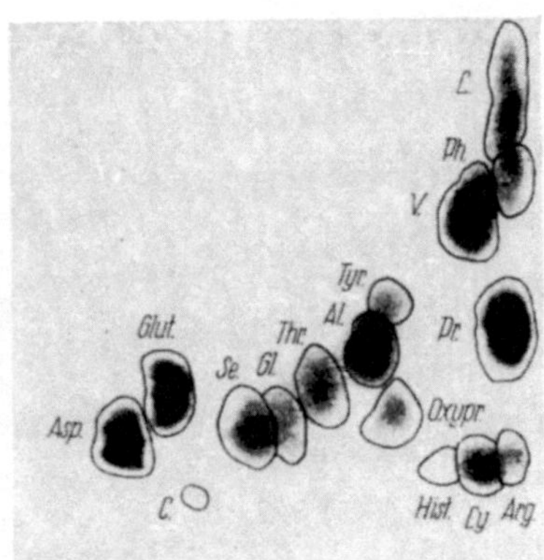

Abb. 4. Chromatogramm von hydrolysierten Wohnröhren. Nachweisreagens: Isatin in Äthanol

Die Annahme, daß Puffs als speziell aktivierte Gene aufzufassen seien, wird weiterhin durch histochemische Befunde unterstützt. Als Speicher für genetische Informationen dient bekanntlich die Desoxyribonukleinsäure. Zur Realisation der genetischen Information wird zunächst eine genspezifische Ribosenukleinsäure gebildet, die über weitere Zwischenträger den Informationsinhalt eines Gens im Stoffwechsel der Zelle zur Wirkung bringt. In den Puffs und Balbiani-Ringen läßt sich mit verschiedenen Färbemethoden ein vermehrtes Auftreten von Ribosenukleinsäure nachweisen (PELLING 1959), während die Desoxyribosenukleinsäure-Menge bei der Puffbildung konstant bleibt (RUDKIN 1955). Mit Hilfe der autoradiographischen Technik lassen sich diese Ergebnisse bestätigen und noch weiter präzisieren. Wird der Zelle markiertes Uridin zum Einbau in die Ribosenukleinsäure angeboten, so kann das aktive Nukleosid auch bereits nach kurzen Inkubationszeiten an den Puffs und Balbiani-Ringen durch seine Strahlung nachgewiesen werden (PELLING 1962). Die übereinstimmenden und sich ergänzenden cytomorphologischen, genetischen und biochemischen Befunde lassen sich zwanglos als differentielle Aktivität der Gene in den einzelnen Organen und Entwicklungsstadien erklären und vermitteln uns eine Vorstellung von der Funktion des genetischen Materials und der Realisierung seines Informationsinhaltes.

Summary

In 1952 BEERMANN has proved that in different organs of *Chironomus*, e. g. salivary glands, malpighian tubules and the different parts of the gut, different patterns of puffs and balbiani-rings can be found. Since then, this finding has been confirmed in other species of the *Diptera*. The structure of the giant chromosomes, the sequence of bands and interbands is constant and characteristic for the species, but on the basis of this sequence a pattern of puffs and balbiani-rings is formed which is related to the specific function or the developmental stage of the special organ. The puffs and balbiani-rings are considered to be physiologically active genes or groups of genes which determine the character and the special function of the different cell types.

Cytological investigation of the giant chromosomes of the salivary gland of *Acricotopus lucidus* have shown, that the three lobes (anterior, main and side lobe) of the salivary gland (Abb. 1) of larvae and prepupae have different patterns of puffs and balbiani-rings. It was additionally observed, that the balbiani-rings of the anterior lobe show a regression during the transition from the larval to the prepupal state.

Because the relation between the presence of puffs and balbiani-rings and the particular physiologic character of the cells is very obvious, it seemed tempting in *Acricotopus* to look for differences in the chemical composition of the different lobes of the salivary gland and their secretions. The chromatographic analysis has revealed that the three lobes differ in their amino acid composition. In the main lobe (Abb. 3) and in the side lobe hydroxyproline is present, against that in the anterior lobe (Abb. 2) this amino acid could not be found. Besides this, it has been proved that carotinoids are accumulated in the anterior lobe (Abb. 5) of the prepupae.

Literaturzusammenstellung

Clever, U., und P. Karlson, 1960: Induktion von Puff-Veränderungen in den Speicheldrüsenchromosomen von *Chironomus tentans* durch Ecdyson. Exp. Cell Res. **20**, 623–626.

Baudisch, W., 1963a: Chemisch-Physiologische Untersuchungen an den Speicheldrüsen von *Acricotopus lucidus*. 100 Jahre Landwirtschaftliche Institute der Universität Halle, S. 152–159.

Baudisch, W., 1963b: Aminosäurezusammensetzung der Speicheldrüsen von *Acricotopus lucidus*. Biol. Zbl. **82**, 351–361.

Beermann, W., 1952: Chromomerenkonstanz und spezifische Modifikationen der Chromosomenstruktur in der Entwicklung und Organdifferenzierung von *Chironomus tentans*. Chromosoma **5**, 139.

Beermann, W., 1961: Ein Balbiani-Ring als Locus einer Speicheldrüsenmutation. Chromosoma **12**, 1–25.

Mechelke, F., 1953: Reversible Strukturmodifikationen der Speicheldrüsenchromosomen von *Acricotopus lucidus*. Chromosoma **5**, 511.

Mechelke, F., 1958: The timetable of physiological activity of several loci in the salivary gland chromosomes of *Acricotopus lucidus*. Prov. of the X. Int. Congr. of Gen. **2**, 185.

Panitz, R., 1964: Hormonkontrollierte Genaktivitäten in den Riesenchromosomen von *Acricotopus lucidus*. Biol. Zbl. **83**, 197–230.

Pelling, C., 1959: Chromosomal synthesis of ribonucleic acid as shown by incorporation of uridine labelled with Tritium. Nature (Lond.) **184**, 655.

Pelling, C., 1962: Tritium in the physical and biological sciences. Vol. 2, p. 327. Wien: International Atomic Energy Agency.

Rudkin, G. T., 1955: The ultraviolet absorption of puffed and unpuffed homologous regions in the salivary gland chromosomes of *Drosophila melanogaster*. Genetics **40**, 593.

FSC www.fsc.org MIX Papier | Fördert gute Waldnutzung FSC® C083411

Zeitfracht Medien GmbH
Ferdinand-Jühlke-Straße 7
99095 Erfurt, Deutschland
produktsicherheit@kolibri360.de